HORMONES AND THE HEART IN HEALTH AND DISEASE

CONTEMPORARY ENDOCRINOLOGY

P. Michael Conn, SERIES EDITOR

HORMONES AND THE HEART IN HEALTH AND DISEASE

Edited by

LEONARD SHARE
University of Tennessee, Memphis, TN

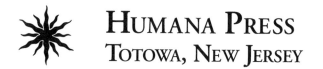

HUMANA PRESS
TOTOWA, NEW JERSEY

Hormones and the heart in health and disease/edited by Leonard Share
    p.   cm.—(Contemporary endocrinology; 20)
    Includes index.
    ISBN 0-89603-726-6 (alk. paper)
    1. Heart—Physiology.   2. Autocrine mechanisms. 3. Atrial natriuretic peptides—Physiological effect.
4. Endothelins—Physiological effect. 5. Hormones—Physiological effect. 6. Catecholamines—Physiological
effect. I. Share, Leonard. II. Series: Contemporary endocrinology (Totowa, NJ); 20.
    [DNLM: 1. Heart—physiology. 2. Peptides—physiology. 3. Hormones—physiology.
WG 202E561 1999]
QP111.4E53 1999
612.1'73—dc21
DNLM/DLC
for Library of Congress   99-10459
                                                                        CIP

PREFACE

The maintenance of arterial blood pressure and the distribution of blood flow to the various organs of the body depends on the control of the pumping action of the heart and of the resistance of the vascular beds in the individual organs in accordance with their metabolic needs. These controls are achieved through the integrated actions of circulating hormones, humoral factors that are synthesized and released in the heart and blood vessels, and the autonomic nervous system. The heart, however, is not only the target for the direct and indirect actions of a number of hormones and humoral factors, it is also an endocrine organ in the traditional sense, synthesizing and secreting into the circulation chemical factors that act at distant sites. In this treatise, *Hormones and the Heart in Health and Disease*, we interpret "endocrinology" broadly and consider traditional hormones as well as autocoids that are secreted by the heart or that act on it. In this overview, the relevant chapters are indicated in parentheses.

The discovery of atrial natriuretic peptide (ANP; atrial natriuretic factor, ANF) in the 1980s indicated that the heart does indeed function as an endocrine organ in the classic sense. ANP (Chapter 1) is synthesized in the heart and secreted into the circulation for actions on the kidney, where it is a potent natriuretic agent, and on the vasculature, where it causes vasodilation. ANP can also affect myocardial contractility.

The heart, among several other organs, can also synthesize the recently discovered peptide humoral factors adrenomedullin (Chapter 2) and urocortin (Chapter 3). Adrenomedullin synthesis is stimulated by volume and pressure overload and may be released into the circulation under these circumstances. Adrenomedullin is a potent vasodilator that can also affect myocardial function. Urocortin is a newly discovered member of the ACTH family of peptides. The demonstration that it causes potent and long-lasting vasodilation and an increase in myocardial contractility suggests that it may be a particularly important cardiovascular hormone.

The heart is the direct target for several circulating hormones. Of particular interest in heart failure is the renin-angiotensin-aldosterone system (Chapter 4). Elevated circulating angiotensin II, as well as angiotensin II produced locally in the heart, can adversely affect myocardial function. This is of particular importance in the failing heart. Elevated plasma concentrations of aldosterone, a mineralocorticoid, as well as glucocorticoids, can also exert negative effects on the heart via structural remodeling and electrolyte disturbances (Chapter 5). The heart can also synthesize corticosteroids, and these may exhibit autocrine and paracrine actions.

The autonomic nervous system plays a major role in determining the pumping action of the heart (Chapter 6). The sympathetic nervous system and catecholamines exert positive inotropic and chronotropic actions on the heart. These effects are opposed by acetylcholine released from vagal nerve endings and neuropeptide Y released from sympathetic nerve endings. Understanding these interactions is key to understanding the participation of the heart in cardiovascular regulation.

Vasopressin is not only the antidiuretic hormone, it is also a potent vasoconstrictor. It has also been demonstrated that vasopressin at physiologically relevant plasma concentrations can decrease heart rate and cardiac output (Chapter 7), and that these actions occur at vasopressin levels that are too low to increase arterial blood pressure. These effects of vasopressin largely result from its central actions on the sympathetic nervous system and on baroreflex sensitivity.

Insulin (Chapter 8) contributes to both the acute and chronic regulation of the mechanical function of the heart. The importance of the long-term actions of insulin on the heart is indicated by the cardiomyopathy that occurs in diabetes mellitus. Much is known about the cellular basis for this action of insulin and about its actions on myocardial metabolism.

The components of the kallikrein-kinin system necessary for the generation of bradykinin are present in the heart and vascular tissue (Chapter 9). Kinins probably act primarily as paracrine agents (local hormones), exerting important cardioprotective actions through the release of various autocoids. The cardioprotective action of angiotensin-converting enzyme (ACE) inhibitors may be due in part to inhibition of the enzymes that degrade kinins. The well-known autocoids, endothelin (Chapter 10), nitric oxide (Chapter 11), and eicosanoids (Chapter 12), are also synthesized in the heart and modulate cardiac performance under physiological and pathophysiological conditions. Endothelin is a potent constrictor of the coronary vasculature and can affect myocardial contractility and hypertrophy. Nitric oxide, on the other hand, is a potent vasodilator. It can also affect myocardial contractility and can influence myocardial metabolism. The synthesis of eicosanoids in the heart can be stimulated by activating both the adrenergic and cholinergic nervous systems and by several circulating and locally generated humoral factors. The eicosanoids exert important modulatory effects on the heart in physiological and pathophysiological circumstances.

It is well known that the incidence of heart disease is lower in premenopausal women than in men. The possibility that estrogen exerts a cardioprotective action is of considerable interest physiologically and clinically (Chapter 13). This cardioprotective effect of estrogen may result in part from its actions on coronary artery endothelium and smooth muscle and on lipid metabolism. On the other hand, there is evidence that testosterone in men is a risk factor for coronary artery disease (Chapter 14). This may be related to the observation that testosterone treatment in men can reduce the plasma concentration of high-density lipoprotein cholesterol.

It is the intent of this treatise to survey and evaluate the hormonal and autocrine factors that modulate cardiac performance in health and disease.

Dr. Jay M. Sullivan, the author of Chapter 13, Estrogen and the Heart, died on February 22, 1999 at the age of 62. He was Chief of the Division of Cardiovascular Diseases of the Department of Medicine at the University of Tennessee, Memphis, and he was known for his work on salt sensitivity in hypertension and the role of estrogen in protecting against cardiovascular disease. He will be missed greatly as a physician and scholar and, for those of us who knew him, as a colleague and friend.

Leonard Share, PhD

CONTENTS

CONTRIBUTORS

CARRIE J. BAGATELL, MD • *Puget Sound Veterans Medical Center, Seattle, WA*

ROBERT D. BERNSTEIN, BA • *Department of Physiology, New York Medical College, Valhalla, NY*

VERNON S. BISHOP, PHD • *Department of Physiology, The University of Texas Health Science Center, San Antonio, TX*

WILLIAM J. BREMNER, MD, PHD • *Department of Medicine, Seattle VA Medical Center, Seattle, WA*

DAVID P. BROOKS, PHD • *Department of Renal Pharmacology, SmithKline Beecham, King of Prussia, PA*

ROGER W. BROWNSEY, PHD • *Department of Biochemistry and Molecular Biology, The University of British Columbia, Vancouver, BC, Canada*

OSCAR A. CARRETERO, MD • *Hypertension and Vascular Research Division, Henry Ford Hospital, Detroit, MI*

SONGCANG CHEN, MD • *Metabolic Research Unit, University of California, San Francisco, CA*

DAVID G. GARDNER, MD • *Metabolic Research Unit, University of California, San Francisco, CA*

HARALAMBOS GAVRAS, MD • *Hypertension and Atherosclerosis Section, Boston University School of Medicine, Boston, MA*

IRENE GAVRAS, MD • *Hypertension and Atherosclerosis Section, Boston University School of Medicine, Boston, MA*

CELSO E. GOMEZ-SANCHEZ, MD • *Harry S Truman Memorial Veterans Hospital, Columbia, MO*

THOMAS H. HINTZE, PHD • *Department of Physiology, New York Medical College, Valhalla, NY*

GABOR KALEY, PHD • *Department of Physiology, New York Medical College, Valhalla, NY*

BRANKA KOVACIC-MILIVOJEVIC, PHD • *Metabolic Research Unit, University of California, San Francisco, CA*

MATTHEW N. LEVY, MD • *Department of Investigative Medicine, Mt. Sinai Medical Center, Cleveland, OH*

FAQUAN LIANG, MD, PHD • *Metabolic Research Unit, University of California, San Francisco, CA*

KAFAIT U. MALIK, PHD, DSC • *Department of Pharmacology University of Tennessee, Memphis, TN*

CLIVE N. MAY, PHD • *Howard Florey Institute of Physiology and Medicine, University of Melbourne, Parksville, Australia*

JOHN H. MCNEILL, PHD • *Department of Pharmaceutical Sciences, The University of British Columbia, Vancouver, BC, Canada*

ELIOT H. OHLSTEIN, PHD • *Department of Cardiovascular Pharmacology, SmithKline Beecham, King of Prussia, PA*

DAVID G. PARKES, PHD • *Department Physiology, Amylin Pharmaceuticals Inc., San Diego, CA*

FABIO A. RECCHIA, MD, PHD • *Department of Physiology, New York Medical College, Valhalla, NY*

BRIAN RODRIGUES, PHD • *Department of Pharmaceutical Sciences, The University of British Columbia, Vancouver, BC, Canada*

WILLIS K. SAMSON, PHD • *Department of Physiology, University of North Dakota School of Medicine and Health Sciences, Grand Forks, ND*

MAX G. SANDERFORD, MS • *Department of Physiology, The University of Texas Health Science Center, San Antonio, TX*

LEONARD SHARE, PHD • *Department of Physiology, The University of Tennessee, Memphis, TN*

JAY M. SULLIVAN, MD (DECEASED) • *Department of Medicine, Division of Cardiovascular Diseases, The University of Tennessee, Memphis, TN*

SUBODH VERMA, PHD • *Department of Pharmaceutical Sciences, The University of British Columbia, Vancouver, BC, Canada*

1

Natriuretic Peptides and the Heart

David G. Gardner, Branka Kovacic-Milivojevic,
Faquan Liang, and Songcang Chen

Contents

In 1981 DeBold et al. *(1)* made a seminal observation that opened an entirely new field of investigation in cardiovascular research. They found that injection of atrial, but not ventricular, extracts into test animals resulted in a natriuretic diuresis and reduction in intravascular volume. This activity was originally termed atrial natriuretic factor, and later, atrial natriuretic peptide (ANP), following its isolation and characterization. ANP is a member of a family of peptides, each encoded by a different gene (Fig. 1). The sites of production of these peptides and, to some degree, their functional activity are typically unique for each member of the group. This chapter will focus on the molecular and cellular mechanisms that govern the production and activity of the natriuretic peptides (NP), with particular emphasis on the heart.

STRUCTURE AND PROCESSING OF NATRIURETIC PEPTIDES

cDNA clones for rat, human, dog, pig, hamster, and rabbit ANP have been isolated. The mRNA transcript for each of these is approx 1 kb in size, encoding a proANP precursor molecule of 126–128 amino acids. Processing of human proANP occurs primarily between Arg_{98} and Ser_{99}, thereby generating a 98-amino-acid amino terminal

From: *Contemporary Endocrinology: Hormones and the Heart in Health and Disease*
Edited by: L. Share © Humana Press Inc., Totowa, NJ

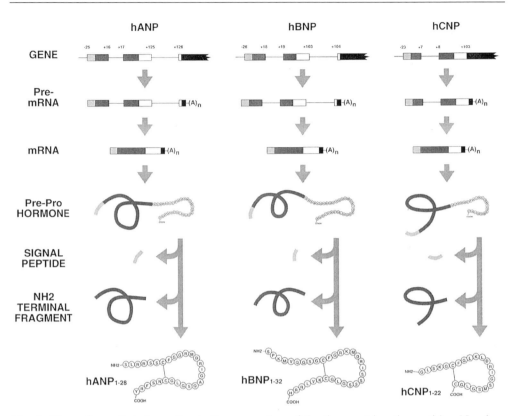

Fig. 1. Flow of genetic information in the generation of the three natriuretic peptides. Numbers describe the amino acids at the exon borders in the human precursor protein. They are numbered relative to the first amino acid in the prohormone molecule. The light-shaded region in the mRNA and preprohormone defines the sequence (nucleotide and amino acid, respectively) encoding the signal peptide. The dark-shaded region denotes the amino terminal fragment of the prohormone and the open box denotes the mature natriuretic peptide sequence. The solid box identifies the combined 3' untranslated and 3' flanking regions. The primary amino acid structure for each peptide, using conventional single-letter nomenclature, is provided at the bottom of the figure. Reproduced in a modified form from ref. *296* with the permission of the publisher (LeJacq Communications, Inc.).

fragment and a 28-amino-acid carboxy-terminal peptide, which represents the predominant circulating form of ANP found in plasma. ANP sequence is highly conserved in evolution. The rat and human peptides, for example, are entirely homologous, except at position 12 (Met in human and Ile in rat).

ProANP is encoded by a single copy gene in the mammalian genome. Genomic clones for the rat, human, mouse, and bovine homologs have been isolated and sequenced. Their structure is simple and highly conserved across species. Coding sequence (i.e., that transcribed into the mature mRNA) is confined to three exons separated by two introns over a total length of 2–3 kb. The first exon of the rat gene harbors the 5'-untranslated region and the first 16 amino acids of the preprohormone (preproANP). The second contains most of the proANP coding sequence found in the mature protein. The third exon encodes the tripeptide Tyr-Arg-Arg preceding an in-frame stop codon and the 3'-untranslated region. The Arg-Arg dipeptide is not found in either the human or the dog proANP sequence. It is removed from the rat sequence shortly after synthesis of the protein, and its function remains unknown.

cDNAs for human, porcine, mouse, hamster, and rat B type NP (BNP), and for porcine, bovine, rat, frog, and human C type NP (CNP), have been isolated and fully characterized. Human proBNP is 108 amino acids in length. Processing of this precursor between Arg_{76} and Ser_{77} releases a mature BNP molecule containing 32 amino acids *(2)*. ANP and BNP share a considerable degree of sequence homology, but BNP sequence homology among species is quite limited. Human proCNP is produced as a 103-amino-acid protein. It is processed between Lys_{81} and Gly_{82} and between Arg_{50} and Asp_{51}, to generate mature peptides of 22 and 53 amino acids *(3)*.

Genomic sequence for proBNP and proCNP are, like ANP, present as single copies in the mammalian genome. Also, like ANP, they contain the bulk of their coding sequence in the first two exons. ProCNP, in fact, lacks the third exon entirely, reflecting the elimination of the carboxy-terminal extension that is encoded in the third exon of proANP and proBNP. This serves to truncate the CNP peptide at the distal cysteine residue of the cystine bridge, which is known to be critical for the activity of each of the NPs. Genomic clones for rat, mouse, human, and dog BNP, and for mouse, porcine, and human CNP, have been identified and partially sequenced.

Each of the peptides described above is encoded in the carboxy terminus of a larger prohormone. Processing of proANP to ANP is thought to occur at, or shortly after, the secretory event. The amino terminal portion of the proANP precursor (proANP 1–98) circulates at concentrations that exceed those of ANP in plasma. These levels increase dramatically in clinical states associated with congestive heart failure (CHF) and myocardial hypertrophy. Controversy exists as to whether the amino terminal portion of the prohormone, or fragments thereof, possesses biological activity in the cardiovascular or renal systems. Data have been presented suggesting that proANPs 1–30, 31–67, and 79–98 each have significant blood-pressure (BP)-lowering and diuretic properties *(4)* in vivo. ProANP$_{1-30}$ and proANP$_{31-67}$ have been shown to be natriuretic; proANP$_{79-98}$ is purported to be kaliuretic. The natriuretic properties of proANP$_{31-67}$ have been linked to the generation of prostaglandin E_2 *(5)*, a signaling mechanism, which is obviously distinct from that employed by ANP itself. The physiological relationship of the proANP fragments to the maintenance of volume homeostasis remains undetermined.

CARDIAC EXPRESSION OF NATRIURETIC PEPTIDE GENES

The NPs each display a unique pattern of tissue-specific expression that contributes to their respective roles in regulating cardiovascular homeostasis. ANP, the prototype of the group, is synthesized predominantly in the cardiac atria. Ventricular ANP is expressed at <5% of that found in atria, and is concentrated in the subendocardial region in areas in and surrounding the cardiac conduction system *(6)*. Of note, ventricular ANP gene expression is increased in the developing fetus and neonate *(7)*. This expression falls off in the weeks to months following birth, to reach the low levels that are found in the quiescent adult ventricle.

Nomenclature aside, the primary site of BNP production is the heart, in which it is expressed in both atrial and ventricular myocytes, although atrial expression does not predominate as it does with ANP *(8)*. Ventricular expression is on the order of one-third of that seen in the atria; as noted above, the ratio for ANP is on the order of 20–50:1. BNP was originally identified in porcine brain *(9)*, but subsequent work failed to confirm the presence of BNP in the brains of other species. Even in porcine brain, it is rather diffusely distributed, and is not concentrated in cardiovascular control centers, implying that it is unlikely to play a major role in the central regulation of cardiovascular homeostasis. CNP, though important in a number of organ systems, is produced at relatively low levels in the heart, and will not be dealt with further here.

There are a number of laboratories have been actively involved in identifying the molecular determinants (i.e., *cis*-acting regulatory elements and *trans*-acting nuclear proteins) that control expression of the NP genes. Two independent approaches have been employed to identify functional *cis*-acting genomic elements. The first involves the generation of chimeric plasmids linking 5' flanking sequence (5' FS), containing regulatory elements from the NP gene of interest, to a reporter gene (e.g., firefly luciferase or bacterial chloramphenicol acetyl transferase) that is typically not expressed in mammalian cells. These are introduced into cultured cardiac myocytes (e.g., neonatal rat cardiac myocytes or transformed myocardial cells in continuous culture) using a variety of techniques. Cells are then cultured for a fixed period of time, cell extracts are generated, and reporter activity quantified. The inference is that the levels of reporter activity in the extracts are an indirect measure of the promoter activity in the NP segment placed immediately upstream.

Seidman et al. *(10)* first demonstrated that *cis*-acting elements in the 5' FS of the rat ANP gene were capable of conferring tissue-specific expression upon a neutral reporter (in this case, CAT-coding sequence). A construct containing more than 3000 bp of rat ANP 5' FS drove expression of the CAT reporter selectively in atrial, and, to a much lower extent, ventricular cardiac myocytes. A subsequent study from the same group indicated that this preferential expression could be demonstrated with as little as 609 bp of rat ANP 5' FS *(11)*. Knowlton et al. *(12)* reported similar findings. In their hands, 3003 bp of rat ANP 5' FS, linked to a luciferase reporter, conveyed selective expression in ventricular cardiac myocytes. Truncation of the 5' FS to −638 preserved the selectivity of tissue-specific expression, although, as with the Seidman study *(10)*, basal expression of the reporter was reduced.

LaPointe et al. *(13)*, working with the human (h) ANP gene promoter, demonstrated atrial-specific expression with as few as 410 bp of 5' FS upstream from the reporter. As noted for the rat gene, appending additional 5' FS to the construct led to further amplification of promoter activity *(14)*. Wu et al. went on to show that a 68-bp segment of DNA, positioned between −400 and −332 relative to the transcription start site, contributed significantly to the atrial-specific expression of this promoter *(14)*. This was based on the loss of reporter activity in the deletion analysis as the 5' border in the native promoter was truncated across this region, and on the ability of this segment to activate a neutral viral thymidine kinase promoter in transfection studies. Subsequent studies showed that this DNA segment associates with nuclear protein(s) present in cardiocyte extracts in a sequence-specific fashion *(15)*.

McBride et al. *(16)* subsequently identified a pair of cardiac myocyte-specific elements (MSEs) positioned around −370 and −190, respectively, in the rat ANP gene. As discussed below, these MSEs appear to represent functional targets for the transcription factor activator protein-1 (AP-1). A subsequent study from this group *(17)* showed that a DNA segment spanning the region from −700 to −136 activated a contiguous core promoter in cardiac myocyes; deletion of this segment from the rat ANP gene resulted in a decrease in transcriptional activity. The same deletion mutants that were inactive in cardiac myocytes were active in nonmyocytes (primarily fibroblasts) from the same neonatal hearts. This would suggest that this element functions as a regulatory switch, selectively activating rat ANP gene expression in the myocyte while extinguishing expression in the neighboring nonmyocytes. A similar element appears to be present in the proximal ANP gene promoter. Progressive deletions in the 5' FS of the hANP gene result in decreased reporter activity in cardiac myocytes, while significantly stimulating activity in independently cultured fibroblasts *(15)*.

The enhancer positioned between −700 and −136 in the rat ANP gene contains several independent transcriptional regulatory elements, including an AT-rich region and a CArG motif (i.e., $CC[A/T]_6GG$). The latter is purported to play an important role in determining tissue-specific, as well as stage-specific, expression of the rat ANP gene. Constructs harboring this motif were more active in cardiac myocytes vs nonmyocytes, and in myocytes collected from 4-d vs 1-d-old animals. The same CArG element forms high-affinity complexes with myocyte nuclear protein(s). This complex competed with homologous CArG sequence, but not with that from the c-*fos* serum response element *(17)*, implying that the involved protein is not the ubiquitously expressed serum response factor (SRF), but rather a related protein specifically tied to myocardial gene expression. This interpretation is controversial and somewhat at odds with the data of Sprenkle et al. *(18)*, who concluded, after completion of a similar analysis, that the protein in question was, in fact, SRF.

Durocher et al. *(19)* recently identified Nkx-2.5, a member of the NK2 family of homeodomain proteins that is expressed at an early stage in precardiac cells, as a transcriptional activator of the rat ANP gene. Two Nkx-2.5 binding sites, collectively referred to as the Nkx-2.5 response element (NKE), were identified in the proximal rANP promoter. The NKE was sufficient to confer cardiac-cell-specific activity to a minimal TATA-containing promoter, and was required for induction of the ANP promoter by Nkx-2.5 in heterologous cells. As noted by the investigators, the NKE-dependent contribution to ANP-promoter activity was both chamber- and developmental-stage-specific, raising the possibility that it may play a role in chamber specification. Durocher et al. *(20)* went on to show that Nkx-2.5 interacts with GATA-4, a transcription factor previously shown to stimulate the rat ANP promoter *(21)*, to effect a synergistic activation of transcription. This interaction appears to involve direct physical contact between Nkx-2.5 and GATA-4, possibly effecting a disinhibition of regulatory domains in the Nkx-2.5 protein.

A second approach to the study of tissue-specific expression involves the use of transgenic mice. Here, as in the transfection studies, ANP-promoter-driven reporter constructs have been used to identify key transcriptional regulatory elements in the gene(s). Instead of introducing them into differentiated cardiocytes in culture, however, the reporters are introduced into the genome of the fertilized egg and reporter gene expression, as an index of promoter activity, is followed in somatic tissues (e.g., heart) throughout development and into adulthood. Field et al. *(22)* introduced a construct linking 500 bp human ANP gene 5' FS to the SV40 T-antigen coding sequence into transgenic mice. Expression of the transgene, inferred from expression of T-antigen and the development of hyperplastic nodules within the myocardium, was atrial specific. T-antigen expression was much lower in the ventricular myocardium, and the hyperplastic nodules much rarer. A similar study from Seidman et al. *(23)* showed that chimeric reporters, linking up to 2400 bp rat ANP 5' FS to CAT coding sequence, were also selectively expressed in the atrial myocardium. CAT expression in the adult atria was approx 4000 times that seen in ventricular tissue. Knowlton et al. *(24)* published a similar analysis of −3003 rat ANP luciferase expression in transgenic mice. As seen with the previous studies, expression of the transgene was predominantly confined to the atria of the adult mouse.

Considerably less is known about the determinants of BNP gene expression. In neonatal rat ventriculocytes, expression of this gene is heavily dependent on the presence of specific GATA *(21,25)* and M-CAT *(26,27)* motifs in the proximal promoter. Grepin et al. *(21)* has described a putatively cardiac-specific member of the GATA gene family (i.e., GATA-4) that associates with the GATA binding sites in the BNP promoter with high affinity and specificity. Forced expression of the GATA-4 protein in HeLa cells results in *trans*-activation of a rBNP-promoter-driven luciferase reporter *(21)*; inhibition of GATA-4 expression blocks differentiation of cardiac muscle cells from a pluirpotent P19 embryonal carcinoma cell line *(28)*. At least one of the two GATA motifs, located between −100 and the transcription start site, is required for GATA-4-inducible expression of the rBNP gene *(25)*. A smaller activation of the rANP promoter was also observed *(21,24)* following overexpression of GATA-4. LaPointe et al. *(26)* identified a region between −127 and −111 that appeared to be critical for expression of the hBNP gene promoter in either atrial or ventricular myocytes. A readily recognizable M-CAT sequence (TCATTCCC) was positioned in this segment, suggesting that the transcription-enhancement factor(s) (e.g., TEF-1), the cognate binding protein(s) for the M-CAT sequence, is important for maintenance of basal transcriptional activity of this gene. This was confirmed for the rat gene by Thuerauf and Glembotski *(27)*. Selective mutagenesis of a similarly positioned M-CAT sequence resulted in a dramatic fall in both basal and phenylephrine-inducible rBNP-promoter activity, as did mutation of the two proximal GATA sites.

REGULATION OF NATRIURETIC PEPTIDE GENES

The NP genes are regulated by a variety of hormones, growth factors, neurotransmitters, and physical stimuli (e.g., electrical or mechanical stimulation), both in vivo and in vitro. Regulation of the family, as a whole, is complex, and the reader is referred to a recent review *(29)* for a more exhaustive treatment of the topic.

A number of hormones and neurotransmitters active at the cell surface have been shown to regulate ANP secretion and/or gene expression. Several of these factors (e.g., endothelin (ET), α-adrenergic agonists, and angiotensin) are known to signal through specific G-protein transducers (primarily Gq) to activate phospholipase Cβ and, consequently, protein kinase C (PKC). These agonists are of particular interest, because they promote the development of a hypertrophic phenotype in cultured neonatal rat cardiac myocytes. This phenotype is characterized by increased protein synthesis, increased cell size, activation of a specific program of gene expression (*see* below), and changes in cytoskeletal architecture. PKC activation, in particular, appears to play a critical role in this process. Phorbol ester, a potent activator of PKC, promotes increases in cell size and protein synthesis, and increases irANP secretion, ANP gene expression, and transcriptional activity in these myocyte cultures *(30)*. In addition, forced expression of PKC α or β leads to direct activation of the rANP promoter in a transiently transfected myocyte model *(31)*.

LaMorte et al. *(32)* explored the signaling mechanism underlying activation of the rANP gene promoter by the α-adrenergic agonist, phenylephrine. They reported that this receptor is linked through the $G_{q,11}$ transducer to phospholipase $C\beta$. A constitutively active $G\alpha_{q,11}$ increased co-transfected rANP gene promoter activity in the absence of exogenous ligand. In addition, microinjection of an antibody directed against $G\alpha_{q,11}$ inhibited the response to exogenous phenylephrine.

Thorburn et al. *(33)* showed that the phenylephrine induction of rANP gene transcription is suppressed by co-transfection of an expression vector encoding a dominant negative Ras protein, implying involvement of this proto-oncogene in the signaling cascade leading from α-adrenergic receptor occupancy to the rANP gene promoter. LaMorte et al. *(32)* showed that activation of the rANP promoter by the constitutively active $G\alpha_{q,11}$ mutant was not affected by the dominant negative Ras mutant. Collectively, these data imply that the α-adrenergic signal traffics through at least two independent pathways, one involving $G\alpha_{q,11}$-dependent activation of phospholipase $C\beta$ and, presumably, PKC, and a second involving the Ras signaling pathway which operates independently of $G\alpha_{q,11}$.

The work of Hunter et al. *(34)* also suggests an important role for the Ras pathway in hypertrophy of the cardiac myocyte. They generated transgenic mice carrying a chimeric gene linking a myosin light-chain gene promoter (MLV-2v) to activated *ras*-coding sequence. Because the MLV-2v promoter is selectively expressed in the cardiac ventricle, overexpression of activated Ras was effectively targeted to this compartment. They found that mice homozygous for the transgene displayed an enlarged, thickened ventricular myocardium exhibiting several of the traditional biochemical markers of hypertrophy, including activation of ANP gene expression. Functional studies demonstrated that these mice also had significant diastolic dysfunction, which impaired cardiac performance. It should be noted, however, that the role of Ras in hypertrophy remains controversial. The work of Abdellatif et al. *(35)* suggests that Ras activates a broad range of gene expression in the cardiac myocyte, not all of which is specifically tied to the hypertrophic phenotype. Furthermore, recent studies from Kovacic-Milivojevic et al. *(36)* indicate that Ras does not uniformly lead to activation of the hypertrophic phenotype under all conditions. Under quiescent conditions such as those employed by Thorburn et al. *(33)*, Kovacic-Milivojevic et al. *(36)* found that activated Ras did, indeed, lead to activation of the hANP gene promoter. However, when the promoter was preactivated (e.g., with ET or by co-transfection with *c-jun*), activated Ras actually decreased hANP promoter activity. This inhibition proved to be selectively extrapolatable to other cardiac-specific promoters, and, mechanistically, was dependent on activation of c-Fos expression by Ras. Thus, although Ras may be permissive for the development of hypertrophy under selected conditions, its overall importance as a mediator of the hypertrophic response remains undefined.

Considerable effort has been devoted to the identification of the *cis*-acting element(s) on the ANP promoter that are responsible for the phenylephrine-mediated induction of transcriptional activity. Ardati and Nemer *(37)* identified a GC-rich, SP-1-like element positioned between -73 and -66 in the rANP gene, which was both necessary and sufficient to confer phenylephrine sensitivity on the core promoter. This element, which they termed phenylephrine regulatory element (PERE), formed a ligand-inducible complex with nuclear proteins found in the cardiac myocyte. Antisera directed against SP-1 did not disrupt the ligand-inducible complex, leading Ardati and Nemer to conclude that the bound protein(s) was similar to, but not identical with, SP-1. More recently, Sprenkle et al. *(18)* have identified a second element in the proximal rANP promoter that also appears to be required for the phenylephrine induction. The element encodes a CArG (i.e., CC(A/T)$_6$GG)-like motif, positioned between −108 and −117, that associates with protein(s) in the myocyte nuclear extracts. Using a combination of oligonucleotide competition and immunoperturbation studies, the authors concluded that the ubiquitous SRF was present in the complex. Site-directed mutagenesis of the CArG motif blocked both phenylephrine induction of a truncated rANP promoter (−134 rANP luciferase) and formation of the SRF–CArG complex. They went on to confirm that mutation of the PERE site described by Ardati and Nemer *(37)* resulted in a similar loss of phenylephrine sensitivity. When either of these mutations, alone or mutation of a second CArG-like motif between −400 and −409, was placed in the context of a longer promoter (i.e., −638 rANP LUC), there was, at best, a modest reduction in promoter activity. However, when any combination of two of the three sites (i.e., either of the CArG elements or the PERE) was mutated, sensitivity to phenylephrine was lost completely. Collectively, the data suggest that regulation of the ANP gene by α-adrenergic agonists is complex. Combinatorial participation of a number of different elements is required for realization of maximal regulatory activity.

There are also several physical factors that control ANP secretion/expression. Repetitive electrical depolarization leads to increased irANP release from isolated rat atria in vitro *(38)*. A similar phenomenon has been noted in cultured neonatal rat ventriculocytes, in which repetitive depolarization leads to an increase in ANP secretion, steady-state ANP mRNA levels, and expression of a rANP-luciferase reporter *(39,40)*. In both the isolated atria and the cultured cell models, hormone release is directly related to the frequency of depolarization, and requires the presence of calcium (Ca) in the extracellular medium, suggesting that Ca entry through voltage-gated channels plays a key role in triggering hormone release under these conditions. In the cultured myocyte scenario, electrical pacing is accompanied by an increase in c-Jun N-terminal kinase (JNK), but not extracellular signal-regulated kinase (ERK) activity *(40)*. Pacing-induced stimulation of the ANP promoter is increased by co-transfection of c-Jun, a substrate for JNK *(41)*. As noted with phenylephrine, proximal serum response factor and Sp-1 binding sites are required for pacing-dependent activation of the promoter.

Mechanical strain (i.e., passive stretch) of the cardiac myocyte is a potent stimulus of ANP secretion/expression in vivo *(42)* and in vitro *(43,44)*. In the former case (as well as with the isolated perfused heart in vitro), stretch is inferred from induced increments of intracardiac pressure or volume. In the latter, it is tied to tension applied to isolated atria or cardiac myocytes cultured on a distensible surface. As with electrical depolarization, stretch-dependent release of irANP from isolated atria is directly related to the strength of the stimulus, and is dependent on the presence of extracellular Ca in the medium. Strain synergizes with a number of nonmechanical stimuli (e.g., ET, phorbol ester, and catecholamines) in stimulating irANP release *(45)*. Inferred strain-dependent stimulation of ANP gene expression has been demonstrated in a number of whole-animal models *(42)*. In vitro, demonstration of strain-activated ANP gene expression has mostly been confined to the cultured cell model *(43,44)*, and, despite several reports of increased steady-state transcript levels following application of the strain stimulus, there have been no reports documenting increased ANP gene transcription. Similarly, examination of available in vivo models has been unsuccessful. Rockman et al. *(46)* banded the aortas of hANPTag-bearing transgenic mice originally developed by Field *(22)*, with the hope of localizing a strain-dependent element(s) within the hANP promoter. Endogenous ANP transcript levels increased significantly in the banded mice; however, there was no increase in reporter activity (i.e., Tag immunoreactivity) in the banded vs control mice. Thus, despite the fact that reporter activity was targeted to the appropriate tissue for expression, strain-dependent regulation was not conferred. Similar studies were carried out by Knowlton et al. *(24)*, using mice bearing either a −3003 rANP luciferase or a −2500 rANP CAT transgene, with essentially the same result (i.e., a failure of the overloaded ventricle to activate the transgenic promoter). Three conclusions can be drawn from these studies. First, those *cis*-acting elements responsible for conferring tissue-specific expression upon the ANP promoter are not sufficient for conferring sensitivity to hemodynamic overload. Second, by inference, either the overload-sensitive elements are located in genomic sequence outside that included in the transgenic reporter constructs, or overload-dependent activation of the ANP gene operates through other than a transcriptional locus. Third, those *cis*-acting elements that have been linked to receptor-mediated hypertrophy in vitro (primarily within the proximal few hundred base pairs of the rANP gene 5' FS) are not sufficient to signal overload-induced activation of the ANP gene in vivo.

Liang et al. *(47)* and Sawada et al. *(48)* have recently documented activation of irBNP secretion, increases in BNP mRNA levels, and, notably, stimulation of the hBNP gene promoter by mechanical strain. Application of strain increased both ERK and stress-activated protein kinase (SAPK)/JNK activity in these cultured myocytes. The pattern of pharmacological inhibition of strain-activated promoter activity more closely followed that of ERK vs SAPK inhibition; however, co-transfection of a dominant negative mutant for either SAPK kinase (SEK) or kinase ERK (MEK), the regulatory kinases lying just upstream from SAPK and ERK, respectively, resulted in suppression of the strain response. Taken together, these data imply roles for both the ERK and SAPK pathways in signaling strain-dependent activation of the hBNP promoter.

The BNP gene transcript has a shorter half life than that for ANP *(49,50)*, a property that is thought to reflect the presence of destabilization sequences (i.e., UUAUU) in the 3' untranslated region of the former. This reduced half-life would be predicted to shorten the time required for a given stimulus to elicit a steady-state induction of transcript levels (i.e., BNP mRNA levels should come to equilibrium earlier than ANP). This property has led several investigators to speculate that BNP may serve a unique early response function *(49,51)*, which is designed to counteract drastic perturbations in cardiovascular homeostasis. Phenylephrine has been shown to increase the half-life of the BNP mRNA, thereby amplifying the effects of transcriptonal activation *(49,50)*. Mechanical strain, on the other hand, has no effect on the half-life of the BNP transcript *(47)*. The role of regulation of transcript stability in controlling BNP mRNA levels in an in-vivo setting, and the importance of the destabilization sequences, alluded to above, in determining this stability have yet to be addressed.

EXPRESSION OF NATRIURETIC GENES IN CARDIAC HYPERTROPHY, HEART FAILURE, AND MYOCARDIAL INFARCTION

There is an abundant literature documenting elevations in NP gene expression in a variety of experimental models and clinical paradigms associated with cardiac hypertrophy *(42,52)*, myocardial infarction (MI) *(53)*, and CHF *(54)*. In each case, this is associated with elevated plasma levels of the NP. The common denominator in each of these conditions is activation of myocyte growth or hypertrophy (because cardiac myocytes are terminally differentiated, increased cell number or hyperplasia does not occur after

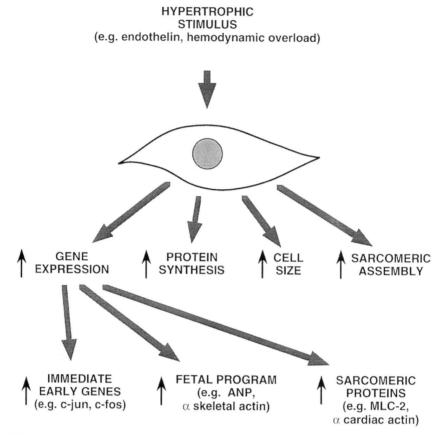

Fig. 2. Phenotypic features of the hypertrophic response in the neonatal rat cardiac myocyte. MLC-2 stands for myosin light chain 2.

the first few weeks of life), as the heart attempts to deal with the aberrant hemodynamics attendant to each of these conditions.

Although myocardial hypertrophy is obviously a condition that can only be reproduced accurately in the intact animal, primary cultures of neonatal rat cardiac myocytes respond to a number of biochemical and physical stimuli with a hypertrophic response that approximates that which occurs in vivo. This response includes an increase in cell size, increased protein synthesis, reorganization of sarcomeric structures, and activation of gene expression (*55*; Fig. 2). The latter appears in successive waves or clusters that are temporally and, perhaps, mechanistically related to one another.

The first wave of expression activates members of the immediate early gene family, which encode products like c-Jun, c-Fos, c-Myc, Jun B, Fra, and Egr-1. These proto-oncogene products, many of which are transcription factors, increase within a matter of minutes. In some cases, the induction returns to basal levels quickly (e.g., within 30–90 min for c-Jun and c-Fos), but in others the induction is more protracted.

The second wave of expression includes a family of genes of the so-called fetal gene program or embryonic repertoire. Included within this group are the genes for ANP, α-skeletal actin, and β-myosin heavy chain (MHC). These genes are typically expressed only in the late fetal and early neonatal periods in the healthy ventricular myocardium. Expression decays rapidly in the weeks to months following birth. Reactivation of these genes in the ventricular myocardium takes place following application of the hypertrophic stimulus in vivo or in vitro. The duration of this reactivated expression is variable. α-skeletal actin returns to baseline within a few days, despite continued application of the hypertrophic stimulus, and ANP remains elevated as hypertrophy progresses. The physiological rationale for reactivation of the fetal gene program has not been worked out. In the case of β-MHC, it may improve cardiac performance by substituting the slower, more energy-efficient, V_3 for the V_1 MHC isoform in the sarcomere. In the case of the NP, it may reflect a counterregulatory mechanism to decompress the central circulation through a combination of vasorelaxation and volume contraction. Alternatively, the NP may serve as an autocrine brake on the hypertrophic process itself, by opposing stimuli to myocyte growth *(56)* and fibroblast replication *(57)*.

The final wave of gene expression involves those genes that encode the structural proteins of the sarcomere and other components of the cellular machinery. These proteins (e.g., α-cardiac actin and myosin light chain-2) contribute to the infrastructure of the myocyte, and ultimately lead to the most visible component of the hypertrophic process in the myocyte.

Expression of the BNP gene is activated under many of the same conditions in which activation of the ANP gene is observed (e.g., hypertension, CHF, and following MI). Plasma BNP levels are typically modest in the basal state, but they increase dramatically in CHF and can actually exceed those of ANP in later stages of the disease (e.g., New York Heart Association Class IV failure) *(58)*. BNP also appears to be activated sooner than ANP in experimental paradigms associated with hypertrophy *(49,51)*, a feature that may be ascribed to rapid transcriptional induction and the relatively short half-life of the transcript. Collectively, these data imply that BNP may be of particular importance early in the response to hypertrophic stimuli, and at later stages of the disease process, in which it may come to dominate circulating NP activity.

Considerable interest has developed recently in the use of plasma BNP *(59)*, ANP *(59,60)*, and amino-terminal proANP *(59,61)* immunoreactivity as an index of cardiac dysfunction early in the development of myocardial disease. Each has been found to be useful in this regard; however, in a recent direct comparison of the three measurements, BNP appeared to be most efficacious *(59)*. Early analyses suggest that plasma BNP measurements are as effective as measurements of ejection fraction in assessing cardiac function. Although one clearly sacrifices potentially useful information (e.g., evidence of wall-motion abnormalities or valvular dysfunction) in relying exclusively on plasma BNP levels, the lower cost of the BNP measurements make them attractive (vs echocardiography or radionuclide measurements) in serially monitoring individual patients for evidence of disease progression.

The sequential activation of the immediate early gene family and the fetal gene program may have a mechanistic as well as temporal link. Kovacic-Milivojevic and Gardner *(62)* showed that transient overexpression of c-Jun, together with low levels of c-Fos, led to increased expression of a co-transfected hANP CAT reporter. The increase in promoter activity required the presence of a 12-*O*-tetradecanoylphorbol 13-acetate (TPA) response element (TRE) located between −241 and −235 in the hANP promoter. TREs have been shown to function in many systems through association with heterodimeric complexes of c-Jun and c-Fos. Similar TRE-dependent activation of α-skeletal actin, another component of the fetal gene program, has been reported *(63)*. These data help to solidify the putative link between the immediate early gene response and subsequent activation of the fetal program.

Individual Jun/Fos family members regulate hANP gene-promoter activity in very unique ways. As noted above, low levels of c-Fos in the presence of c-Jun activates the promoter; however, as c-Fos levels are increased, a dose-related suppression, rather than activation, of the promoter is observed *(62)*. The suppression is not dependent on the presence of the TRE in the promoter, but, appears to localize to a promoter segment positioned between −210 and the transcription start site.

Fra 1, a homolog of c-Fos, amplifies c-Jun activity over a broad dose range, and does not display the inhibitory activity of c-Fos *(64)*. By exchanging various regions of the c-Fos protein with those from Fra 1, Kovacic-Milivojevic and Gardner *(64)* were able to localize the c-Fos-dependent suppressive activity to the amino and carboxy termini of that molecule.

Jun B, a weak functional homolog of c-Jun in other systems, effected a dose-dependent activation of hANP gene-promoter activity in transfected neonatal rat cardiocytes *(65)*. In atriocytes, as expected, Jun B was considerably less active than c-Jun in this regard, and, when it was added, together with c-Jun, there was an intermediate level of activation (i.e., between that obtained with either c-Jun or Jun B alone), presumably reflecting competition by Jun B for c-Jun binding sites on the promoter. In ventriculocytes, on the other hand, the combination of c-Jun and Jun B led to a synergistic activation of the promoter, implying that mixed homodimeric pairs of these Jun family proteins possess highly unique properties in this particular context, which could prove to be important physiologically.

Nevertheless, the role of the AP-1 complex (i.e., mixed hetero- and homodimeric combinations of the c-Jun and c-Fos family members) in regulating the ANP gene promoter remains controversial. McBride et al. *(16)* reported that overexpression of either c-Jun or c-Fos resulted in suppression of a co-transfected rANP promoter-driven growth hormone reporter. Two MSEs (*see* section "Cardiac Expression of Natriuretic Peptide Genes") positioned between −370 and −190 in the rat promoter were required for the effect. The discrepancy between these findings and those of Kovacic et al. *(61,64,65)* remain unexplained.

Activation of the various mitogen-activated protein kinase (MAPK) cascades has been linked to the increase in ANP gene expression and the onset of hypertrophy in the cultured neonatal rat myocyte model. The Ras/Raf/MEK/ERK pathway was the first of the MAPK pathways to be invoked as playing a role in the signaling mechanism leading to hypertrophy. ET *(66)*, angiotensin II *(67)*, fibroblast growth factor *(66)*, phenylephrine *(68)*, and mechanical strain *(47,69,70)* have each been shown to increase ERK activity in these cells.

Angiotensin II *(71)* and mechanical strain *(69)* have been shown to activate p21 Ras and, as noted above, Ras appears to participate in the phenylephrine-dependent induction of ANP gene expression *(32,33)*. Selective overexpression of an activated Ras in the ventricular myocardium of transgenic mice leads to a phenotypic picture suggestive of hypertrophy *(34)*.

Activated Raf also promotes development of the hypertrophic phenotype, including stimulation of ANP gene-promoter activity. Dominant negative Raf mutants interfere with phenylephrine-dependent induction of this promoter *(72)*. In addition, several agonists with hypertrophic activity in cultured myocytes (e.g., ET, fibroblast growth factor, and phorbol ester) increase Raf activity (i.e., c-Raf and/or Raf A) in these cells *(73)*.

Constitutively active ERK and MEK (MAPK kinase) each stimulate a co-transfected rANP-luciferase reporter *(74)*, and, when used together, a synergistic activation is observed. Dominant negative mutants of ERK or MEK suppress activation of the ANP gene promoter by phenylephrine *(68,74)* and mechanical strain *(47)*, or by activated Raf *(72)*, lending further support to the link between the hypertrophic phenotype and the ERK signaling cascade.

These data, coupled with the well-documented association of a variety of hypertrophic stimuli *(66,69,70)* with increased cellular ERK activity, suggest that the Ras/Raf/MEK/ ERK cascade may play an important role in the signaling mechanism leading to hypertrophy. However, this hypothesis remains highly controversial. Post et al. *(75)* recently provided data that appear to dissociate activation of ERK from receptor-mediated hypertrophy in neonatal cardiac myocytes. They identified several agonists (i.e., carbachol or adenosine triphosphate) that activate ERK very effectively, but fail to stimulate ANP gene promoter activity or other phenotypic markers of hypertrophy. Furthermore, neither the MEK inhibitor, PD098059, nor a dominant negative mutant of MAPK suppressed phenylephrine-dependent rANP promoter activity, in their hands. Thorburn et al. *(76)* reported that the protein kinase MEKK1 increased both ERK and SAPK/JNK activity in cultured neonatal myocytes; however, although activation of the SAPK cascade activated ANP promoter activity, activation of the ERK pathway(s) suppressed it.

Other studies have suggested the involvement of the small G protein Rho *(76,77)* in the transcriptional response to hypertrophy. In the study of Sah et al. *(77)*, dominant negative Rho (N19RhoA) reduced the induction of ANP promoter activity by phenylephrine, and virtually abolished that induced by activated $G\alpha_q$; however, the response to activated Ras was unaffected. Taken together, these data imply that Ras and Rho function independently and synergistically to increase ANP promoter activity.

The JNKs are clearly activated by mechanical strain *(47)*, Ca ionophore *(40)*, electrical pacing *(40)*, and ET *(78)* in cultured ventriculocytes. Each of these is associated with enhanced ANP and/or BNP promoter activity. In the case of the Ca ionophore and electrical pacing, the ERKs are not activated. Dominant negative SEK (JNK kinase), like dominant negative MEK, suppresses strain-dependent activation of the hBNP gene promoter *(47)*. Thus, the collective data available at this point support participation of the SAPK/JNK and Rho-dependent pathways in the transcriptional response to hypertrophy. Support for the ERK pathway is more mixed, but it clearly plays an important role, at least with selected hypertrophic agonists. Better definition of the crosstalk among these various pathways with the development of hypertrophy, will assist in identifying a explanation for the discrepant experimental findings.

DIRECT EFFECTS OF NATRIURETIC PEPTIDES IN THE HEART

The NPs exert their biological effects through association with high-affinity receptors present on the surface of target cells. The biologically active receptors (NPR-A and NPR-B) share ~60% overall identity at the amino acid level *(79)*. Each consists of an extracellular ligand-binding domain that is covalently linked, through a regulatory kinase-like domain, to a guanylyl cyclase catalytic core at its carboxy terminus. Interaction of the ligand with the extracellular portion of the receptor leads to activation of cyclase, and increased cellular cyclic guanine monophosphate (cGMP) levels. It is thought that the increase in cyclase activity may result from transient inactivation of an inhibitory activity originating in the kinase-like domain. NPR-A binds ANP and BNP with near-equal affinity; CNP binds with much lower affinity. NPR-B recognizes CNP as its primary ligand and binds only poorly to ANP and BNP.

A third type of receptor, NPR-C, is believed to function primarily in a clearance mode, removing circulating ligand (it binds ANP, BNP, and CNP, as well as a number of structurally inactive NP analogs, with near-equivalent affinity) from the extracellular space, internalizing and degrading it. A number of studies have suggested that NPR-C may possess an additional signaling function independent of that linked to NPR-A and -B *(80)*, although this remains controversial.

Receptors for the NPs have been identified in myocardium *(81)*, and in cultured rat ventricular myocytes in vitro *(82)*. This has been confirmed by independent analyses of NPR transcript levels *(81,82)*. Myocyte cultures display relatively low levels of NP-binding activity, and respond weakly to the NPs with increased cGMP accumulation *(82)*. Cultured cardiac mesenchymal cells (i.e., primarily fibroblasts) also display NP-binding activity (primarily NPR-C), and NP-dependent activation of cGMP accumulation (NPR-A and NPR-B) is somewhat stronger than in myocytes *(57,82)*. Transcripts for all three receptor subtypes have been identified in cultured cardiac mesenchymal cells *(57)*. These cells respond to treatment with NPs with a decrease in agonist-stimulated ^{3}H-thymidine incorporation and cell number *(57)*; these effects are mimicked by cGMP analogs with agonist activity, as well as by ligands with selective affinity for NPR-C. These data imply that the antimitogenic activity of the NPs in cardiac mesenchymal cells is mediated through a combination of A, B, and C receptors.

Because of the well-documented effects of the NPs in mesenchymal cell cultures, the significance of the low-level effects seen in myocyte cultures, which are typically contaminated to some degree with cardiac mesenchymal cells, comes into question. However, several recent studies suggest that the NPs do exert direct effects on the myocytes themselves. A number of laboratories have shown that ANP reduces cyclic AMP levels and adenylyl cyclase activity in cultured atrial and/or ventricular myocytes *(83,84)*. Clemo et al. *(85)* have shown that ANP decreases cell volume of isolated rabbit atrial and ventricular myocytes, presumably through inhibition of Na^+–K^+–$2Cl^-$ co-transport. McCall and Fried *(86)* demonstrated that atriopeptin II reduces contractility and Ca influx in cultured neonatal myocytes. Meulemans et al. *(87)* have shown that atriopeptin III induces early relaxation in isolated mammalian papillary muscle; however, this effect was endocardial-dependent, implying a paracrine interaction (e.g., nitric oxide-dependent) between the endothelial and myocardial cells. In addition, a small number of studies have implied the existence of a short-loop negative feedback mechanism wherein the cardiac NPs (i.e., ANP and BNP) feedback at the level of the myocyte, to directly regulate their own synthesis and secretion *(88)*. Unfortunately, most of these are in vivo studies that do not exclude independent effects of hemodynamic changes triggered by NP administration; however, Nachshon et al. *(89)*, using an in vitro cultured myocyte system, showed that cGMP analogs with agonist activity reduce irANP secretion, but that the NP receptor antagonist HS-142-1 had the opposite effect. More recently, Wu et al. *(56)* demonstrated that treatment of myocyte cultures with ANP resulted in increased apoptosis in this cell population. The implications of this finding, vis-a-vis cardiac hypertrophy and failure, remain to be determined.

USE OF TRANSGENIC ANIMALS TO INVESTIGATE THE NATRIURETIC PEPTIDE SYSTEM IN THE INTACT ANIMAL

Transgenic animals have provided useful tools for the investigation of selective amplification or inhibition of specific gene products in vivo. They are particularly valuable in evaluating the effects of such perturbations during development, when key organ systems assemble and begin to function.

Steinhelper et al. *(90)* produced a mouse that overexpressed the mouse proANP cDNA under control of the transthyretin gene promoter. Transthyretin is a protein that is selectively produced in, and secreted from, the hepatocytes of the liver. Transgenics display high circulating levels of ANP immunoreactivity in plasma. A portion of this is low mol wt material similar in size to mature ANP (~3000 kDa); the remainder appears to be the unprocessed prohormone. The presence of mature ANP in plasma, if it is processed appropriately, is, to some degree, unexpected. ProANP is thought to be processed by a particulate enzyme (i.e., membrane-bound or confined to secretory vesicles). One would not, a priori, anticipate finding such activity in the hepatocyte, which typically lacks secretory granules and employs the constitutive, rather than the regulated, secretory pathway. This raises the possibility that proANP may be processed to some extent in the extracellular compartment. What immunoreactive ANP circulates in these animals appears to be bioactive, because the mice are clearly hypotensive relative to their nontransgenic littermates. These data lend support to the notion that chronic elevations in circulating ANP levels lead to significant perturbations in cardiovascular function, including effects on blood pressure (BP), despite activation of counterregulatory systems, which one might expect to blunt these effects. A number of additional studies *(91)* have documented that these transgenic mice have distinct, though at times subtle, abnormalities in cardiovascular and renal function, which undoubtedly reflect the tonically elevated levels of ANP bioactivity in plasma.

A parallel study was reported by Ogawa et al. *(92)* who linked the human serum amyloid P component promoter to the mouse BNP cDNA coding sequence, and introduced the chimeric construct into a transgenic mouse. As one might anticipate, these mice are hypotensive and display elevated circulating levels of BNP and cGMP.

The alternative approach of embryonic deletion or knock-out of specific genes of interest has provided important insights into the effects of suppression of the NP system(s) in the intact animal. John et al. *(93)* sequentially inactivated both alleles of the mouse ANP gene. Mice homozygous for the deletion display no detectable irANP in plasma, and are hypertensive on normal rat chow. Mice heterozygous for the deletion (i.e., one normal allele and one missing allele) have normal circulating ANP levels and normal BP on the standard rat chow; however, when placed on a high salt diet (8% NaCl), a maneuver that would be predicted to stress the NP system, they become hypertensive.

Lopez et al. *(94)* recently reported that knock-out of the type A NP receptor (NPR-A) gene results in a heterozygote with sustained hypertension that does not display salt sensitivity. Because NPR-A is thought to represent the cognate ligand for ANP, it is not clear why these knock-outs (i.e., NPR-A vs ANP) do not demonstrate a similar phenotype. The most likely explanation is that a second NP (e.g., BNP), capable of interacting with NPR-A, is increased in the ANP gene-deleted mice. This peptide might be capable of partially compensating for the loss of ANP reserve in the heterozygotes, until the added stress of the high salt diet is introduced. The availability of the second peptide in the receptor knock-outs would not be predicted to have much effect, because ANP is plentiful, though not elevated *(94)*, in this situation. Kishimoto et al. *(95)* have gone on to show that ANP is acting almost exclusively through NPR-A in the intact animal, because the homozygous knock-outs display no response to either exogenous or endogenous elevations in ANP. The homozygotes do, however, respond to salt loading appropriately, with increased urinary sodium excretion. Thus, other mechanisms (e.g., pressure natriuresis or suppression of the renin–angiotensin system) can compensate for the lack of ANP activity in the kidney, albeit at the expense of an elevated BP.

ACKNOWLEDGMENTS

Supported by HL 45637 and HL 35752 from the National Institutes of Health. The authors are grateful to Karl Nakamura for assistance with preparation of the figures.

REFERENCES

1. de Bold AJ, Borenstein HB, Veress AT, Sonnenberg H. Rapid and potent natriuretic response to intravenous injection of atrial myocardial extract in rats. Life Sci 1981;28:89–94.
2. Kojima M, Minamino N, Kangawa K, Matsuo H. Cloning and sequence analysis of cDNA encoding a precursor for rat brain natriuretic peptide. Biochem Biophys Res Commun 1989;159:1420–1426.
3. Tawaragi Y, Fuchimura K, Tanaka S, Minamino N, Kangawa K, Matsuo H. Gene and precursor structures of human C-type natriuretic peptide. Biochem Biophys Res Commun 1991;175:645–651.
4. Vesely DL, Douglass MA, Dietz JR, Gower WR Jr, McCormick MT, Rodriguez-Paz G, Schocken DD. Three peptides from the atrial natriuretic factor prohormone amino terminus lower blood pressure and produce diuresis, natriuresis, and/or kaliuresis in humans. Circulation 1994;90:1129–1140.
5. Gunning ME, Brady HR, Otuechere G, Brenner BM, Zeidel ML. Atrial natriuretic peptide(31-67) inhibits Na+ transport in rabbit inner medullary collecting duct cells. Role of prostaglandin E2. J Clin Invest 1992;89:1411–147.
6. Anand-Srivastava MB, Thibault G, Sola C, Fon E, Ballak M, Charbonneau C, et al. Atrial natriuretic factor in Purkinje fibers of rabbit heart. Hypertension 1989;13:789–798.
7. Wei YF, Rodi CP, Day ML, Wiegand RC, Needleman LD, Cole BR Needleman P. Developmental changes in the rat atriopeptin hormonal system. J Clin Invest 1987;79:1325–1329.
8. Gerbes AL, Dagnino L, Nguyen T, Nemer M. Transcription of brain natriuretic peptide and atrial natriuretic peptide genes in human tissues. J Clin Endocrinol Metab 1994;78:1307–1311.
9. Sudoh T, Kangawa K, Minamino N, Matsuo H. New natriuretic peptide in porcine brain. Nature 1988;332:78–81.
10. Seidman CE, Wong DW, Jarcho JA, Bloch KD, Seidman JG. Cis-acting sequences that modulate atrial natriuretic factor gene expression. Proc Natl Acad Sci USA 1988;85:4104–4108.
11. Rosenzweig A, Halazonetis TD, Seidman JG, Seidman CE. Proximal regulatory domains of rat atrial natriuretic factor gene. Circulation 1991;84:1256–1265.
12. Knowlton KU, Baracchini E, Ross RS, Harris AN, Henderson SA, Evans SM, Glembotski CC, Chien KR. Co-regulation of the atrial natriuretic factor and cardiac myosin light chain-2 genes during alpha-adrenergic stimulation of neonatal rat ventricular cells. Identification of cis sequences within an embryonic and a constitutive contractile protein gene which mediate inducible expression. J Biol Chem 1991;266:7759–7768.
13. LaPointe MC, Wu JP, Greenberg B, Gardner DG. Upstream sequences confer atrial-specific expression on the human atrial natriuretic factor gene. J Biol Chem 1988;263:9075–9078.
14. Wu J, LaPointe MC, West BL, Gardner DG. Tissue-specific determinants of human atrial natriuretic factor gene expression in cardiac tissue. J Biol Chem 1989;264:6472–6479.
15. Wu JP, Kovacic-Milivojevic B, Lapointe MC, Nakamura K, Gardner DG. Cis-active determinants of cardiac-specific expression in the human atrial natriuretic peptide gene. Mol Endocrinol 1991;5:1311–1322.
16. McBride K, Robitaille L, Tremblay S, Argentin S, Nemer M. Fos/jun repression of cardiac-specific transcription in quiescent and growth-stimulated myocytes is targeted at a tissue-specific cis element. Mol Cell Biol 1993;13:600–612.
17. Argentin S, Ardati A, Tremblay S, Lihrmann I, Robitaille L, Drouin J, Nemer M. Developmental stage-specific regulation of atrial natriuretic factor gene transcription in cardiac cells. Mol Cell Biol 1994;14:777–790.
18. Sprenkle AB, Murray SF, Glembotski CC. Involvement of multiple cis elements in basal- and alpha-adrenergic agonist-inducible atrial natriuretic factor transcription. Roles for serum response elements and an SP-1-like element. Circ Res 1995;77:1060–1069.

19. Durocher D, Chen CY, Ardati A, Schwartz RJ, Nemer M. The atrial natriuretic factor promoter is a downstream target for Nkx-2.5 in the myocardium. Mol Cell Biol 1996;16:4648–4655.

20. Durocher, D, Charron F, Warren R, Schwartz RJ, Nemer M. The cardiac transcription factors Nkx2-5 and GATA-4 are mutual cofactors. EMBO J 1997;6:5687–5696.

21. Grepin C, Dagnino L, Robitaille L, Haberstroh L, Antakly T, Nemer M. A hormone-encoding gene identifies a pathway for cardiac but not skeletal muscle gene transcription. Mol Cell Biol 1994;14: 3115–3129.

22. Field LJ. Atrial natriuretic factor-SV40 T antigen transgenes produce tumors and cardiac arrhythmias in mice. Science 1988;239:1029–1033.

23. Seidman CE, Schmidt EV, Seidman JG. cis-dominance of rat atrial natriuretic factor gene regulatory sequences in transgenic mice. Can J Physiol Pharmacol 1991;69:1486–1492.

24. Knowlton KU, Rockman HA, Itani M, Vovan A, Seidman CE, Chien KR. Divergent pathways mediate the induction of ANF transgenes in neonatal and hypertrophic ventricular myocardium. J Clin Invest 1995;96:1311–1318.

25. Thuerauf DJ, Hanford DS, Glembotski CC. Regulation of rat brain natriuretic peptide transcription. A potential role for GATA-related transcription factors in myocardial cell gene expression. J Biol Chem 1994;269:17,772–17,775.

26. LaPointe MC, Wu G, Garami M, Yang X-P, Gardner DG. Tissue-specific expression of the human brain natriuretic peptide gene in cardiac myocytes. Hypertension 1996;27:715–722.

27. Thuerauf DJ, Glembotski CC. Differential effects of protein kinase C, Ras, and Raf-1 kinase on the induction of the cardiac B-type natriuretic peptide gene through a critical promoter-proximal M-CAT element. J Biol Chem 1997;272:7464–7472.

28. Grepin C, Robitaille L, Antakly T, Nemer M. Inhibition of transcription factor GATA-4 expression blocks in vitro cardiac muscle differentiation. Mol Cell Biol 1995;15:4095–4102.

29. Gardner D, Wu J, Kovacic-Milivojevic B. Cellular and molecular aspects of the A-type natriuretic peptide. In: Samson WK, Levin ER, eds. Natriuretic Peptides in Health and Disease. Humana, Totowa, NJ, 1997, pp. 71–94.

30. Dunnmon PM, Iwaki K, Henderson S, Sen A, Chien KR. Phorbol esters induce immediate-early genes and activate cardiac gene transcription in neonatal rat myocardial cells. J Mol Cell Cardiol 1990;22:901–910.

31. Shubeita HE, Martinson EA, Van Bilsen M, Chien KR, Brown JH. Transcriptional activation of the cardiac myosin light chain 2 and atrial natriuretic factor genes by protein kinase C in neonatal rat ventricular myocytes. Proc Natl Acad Sci USA 1992; 89:1305–1309.

32. LaMorte VJ, Thorburn J, Absher D, Spiegel A, Brown JH, Chien KR, Feramisco JR, Knowlton KU. Gq- and ras-dependent pathways mediate hypertrophy of neonatal rat ventricular myocytes following alpha 1-adrenergic stimulation. J Biol Chem 1994;269:13,490–13,496.

33. Thorburn A, Thorburn J, Chen SY, Powers S, Shubeita HE, Feramisco JR, Chien KR. HRas-dependent pathways can activate morphological and genetic markers of cardiac muscle cell hypertrophy. J Biol Chem 1993;268:2244–2249.

34. Hunter JJ, Tanaka N, Rockman HA, Ross J, Chien KR. Ventricular expression of a MLC-2v-ras fusion gene induces cardiac hypertrophy and selective diastolic dysfunction in transgenic mice. J Biol Chem 1995;270:23,173–23,178.

35. Abdellatif M, MacLellan WR, Schneider MD. p21 Ras as a governor of global gene expression. J Biol Chem 1994;269:15,423–15,426.

36. Kovacic-Milivojevic B, Zlock DW, Gardner DG. Ras inhibits Jun-activated human atrial natriuretic peptide gene transcription in cultured ventricular myocytes. Circ Res 1997;80:580–588.

37. Ardati A, Nemer M. A nuclear pathway for alpha 1-adrenergic receptor signaling in cardiac cells. EMBO J 1993;12:5131–5139.

38. Schiebinger RJ, Li Y, Cragoe EJ Jr. Calcium dependency of frequency-stimulated atrial natriuretic peptide secretion. Hypertension 1994;23:710–716.

39. McDonough PM, Glembotski CC. Induction of atrial natriuretic factor and myosin light chain-2 gene expression in cultured ventricular myocytes by electrical stimulation of contraction. J Biol Chem 1992; 267:11,665–11,668.

40. McDonough PM, Stella SL, Glembotski CC. Involvement of cytoplasmic calcium and protein kinases in the regulation of atrial natriuretic factor secretion by contraction rate and endothelin. J Biol Chem 1994;269:9466–9472.

41. McDonough PM, Hanford DS, Sprenkle AB, Mellon NR, Glembotski CC. Collaborative roles for c-Jun N-terminal kinase, c-Jun, serum response factor, and Sp1 in calcium-regulated myocardial gene expression. J Biol Chem 1997;272:24,046–24,053.

42. Day ML, Schwartz D, Wiegand RC, Stockman PT, Brunnert HE, Tolunay SR, et al. Ventricular atriopeptin. Unmasking of messenger RNA and peptide synthesis by hypertrophy or dexamethasone. Hypertension 1987;9:485–491.

43. Sadoshima J, Jahn L, Takahashi T, Kulik TJ, Izumo S. Molecular characterization of the stretch-induced adaptation of cultured cardiac cells. An in vitro model of load-induced cardiac hypertrophy. J Biol Chem 1992;267:10,551–10,560.

44. Gardner DG, Wirtz H, Dobbs LG. Stretch-dependent regulation of atrial peptide synthesis and secretion in cultured atrial cardiocytes. Am J Physiol 1992;263:E239–E244.

45. Schiebinger RJ,. Greening KM. Interaction between stretch and hormonally stimulated atrial natriuretic peptide secretion. Am J Physiol 1992;262:H78–H83.

46. Rockman HA, Ross RS, Harris AN, Knowlton KU, Steinhelper ME, Field LJ, Ross J Jr, Chien KR. Segregation of atrial-specific and inducible expression of an atrial natriuretic factor transgene in an in vivo murine model of cardiac hypertrophy. Proc Natl Acad Sci USA 1991;88:8277–8281.

47. Liang F, Wu J, Garami M, Gardner DG. Mechanical strain increases expression of the brain natriuretic peptide gene in rat cardiac myocytes. J Biol Chem 1997;272:28,050–28,056.

48. Sawada Y, Suda M, Yokoyama H, Kanda T, Sakamaki T, Tanaka S, et al. Stretch-induced hypertrophic growth of cardiocytes and processing of brain-type natriuretic peptide are controlled by proprotein-processing endoprotease furin. J Biol Chem 1997;272:20,545–20,554.

49. Hanford DS, Thuerauf DJ, Murray SF, Glembotski CC. Brain natriuretic peptide is induced by alpha 1-adrenergic agonists as a primary response gene in cultured rat cardiac myocytes. J Biol Chem 1994;269:26,227–26,233.

50. Hanford DS, Glembotski CC. Stabilization of the B-type natriuretic peptide mRNA in cardiac myocytes by alpha-adrenergic receptor activation: potential roles for protein kinase C and mitogen-activated protein kinase. Mol Endocrinol 1996;10:1719–1727.

51. Nakagawa O, Ogawa Y, Itoh H, Suga S, Komatsu Y, Kishimoto I, et al. Rapid transcriptional activation and early mRNA turnover of brain natriuretic peptide in cardiocyte hypertrophy. Evidence for brain natriuretic peptide as an "emergency" cardiac hormone against ventricular overload. J Clin Invest 1995;96:1280–1287.

52. Dene H, Rapp JP. Quantification of messenger ribonucleic acid for atrial natriuretic factor in atria and ventricles of Dahl salt-sensitive and salt-resistant rats. Mol Endocrinol 1987;1:614–620.

53. Mendez R, Pfeffer JM, Ortola FV, Bloch KD, Anderson S, Seidman JG, Brenner BM. Atrial natriuretic peptide transcription, storage, and release in rats with myocardial infarction. Am J Physiol 1987;253:H1449–H1455.

54. Saito Y, Nakao K, Arai H, Nishimura K. Okumura K. Obata K, et al. Augmented expression of atrial natriuretic polypeptide gene in ventricle of human failing heart. J Clin Invest 1989;83:298–305.

55. Chien KR, Knowlton KU, Zhu H. Chien S. Regulation of cardiac gene expression during myocardial growth and hypertrophy: molecular studies of an adaptive physiologic response. FASEB J 1991;5:3037–3046.

56. Wu CF, Bishopric NH, Pratt RE. Atrial natriuretic peptide induces apoptosis in neonatal rat cardiac myocytes. J Biol Chem 1997;272:14,860–14,866.

57. Cao L, Gardner DG. Natriuretic peptides inhibit DNA synthesis in cardiac fibroblasts. Hypertension 1995;25:227–234.

58. Mukoyama M, Nakao K, Hosoda K, Suga S, Saito Y, Ogawa Y, et al. Brain natriuretic peptide as a novel cardiac hormone in humans. J Clin Invest 1991;87:1402–1412.

59. Yamamoto K, Burnett JC Jr, Jougasaki M, Nishimura RA, Bailey KR, Saito Y, Nakao K, Redfield MM. Superiority of brain natriuretic peptide as a hormonal marker of ventricular systolic and diastolic dysfunction and ventricular hypertrophy. Hypertension 1996;28:988–994.

60. Davis KM, Fish LC, Elahi D, Clark BA, Minaker KL. Atrial natriuretic peptide levels in the prediction of congestive heart failure risk in frail elderly. JAMA 1992;267:2625–2629.

61. Lerman A, Gibbons RJ, Rodeheffer RJ, Bailey KR, McKinley LJ, Heublein DM. Burnett JC Jr. Circulating N-terminal atrial natriuretic peptide as a marker for symptomless left-ventricular dysfunction. Lancet 1993;341:1105–1109.

62. Kovacic-Milivojevic B, Gardner DG. Divergent regulation of the human atrial natriuretic peptide gene by c-jun and c-fos. Mol Cell Biol 1992;12:292–301.

63. Bishopric NH, Jayasena V, Webster KA. Positive regulation of the skeletal alpha-actin gene by Fos and Jun in cardiac myocytes. J Biol Chem 1992;267:25,535–25,540.

64. Kovacic-Milivojevic B, Gardner DG. Fra-1, a Fos gene family member that activates atrial natriuretic peptide gene transcription. Hypertension 1995;25:679–682.

65. Kovacic-Milivojevic B, Wong VSH, Gardner DG. Selective regulation of atrial natriuretic peptide gene by individual components of AP-1 complex. Endocrinology 1996;137:1108–1117.

66. Bogoyevitch MA, Glennon PE, Andersson MB, Clerk A, Lazou A, Marshall CJ, Parker PJ, Sugden PH. Endothelin-1 and fibroblast growth factors stimulate the mitogen-activated protein kinase signaling cascade in cardiac myocytes. The potential role of the cascade in the integration of two signaling pathways leading to myocyte hypertrophy. J Biol Chem 1994;269:1110–1119.

67. Sadoshima J, Qiu Z, Morgan JP, Izumo S. Angiotensin II and other hypertrophic stimuli mediated by G protein-coupled receptors activate tyrosine kinase, mitogen-activated protein kinase, and 90-kD S6 kinase in cardiac myocytes. The critical role of $Ca(2+)$-dependent signaling. Circ Res 1995;76:1–15.

68. Thorburn J, Frost JA, Thorburn A. Mitogen-activated protein kinases mediate changes in gene expression, but not cytoskeletal organization associated with cardiac muscle cell hypertrophy. J Cell Biol 1994; 126:1565–1572.

69. Sadoshima J, Izumo S. Mechanical stretch rapidly activates multiple signal transduction pathways in cardiac myocytes: potential involvement of an autocrine/paracrine mechanism. EMBO J 1993;12:1681–1692.

70. Yamazaki T, Komuro I, Kudoh S, Zou Y, Shiojima I, Mizuno T, Takano H, et al. Mechanical stress activates protein kinase cascade of phosphorylation in neonatal rat cardiac myocytes. J Clin Invest 1995;96:438–446.

71. Sadoshima J, Izumo S. The heterotrimeric Gq protein-coupled angiotensin II receptor activates p21 ras via the tyrosine kinase-Shc-Grb2-Sos pathway in cardiac myocytes. EMBO J 1996;15:775–787.

72. Thorburn J, McMahon M, Thorburn A. Raf-1 kinase activity is necessary and sufficient for gene expression changes but not sufficient for cellular morphology changes associated with cardiac myocyte hypertrophy. J Biol Chem 1994;269:30,580–30,586.

73. Bogoyevitch MA, Marshall CJ, Sugden PH. Hypertrophic agonists stimulate the activities of the protein kinases c-Raf and A-Raf in cultured ventricular myocytes. J Biol Chem 1995;270:26,303–26,310.

74. Gillespie-Brown J, Fuller SJ, Bogoyevitch MA, Cowley S, Sugden PH. The mitogen-activated protein kinase kinase MEK1 stimulates a pattern of gene expression typical of the hypertrophic phenotype in rat ventricular cardiomyocytes. J Biol Chem 1995;270:28,092–28,096.

75. Post GR, Goldstein D, Thuerauf DJ, Glembotski CC, Brown JH. Dissociation of p44 and p42 mitogen-activated protein kinase activation from receptor-induced hypertrophy in neonatal rat ventricular myocytes. J Biol Chem 1996;271:8452–8457.

76. Thorburn J, Xu S, Thorburn A. MAP kinase- and Rho-dependent signals interact to regulate gene expression but not actin morphology in cardiac muscle cells. EMBO J 1997;16:1888–1900.

77. Sah VP, Hoshijima M, Chien KR, Brown JH. Rho is required for Galphaq and alpha1-adrenergic receptor signaling in cardiomyocytes. Dissociation of Ras and Rho pathways. J Biol Chem 1996;271: 31,185–31,190.

78. Bogoyevitch MA, Ketterman AJ, Sugden PH. Cellular stresses differentially activate c-Jun N-terminal protein kinases and extracellular signal-regulated protein kinases in cultured ventricular myocytes. J Biol Chem 1995;270:29,710–29,717.

79. Koller KJ, Goeddel DV. Molecular biology of the natriuretic peptides and their receptors. Circulation 1992;86:1081–1088.

80. Levin ER. Natriuretic peptide C-receptor: more than a clearance receptor. Am J Physiol 1993;264: E483–E489.

81. Wilcox JN, Augustine A, Goeddel DV, Lowe DG. Differential regional expression of three natriuretic peptide receptor genes within primate tissues. Mol Cell Biol 1991;11:3454–3462.

82. Nunez DJ, Dickson MC, Brown MJ. Natriuretic peptide receptor mRNAs in the rat and human heart. J Clin Invest 1992;90:1966–1971.

83. Anand-Srivastava MB, Cantin M. Atrial natriuretic factor receptors are negatively coupled to adenylate cyclase in cultured atrial and ventricular cardiocytes. Biochem Biophys Res Commun 1986;138:427–436.

84. Cramb G, Banks R, Rugg EL, Aiton JF. Actions of atrial natriuretic peptide (ANP) on cyclic nucleotide concentrations and phosphatidylinositol turnover in ventricular myocytes. Biochem Biophys Res Commun 1987;148:962–970.

85. Clemo HF, Baumgarten CM. Atrial natriuretic factor decreases cell volume of rabbit atrial and ventricular myocytes. Am J Physiol 1991;260:C681–C690.

86. McCall D, Fried TA. Effect of atriopeptin II on Ca influx, contractile behavior and cyclic nucleotide content of cultured neonatal rat myocardial cells. J Mol Cell Cardiol 1990;22:201–212.

87. Meulemans AL, Sipido KR, Sys SU, Brutsaert DL. Atriopeptin III induces early relaxation of isolated mammalian papillary muscle. Circ Res 1988;62:1171–1174.

88. Vesely DL, Douglass, MA. Dietz JR, Giordano AT, McCormick MT, Rodriguez-Paz G, Schocken DD. Negative feedback of atrial natriuretic peptides. J Clin Endocrinol Metab 1994;78:1128–1134.

89. Nachshon S, Zamir O, Matsuda Y, Zamir N. Effects of ANP receptor antagonists on ANP secretion from adult rat cultured atrial myocytes. Am J Physiol 1995;268: E428–E432.

90. Steinhelper ME, Cochrane KL, Field LJ. Hypotension in transgenic mice expressing atrial natriuretic factor fusion genes. Hypertension 1990;16:301–307.

91. Barbee RW, Perry BD, Re RN, Murgo JP, Field LJ. Hemodynamics in transgenic mice with over-expression of atrial natriuretic factor. Circ Res 1994;74:747–751.

92. Ogawa Y, Itoh H, Tamura N, Suga S, Yoshimasa T, Uehira M, et al. Molecular cloning of the complementary DNA and gene that encode mouse brain natriuretic peptide and generation of transgenic mice that overexpress the brain natriuretic peptide gene. J Clin Invest 1994;93:911–921.

93. John SW, Krege JH, Oliver PM, Hagaman JR, Hodgin JB, Pang SC, Flynn TG, Smithies O. Genetic decreases in atrial natriuretic peptide and salt-sensitive hypertension. Science 1995;267:679–681.

94. Lopez MJ, Wong SK, Kishimoto I, Dubois S, Mach V, Friesen J, Garbers DL, Beuve A. Salt-resistant hypertension in mice lacking the guanylyl cyclase-A receptor for atrial natriuretic peptide. Nature 1995; 378:65–68.

95. Kishimoto I, Dubois SK, Garbers DL. The heart communicates with the kidney exclusively through the guanylyl cyclase-A receptor: acute handling of sodium and water in response to volume expansion. Proc Natl Acad Sci USA 1996;93:6215–6219.

2

Adrenomedullin and the Heart

Willis K. Samson

Contents

THE BIOCHEMISTRY
AND MOLECULAR BIOLOGY OF ADRENOMEDULLIN
AND PROADRENOMEDULLIN N-TERMINAL 20 PEPTIDE

Biologic assays employed for screening novel peptides, once sequenced, or even during initial purification attempts, have evolved over the years from whole-animal models to isolated tissue systems in perfusion chambers, and, most recently, to systems employing cultured mammalian cells. The end product of these most recent bioassay systems can be monitored on the basis of cell growth or division, hormone secretion, or even changes in intracellular signaling events. It was using just such a bioassay that Matsuo et al. *(1)*, in 1993, isolated a novel vasoactive hormone, termed adrenomedullin (AM). The peptide stimulated platelet adenylyl cyclase activity, and then, in whole-animal bioassay, was found to be a potent vasodilator *(1)*. This chapter describes the identification of the pharmacologic and physiologic properties of AM and its sibling pair, proadrenomedullin N-terminal 20 peptide (PAMP), with particular focus on production in, and the effects on, the cardiovascular system.

Discovery and Gene Sequencing

The human AM gene was cloned from extracts of a pheochromocytoma *(2)*. Located on chromosome 11, and consisting of four exons and three introns *(3)*, the AM gene encodes a 185 amino preprohormone (Fig. 1). The genetic sequence is well preserved among species, and the level of peptide homology is extensive *(4)*. Recent anaylsis of the human AM gene revealed the presence of two transcription start sites downstream from

From: *Contemporary Endocrinology: Hormones and the Heart in Health and Disease*
Edited by: L. Share © Humana Press Inc., Totowa, NJ

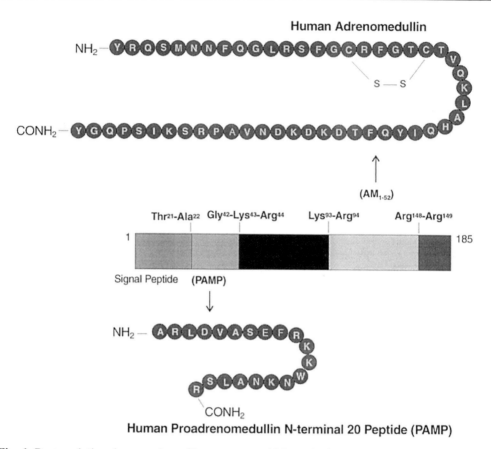

Fig. 1. Postranslational processing of human preproAM results in the production of at least two biologically active peptides, AM and proadrenomedullin N-terminal 20 peptide.

the TATA box. In human aortic endothelial cells (ECs) both the nuclear factor for interleukin-6 expression (NF-IL6) and activator protein-2 (AP-2) consensus sequences have been identified in the promotor region as the functional transcriptional regulatory elements of the human AM gene. Human AM is 52 amino acids in length, contains a single disulfide bond, which is necessary for biologic activity, and is C-terminally amidated *(1)*. Rat AM differs from human in only six positions, and is 50 amino acids in length *(4)*. Human and rat PAMP are both 20 amino acids in length, and differ in only three positions *(1,4)*. Human AM and PAMP are biologically active in the rat.

The first 21 encoded amino acids of the preprohormone represent the signal peptide, and, after their removal by cleavage between the threonine in position 21 and the alanine in position 22, the 164-amino-acid prohormone is further processed to the N-terminally located 20-amino-acid PAMP by enzymatic cleavage between positions 43 (lysine) and 44 (arginine). Further posttranslational processing by cleavage of the lysine–arginine pairing at positions 93 and 94, and the arginine doublet at positions 148 and 149, results in the liberation of AM. These are to date the only posttranslational products of the preproadrenomedullin (preproAM) gene product demonstrated to possess biologic activity, although shortened fragments of AM and PAMP, derived by further enzymatic cleavage, are to some degree also active.

Sites of Adrenomedullin Gene Transcription

PreproAM mRNA has been detected not only in pheochromocytomas and normal adrenal glands (1), but also in human heart, kidney, and lung (5–7); in rat, transcripts have been detected in extracts of adrenal, kidney, lung, heart, spleen, duodenum, liver, submandibular gland, and brain (7–9). ECs cells abundantly transcribe the AM gene (10), as do cardiomyocytes (11). AM-like immunoreactivity has been identified in multiple tissues, most notably adrenal medulla, blood vessels, kidney, anterior pituitary gland, hypothalamus, heart, lung, thyroid gland, submandibular gland, liver, pancreas, stomach, intestine, testis, and choroid plexus (5–7,10–21).

Both AM and PAMP circulate in man, like other vasoactive hormones, in the low pg/mL range (22–24). The plasma half-life of AM is approx 22 min, the volume of distribution in man 900 mL/kg, and the metabolic clearance rate 27.4 mL/kg/min (25). In experimental animals, AM similarly circulates in plasma in the low pg/mL range. Elevated plasma levels of AM have been observed in a number of human pathologies, including pulmonary hypertension (20), heart failure (14), essential hypertension (22,26,27), liver disease with ascites (28), renal failure (24,26,28), thyrotoxicosis (29), and acute asthma (30). These pathologic elevations may reflect tissue damage characteristic of the disease states, or, alternatively, secretion of hormone as a physiologically relevant compensatory mechanism in disease. In septic shock (31,32), elevated plasma levels of AM are directly correlated with an important manifestation of the pathology, which is hypotension.

Transcriptional Regulation and Hormone Secretion

Cultured vascular smooth muscle cells (VSMC) and ECs have served as the preferred models for the study of transcriptional regulation; however, message levels also have been examined in heart following in vivo volume overload (18), and in cultured rat ventricular myocytes (11) during glucocorticoid administration. Proinflammatory factors, such as lipopolysaccharide, interleukin-1, and tumor necrosis factor, are potent stimulators of AM transcription in cultured VSMCs (21), probably through induction of the transciptional factor, NF-IL6. Endotoxin stimulation of AM gene transcription, and AM secretion in vitro, mirror the in vivo situation, in which, in man (31), septic shock is accompanied by high circulating levels of AM. In experimental animals (33), lipopolysaccharide infusion results in significant elevation in plasma AM levels and induction of AM gene expression in aorta, lung, adrenal gland, skeletal and cardiac muscle, ileum/jejunum, brain, kidney, and submaxillary gland. Thus, the vasodilatory effect of endotoxins may be exerted in a wide variety of tissues by recruitment of locally produced AM. Growth factors, including fibroblast growth factor and epidermal and platelet derived growth factors, also stimulate AM mRNA accumulation (21), possibly by activating phospholipase C and protein kinase C, thereby inducing AP-2. Retinoic acid, mineralo- and glucocorticoids, and thyroid hormones also weakly stimulate transcription of the AM gene (15). This effect of thyroid hormones in vitro may be reflected in the observation of elevated plasma AM levels in thyrotoxicosis (29). Negative regulators of AM gene transcription include cyclic adenosine monophosphate (cAMP) and transforming growth factor-β (34). Physical factors, such as shear stress, can increase AM gene transcription (13). Cultured rat astrocytes also express AM mRNA, and expression is stimulated by interferon-γ (35). Finally, nicotinic agents stimulate the release of both AM and PAMP from cultured adrenal medullary cells (17).

THE PHARMACOLOGY OF AM AND PAMP

It became evident, even in initial studies, that the structural homology AM shared with calcitonin gene related peptide (CGRP) had biologic consequence. Indeed, many reports of the pharmacologic effect of AM in whole animals and in tissue assays indicated shared biologic function *(36)*. Some of the actions of AM were blocked by a peptide antagonist of CGRP binding, and the uniqueness of AM's action initially came into question.

Localization and Identification of AM and PAMP Receptors

The CGRP antagonist ($CGRP_{8-37}$) blocks the vasorelaxant effect of AM in several vascular beds, most notably the cerebral arterioles *(37,38)* and mesenteric arteries *(39,40)*. However, the blood-pressure (BP)-lowering effect of iv infusion of AM is not blocked by $CGRP_{8-37}$ *(41,42)*, and the increased renal blood flow observed in isolated kidney or *in situ* tissue preparations is also not blocked by the antagonist *(43,44)*. It is now clear that AM can bind to the $CGRP_1$ receptor with lower affinity than CGRP *(45)*. On the other hand, CGRP has not been reported to bind to the recently characterized AM receptor *(46)*. That AM receptor is coupled (Fig. 2), via a cholera-toxin-sensitive G protein, to adenylyl cyclase and phosholipase C *(47)*. In bovine aortic ECs *(47)*, increased intracellular Ca^{2+} levels result initially from mobilization of intracellular stores by inositol triphosphate (IP_3). A prolonged opening of the ion channel in the plasma membrane also follows AM receptor activation. The increased intracellular calcium levels may contribute to the activation of nitric oxide synthase (NOS) activity. A direct effect of AM binding on NOS activity, via G-protein coupling, has been suggested *(47)*. AM exerts its inhibitory effects on basal and corticotropin-releasing hormone (CRH)-simulated adrenocorticotrophic hormone (ACTH) secretion without activating adenylyl cyclase *(48)*; thus, a second class of receptors, not linked to adenylyl cyclase, probably exists. Further evidence for additional AM receptors, or at least alternative signaling pathways, comes from studies describing the role of adenosine receptors. These receptors transduce, via activation of adenosine triphosphate (ATP)-sensitive K^+ channels, the dilatory effect of AM in coronary vessels *(49)*. The effect of the peptide to dilate rat cerebral arterioles is blocked by both glybenclamide, an inhibitor of ATP-sensitive K^+ channels, and iberiotoxin, an inhibitor of Ca^{2+}-dependent K^+ channels *(41)*, further suggesting involvement of potassium channels in the transduction of AM signaling.

A 90-kDa protein that demonstrates selective affinity for PAMP has been isolated *(50)*; however, little else is known about the receptors that bind the peptide. AM vasodilates, at least in part, via a stimulation of EC NOS activity *(51)*. The vasorelaxant effect of PAMP is apparently not exerted directly on ECs or VSMCs. Instead, PAMP exerts presynaptic inhibition of sympathetic terminals innervating the vessel. PAMP, but not AM, significantly decreased norepinephrine overflow induced by periarterial nerve stimulation *(52)* in perfused rat mesenteric arteries. This effect of PAMP was not blocked by $CGRP_{8-37}$, hexamethonium, or yohimbine, suggesting a direct effect of the peptide on neural membrane polarization state.

Further evidence for a G-protein-mediated signaling mechanisms for PAMP comes from experiments in pheochromocytoma-derived (PC) 12 cells *(53)*. In these cells, PAMP inhibited a voltage-gated Ca^{2+} channel current via a pertussis-toxin-sensitive G protein. These results in transformed cells have physiologic correlates. Addition of exogenous PAMP to cultures of normal adrenal medullary cells, prior to nicotinic stimulation,

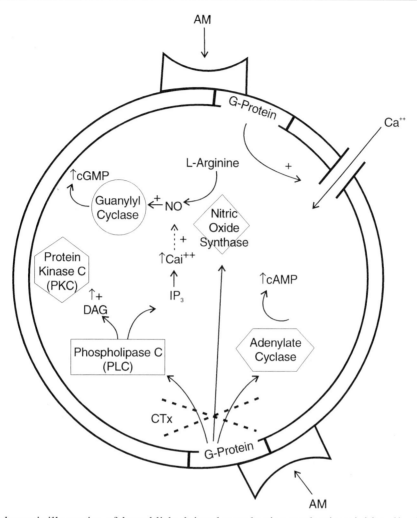

Fig. 2. Schematic illustration of the published signal transduction mechanisms initiated by AM and PAMP PTx, pertussis toxin; CTx, cholera toxin; cGMP, cyclic guanosine monophosphate; cAMP, cyclic adenosine monophosphate; NO, nitric oxide; DAG, diacyl glycerol; IP$_3$, inositol triphosphate.

resulted in significantly attenuated catecholamine release *(17)* that was not caused by a blockade of voltage-dependent Ca^{2+} channels or voltage-dependent Na^+ channels. Carbachol stimulates the release of catecholamines and the peptides AM and PAMP from adrenal medullary cells. Thus, PAMP may act in a paracrine fashion to limit catecholamine secretion from the gland.

Cardiovascular Actions of AM and PAMP in Humans

Not all of the renal and cardiovascular effects of AM originally observed in animal models have been confirmed in human infusion trials. When AM was infused at either 2 or 8 ng/kg/min *(54)*, significant reductions in mean arterial pressure were observed. Sympathetic nervous system (SNS) activity, renin secretion, and renal function did not change. Those authors hypothesized that the threshold for vascular actions of AM in humans may be lower than that for either the endocrine or renal effects. This might explain why renal and endocrine effects of AM, observed in animal models, were not obtained in this human infusion trial. As in animal studies, the vascular effect of AM appears to be mediated via activation of nitric oxide (NO) production, because pretreatment with a false substrate for NOS, N-G-monomethyl-L-arginine, blocked the ability of AM to increase forearm blood flow in normal human volunteers *(55)*. In another study, plasma AM levels were raised in healthy volunteers to concentrations over 40 times normal *(25)*. At this infusion rate (13.4 pmol/kg/min) a significant decrease in diastolic BP and a concomitant increase in pulse rate were observed. Of all the hormones examined, including pituitary and adrenal factors, only plasma levels of prolactin were significantly altered, and it could be that this was an artifact of the infusion protocol. This study provides convincing argument that AM must act as a local paracrine factor in the blood vessels, because the concentrations necessary to affect significant changes in cardiovascular parameters greatly exceed levels attained even under most pathologically elevated conditions.

Thus, neither AM nor PAMP may act physiologically as circulating hormones. Instead, their local, paracrine, or autocrine actions may be of primary importance, and elevated circulating levels observed in a wide spectrum of human pathologies may only represent spillover into the bloodstream during increased *in situ* production and secretion. Indeed, production of AM in kidney, particularly in glomerulus and tubule, predicts a local action, and thus the levels attained in iv infusion studies may not recapitulate physiologic tissue exposure. Still, it is difficult to rule out effects of circulating hormone more in the physiologic range, because, in all whole-animal studies, rapid compensatory mechanisms can come into play, or, alternatively, normal compensatory mechanisms may be interrupted by the peptide infused. This appears to be the case for AM, because the normal sympathetic response to hypotension is buffered by a direct affect of the peptide to desensitize the baroreceptor *(56)*. Also, these peripheral infusion studies cannot mimic the patterns of potential hormone secretion that may occur in vivo. Thus, results from animal studies, which might not be obtained in human trials, should not be ignored. Indeed, one of the most therapeutically promising effects of AM, extensively reported in a variety of species (vide infra), diuresis/natriuresis, has yet to be seen in humans.

Vascular Actions

In addition to causing prolonged hypotension, primarily because of generation of NO in the vasculature *(51,55)*, AM also inhibits the production of procontractile factors, particularly endothelin *(57)*. The vasorelaxant effect of AM is attenuated in endothelium denuded isolated artery segments *(58)*, indicating that circulating AM acts primarily on ECs, in which receptors for the peptide have been demonstrated *(59)*. However, residual activity remains, probably reflecting the ability of AM to stimulate adenylyl cyclase activity in the smooth muscle itself *(60)*. The effect of AM on NO production in ECs is not affected by $CGRP_{8-37}$; however, the action to elevate cAMP levels in VSMCs is blocked by the CGRP antagonist *(60)*. The inability of the CGRP antagonist to block the vasorelaxant effect of AM in some vascular beds may only reflect, then, the potent effect of AM on EC NO production, and possibly cAMP accumulation *(58)*, and not its action in VSMCs, which can be blocked by $CGRP_{8-37}$. Through mechanisms not yet completely elucidated, AM has also been demonstrated to decrease calcium mobilization and calcium sensitivity of the contractile elements in VSMCs *(61)*.

A role for locally produced AM in the prevention of pathologic vascular remodeling has been hypothesized. AM exerts antigrowth effects in the vasculature *(62,63)* and kidney *(64)*. In addition to preventing VSMC proliferation in culture, antimigratory effects have been demonstrated. Thus, AM may protect against the development of atherosclerosis or restenosis. In ECs, AM acts as a survival factor, suppressing apoptosis *(65)*.

Renal Actions

Diuretic and natriuretic effects of AM in the kidney are the result of both increased renal blood flow and direct tubular actions *(66–68)*. The threshold for natriuresis and decreased distal fractional sodium reabsorption is lower than that for changes in renal blood flow *(67)*. As a result, tubular effects seem to occur before significant changes in blood flow or glomerular filtration, suggesting the importance of paracrine actions of AM in the tubule. AM gene products and AM immunoreactivity have been reported in glomerulus, cortical collecting duct, and outer and inner medullary collecting ducts, but not in medullary thick ascending limb or proximal convoluted tubule *(69)*. In isolated tissue segments where message is found, AM elevates cAMP accumulation *(69)*. Additionally, AM increased osmotic permeability of the inner medullary collecting duct, further establishing a direct tubular site of action *(69)*. The tubular effects of AM are complemented by hypothalamic actions to inhibit arginine vasopressin (AVP) release *(70)*, and by adrenal effects to inhibit aldosterone secretion *(71,72)*.

AM may affect glomerular filtration by a variety of mechanisms. The peptide lowers renal vascular resistance, via a prostaglandin-dependent mechanism *(73)*, and inhibits mesangial cell proliferation *(64,74)*. Although the tubular effects may be exerted via the $CGRP_1$ receptor, the glomerular effects are not blocked by the CGRP antagonist *(75)*.

AM may also affect the endocrine function of the kidney. Originally, it was thought that the ability of AM to stimulate renin secretion was solely the result of the hypotensive effect of the peptide. Those in vivo studies could not, however, rule out nonreflexive actions of AM. A direct action of AM to stimulate renin production and release, via a cAMP-dependent mechanism, has been demonstrated in isolated, perfused rat kidneys and primary cultures of mouse juxtaglomerular granular cells *(76)*. Thus, in experimental models, the hallmark renal effects of AM include actions on renal perfusion pressure, glomerular filtration, tubular handling of sodium, and a direct action on renin secretion.

Adrenal Actions

The preproAM gene is transcribed not only in chromaffin cells, but also in cells of the superficial adrenal cortex. There, significant actions of the preproAM-derived peptides have been demonstrated. Release of aldosterone from cultured glomerulosa cells *(72)*, under angiotensin II (ANG II)-stimulated, but not basal, conditions, is inhibited by AM, and even more potently, and at lower doses, by PAMP. Although the effect of AM is blocked by the CGRP antagonist *(72)*, that of PAMP is not *(77)*. These in vitro results have been confirmed in vivo in two unique models of sodium dishomeostasis *(72)*, in which elevated aldosterone levels in rats on a low-sodium diet, and in nephrectomized rats, were significantly suppressed by iv infusion of AM. The ability of AM infusion to lower plasma cortisol levels in conscious sheep, on the other hand, may not result from a direct adrenal action, because the peptide suppresses ACTH secretion in vivo *(78)*, and from dispersed anterior pituitary cells in vitro *(48)*. Direct effects of AM and PMP on mineralocorticoid secretion have been demonstrated, but any lowering of cortisol levels observed in vivo may reflect a pituitary site of action of the peptides, and not direct cortical effects in adrenal gland.

Direct Cardiac Actions

Elevations in circulating AM levels in human disease states characterized by volume or pressure overload *(14,20,22,26,27)* suggest, as is the case for the natriuretic peptides *(79)*, cardiac production and secretion of the preproAM-derived peptides. Indeed, the gene is transcribed in myocytes *(11)*, cells in which AM exerts an autocrine/paracrine action *(12)*. Regulation of gene expression by glucocorticoids *(11)* and physical *(80)*, and possibly genetic *(81)* factors has been reported. As in the peripheral vasculature *(62,63)* and kidney *(64)*, AM may act in heart to inhibit cell growth and hypertrophy. In cultured cardiomyocytes, AM increases early gene expression *(82)*, and downregulates transcription of the ANP gene *(83)*. It is a potent inhibitor of ANG II-stimulated protein synthesis in cultured myocytes *(12)* and coronary artery smooth muscle cell migration *(63)*, and thus may play an important role in the prevention of cardiac growth and coronary vessel remodeling.

Direct procontractile effects of AM have been observed in isolated heart preparations *(84)*. In conscious sheep, the hypotensive effect of iv infusion of AM was accompanied by concomitant increases in heart rate (HR), cardiac output, and force of cardiac contractility. Originally, this suggested a baroreceptor-mediated activation of sympathetic function *(78,85)*; however, when the fall in BP was held to a minimum, increased cardiac contractile function was still observed *(85,86)*. In addition, evidence that AM actually dampens baroreceptor function was obtained in conscious rabbits, in which the sympathetic response to the fall in BP caused by AM was less than that occurring in response to a similar drop in pressure caused by sodium nitroprusside *(56)*. The direct cardiac effect of AM, independent of the involvement of the autonomic nervous system, was established in studies in conscious sheep *(87)*. First, the increased contractile function observed following a hypotensive dose of AM was not prevented by prior blockade of α- or β-adrenergic receptors. Second, during muscarinic blockade, the increases in contractility, HR, and cardiac output, in fact, were enhanced. These actions in heart may be cardioprotective, preventing cardiovascular collapse in the face of extreme hypotension in such states as septic shock, when plasma levels of AM rise rapidly, and are maintained at supraphysiologic levels until the resolution of the inflammatory stimulus *(29,33)*. As discussed below, some of the central nervous system (CNS) actions of both AM and PAMP complement these cardioprotective effects, assuring maintenance of cerebral perfusion, even during acute hypotensive episodes.

Recently, a potential therapeutic use of AM was identified in an ovine model of heart failure *(88)*. In these animals, AM infusion caused significant decreases in peripheral resistance, mean arterial pressure, left atrial pressure, and circulating aldosterone levels. Cardiac output increased, as did urinary sodium excretion. It remains to be seen if AM can reduce the pressure and volume stress of heart failure in other animal models of the disease; however, these findings suggest that, under conditions of exaggerated pressure and volume that lead to heart failure, AM may play an ameliorative role.

Effects in Lung

Potent vasodilatory effects of AM in the pulmonary circulation of the normoxic rat, via NO-dependent and prostaglandin-independent mechanisms, have been demonstrated *(89)*. This was most prominent in the smaller arterioles, and was not blocked by $CGRP_{8-37}$ *(90)*. The ability of AM to relax precontracted pulmonary arterial rings *(91)* may have physiologic relevance. Increased AM levels in the pulmonary circulation of patients with pulmonary hypertension *(92)* may act to reduce pulmonary vascular resistance *(93)*. A role in the prevention of airway inflammation is suggested by the ability of AM to inhibit cytokine-induced neutrophil chemoattractant release from alveolar macrophages *(94)*. Finally, plasma levels of AM in patients with asthma are significantly elevated *(30)*. This may reflect a compensatory recruitment of the peptide to counteract bronchoconstriction, because AM can inhibit bronchoconstriction in response to acetylcholine and histamine *(91)*.

Central Nervous System Actions

Immunocytochemistry and radioimmunoassay studies have detected AM in a variety of CNS sites, most notably the hypothalamus, thalamus, and brain stem. AM-positive neurons were localized to the paraventricular (PVN) and supraoptic nuclei *(9)*, as well as the infundibular nucleus in the medial basal hypothalamus *(6)*. Abundant neuronal staining for AM is present in both magnocellular (projecting to posterior pituitary gland) and parvocellular (projecting to other CNS sites, including median eminence and brainstem) elements of the PVN. This suggests effects of AM on neuroendocrine function (parvocellular elements), or, because of the magnocellular localization, an autocrine or paracrine action on AVP release. In conscious sheep *(78)* under euvolemic and normosmotic conditions, intracerebroventricular (icv) injection of AM did not significantly alter AVP release. Furthermore, ACTH levels remained unchanged, indicating a failure to alter hypothalamic, neuroendocrine mechanisms controlling corticotroph function. However, when plasma AVP levels were elevated in rabbits by hypovolemia or hypernatremia *(70)*, icv administration of AM decreased plasma AVP levels. Thus, AM may act centrally to inhibit AVP secretion, the effect being manifest only under conditions of high secretory activity.

AM binding has been described in both hypothalamus and brainstem *(46)*, and neuronal *(95)*, as well as glial *(96)*, sites of action have been reported. The peptide exerted profound effects on cerebral blood flow (CBF) *(37)*, suggesting receptors on cerebral blood vessels as well. Because the CGRP antagonist blocks the vasodilatory effect of AM *(41)*, the vascular effects of AM in brain may be caused by an action on the shared CGRP receptor. Nevertheless, the potent vasodilatory effect of AM may reflect an important role for endogenous peptide. The decrease in CBF, normally seen following middle cerebral artery occlusion *(97)*, was blocked by prior icv administration of AM in the spontaneously hypertensive rat. Total CBF also increased. Thus, the peptide may prevent ischemic brain damage by increasing collateralization. AM may play an important antimitogenic role in glia *(96,98)*, as has been hypothesized for another locally produced vasodilatory peptide, atrial natriuretic peptide *(99)*.

Significant, dose-related, inhibitory actions of AM on water drinking *(100)* and salt appetite *(101)* complement the natriuretic and diuretic effects of AM in the kidney. These CNS effects were independent of CGRP receptors, and were not, in the effective dose range, caused by a nonspecific inhibition of appetitive behaviors. This is significant, because the structural homolog, CGRP, when administered centrally at high doses *(102)*, inhibits food intake. It has been reported that microgram doses of AM can significantly inhibit fasting-induced food intake *(103)*. However, using more physiologically relevant doses (low- to mid-nanogram), the author has not observed any significant effects of AM on food intake under fasted or ad libitum feeding conditions. The doses of AM we employed were those that significantly inhibit water and salt appetites *(100,101)* and stimulate SNS function *(104)*, and were more in the apparent physiologic range *(8)*. The ED_{50} for AM's inhibition of water drinking (100–200 ng) is only one order of magnitude greater than the levels measured in harvested CNS tissues (8). In order to demonstrate a significant effect on food intake, 10 μg of AM had to be injected icv (103). Thus, the high dose of AM employed may indicate a pharmacologic interaction with CGRP receptors, which might not have physiologic relevance.

The very first evidence for a physiologic role for AM (101) came from CNS studies. The author and others have employed a model of isotonic hypovolemia to study the roles of a variety of CNS peptides on ingestive behaviors (105,106). This model demonstrated that exogenous AM can significantly, and in a dose related fashion, inhibit salt appetite (101). Animals made hypovolemic by polyethylene glycol administration (105,106) were pretreated with either normal rabbit serum (NRS) or anti-AM antiserum, icv, prior to returning drinking bottles containing tap water or 0.3 M NaCl to the cages. The expected, robust drinking of tap water and saline occurred in rats pretreated with NRS. Pretreatment of hypovolemic rats with anti-AM antiserum resulted in a significant stimulation of saline intake, which was apparent for 5 h of testing (101). Cumulative fluids intake (tap water + saline) was also significantly increased over this period. Within 24 h, the antiserum-injected animals had fully recovered, consuming over that period the same amounts of water and saline as NRS-injected controls. Thus, a significant, physiologically relevant role in the CNS regulation of sodium, and therefore volume, homeostasis has been established for centrally produced AM.

Does PAMP in brain, as in the periphery, exert similar actions to those of AM? When injected in doses similar to those for AM, PAMP did not significantly affect thirst (water drinking) or salt appetite (saline drinking). In another experimental paradigm, central administration of AM, but not PAMP, was found to inhibit gastric emptying (107). The physiologic relevance of this effect of AM is not yet clear, but those studies did indicate that the CNS effect of AM was mediated via activation of the adrenal gland, since both adrenalectomy and β-adrenergic blockade abolished the effect.

Within the CNS, AM and PAMP act in similar fashion to activate the SNS (104). An apparent, physiologic paradox was reported in 1994 (108), when icv injections of AM in urethane-anesthetized rats were demonstrated to be hypertensive. Arterial pressure rose gradually over 20 min, and remained elevated for up to 2 h. A more transient elevation in abdominal sympathetic discharge was also observed. Pretreatment with the CGRP antagonist blocked both the hypotensive effect of AM in the periphery and the hypertensive effects when given centrally. In Inactin-anesthetized (Research Biochemicals International, Natick, MA) rats, the author had not observed significant changes in BP following icv injection of AM in doses that were biologically active (appetitive behaviors) in conscious animals (100). Doses were less than those reported to be hypertensive in the urethane-anesthetized rats (108). Subsequently, Ferguson et al. (95) were able to demonstrate direct effects of AM on neuronal firing rates of cardiovascular regulatory elements of the area postrema in slice preparations. Thus, it was possible to demonstrate CNS actions of AM to control sympathetic outflow, and therefore HR and blood (104,109). Choice of anesthetic employed might have, in the initial studies, determined the responsiveness of the animal to centrally administered AM. As a result, it was clear that these studies had to be conducted in the unanesthetized animal, in order to avoid the potential artifact of anesthetics.

Therefore, the focus switched to unanesthetized animals, and, indeed, in conscious, unrestrained rats, both AM and PAMP are hypertensive when administered into the cerebroventricular system *(104)*. The author cannot speculate on the exact site of action of the peptides, because both lateral ventricle and fourth ventricle administrations significantly elevate mean arterial pressure. CGRP, when injected in similar doses 3–300 pmol, did not significantly alter BP or HR in these conscious, unrestrained animals. Therefore, it is unlikely that the effect of AM on BP was mediated via an action on CGRP receptors. Additionally, pretreatment with the CGRP antagonist failed to significantly alter the hypertensive effect of AM or PAMP.

In all experiments, ANG II (100 pmol) was also injected icv and the hypertensive actions of PAMP and AM compared to that of ANG II *(104)*. The actions of AM and PAMP were dose-related and transient, having abated by 10 min postinjection. The onset and pattern of the transient elevation of BP was quite similar to the central hypertensive action of ANG II. Like ANG II, the hypertensive effects of AM and PAMP could be blocked by pretreatment (iv) with the α-adrenergic blocker, phentolamine, suggesting that both AM and PAMP act within brain to stimulate SNS function. The author then hypothesized that, because of these similarities, both proAM-derived peptides might act centrally via recruitment of endogenous ANG II. To test this hypothesis, the ANG II receptor blocker, saralasin, was employed. In all animals, icv injections of AM or PAMP and ANG II, resulted in significant increases in BP prior to saralasin treatment. Following angiotensin receptor blockade, however, none of these peptides significantly altered mean arterial BP. These results strongly suggest that AM and PAMP act on neural systems that converge on cells receptive to endogenous ANG II. There is no evidence that AM or PAMP can bind to the ANG II receptor. Therefore, the author suggests that the actions of the peptides are exerted upstream to the ANG II synapse.

The author has demonstrated that AM and PAMP exert significant hypertensive actions in the brains of conscious rats, and hypothesizes that the CNS actions of AM and PAMP are cardioprotective, counteracting either the volume-unloading actions of the peptides in the periphery or acting in general to protect against hypotensive crisis. This would provide a margin of safety that would protect against circulatory collapse in situations when elevated plasma levels of peptide, such as septic shock *(31)*, might precipitously lower venous return. A similar situation exists in the heart, in which the peripheral hypotensive effects of at least AM are counterbalanced by the positive inotropic effects of the peptide in the myocardium *(84,87)*. What stimuli activate the neurons containing AM and PAMP are not known, nor, for that matter, what might control expression of the AM gene products in brain. Those are important issues that require immediate attention, in order to determine the physiologic relevance of these sympathostimulatory effects of the preproAM-derived peptides.

Pituitary Actions

AM-like immunoreactivity is present in pituitary gland extracts *(8)*, particularly extracts of the anterior lobe *(7)*. Because abundant staining for AM immunoreactivity can be detected in magnocellular cells of the paraventricular nucleus, it is assumed that the posterior lobe also contains AM *(9)*. Labeled AM binds to pituitary cell membranes *(46)*, but this may not represent a unique AM binding site, because both CGRP and islet amyloid polypeptide can competitively displace labeled AM. The phenotypic identity of anterior pituitary cells to which AM can bind is unknown at present. Functional studies, however, have identified the corticotroph as the most likely cell type in the anterior lobe to bear AM receptors. In sheep, peripheral *(85)*, but not central *(78)*, AM infusion resulted in profound suppression of plasma ACTH levels. This occurred even in the face of baroreceptor activation, suggesting a direct pituitary site of action. Cell culture studies have verified this direct pituitary site of action. In dispersed anterior pituitary cells, AM exerted a dose-related, significant inhibition of basal and CRH-stimulated adrenocortico-trophic hormone (ACTH) secretion *(48)*. The signaling mechanism that transduces this effect of AM remains unknown, but the effect was not mediated via activation of adeny-late cyclase, guanylyl cyclase, or NOS, and was not blocked by the CGRP antagonist. The effect appears selective for the corticotroph, because neither growth hormone nor lutein-izing hormone secretion were significantly altered by AM.

The rat pituitary gland has been reported to contain 1.12 fmol AM/mg wet wt *(8)*. This would predict that about 50–100 pg AM are present in the gland (which, in adult donors, weighs approx 10 mg). The ED_{50} for the inhibitory effect of AM on ACTH secretion (10–100 pM) translates to 57.3–573 pg AM. Thus, in dispersed pituitary cells, physiologically relevant levels of AM exert significant inhibitory effects on both basal and CRH-stimulated ACTH secretion. This suggests a physiological role for AM in the neuroendocrine regulation of corticotroph function.

Basal, but not CRH-stimulated, ACTH secretion in vitro is also inhibited by PAMP in doses ranging from 0.1 to 10 nM. The effect is completely reversed by 100 nM glybenclamide, suggesting an action of the peptide on ATP-sensitive K^+ channels *(110)*. Thus, it appears that in anterior pituitary gland, as in the vasculature and adrenal cortex, proAM-derived peptides may exert physiologically relevant actions via parallel mecha-nisms, ensuring accurate control of cellular function. These pituitary actions of AM and PAMP may complement effects of the peptide in the adrenal gland and kidney. Because the anterior pituitary gland is not behind the blood–brain barrier, these pharmacologic effects in dispersed, cultured cells may reflect actions exerted by either locally produced peptides or those brought to the gland by the general circulation, particularly under high secretion states.

SUMMARY

Two biologically active peptides are encoded by the AM gene. Both exert hypotensive actions in the peripheral vasculature, albeit by apparently differing mechanisms. One of these, AM, also exerts potent natriuretic and diuretic effects in experimental animals, and both AM and PAMP are potent inhibitors of aldosterone secretion (Fig. 3). The renal and adrenal actions of AM are matched by effects of AM in brain to inhibit salt and water intakes, and by both peptides in pituitary to inhibit ACTH secretion. Cardioprotective actions of AM are exerted directly on the heart to increase coronary perfusion and contractility. In brain, AM exerts similar vasodilatory effects, increasing collaterali-zation. Both AM and PAMP act in brain, via angiotensinergic neural systems, to stimu-late SNS function, providing additional cardioprotection to that exerted in the heart. These cardioprotective actions may play an important role in the prevention of vascular collapse or prolonged hypotensive crisis.

ACKNOWLEDGMENTS

The outstanding technical assistance of Tonya Murphy is recognized, as is the Max Baer Heart Fund, from the Dakota Aerie of the Fraternal Order of Eagles, which supports these studies on the physiology of the proadrenomedullin-derived peptides.

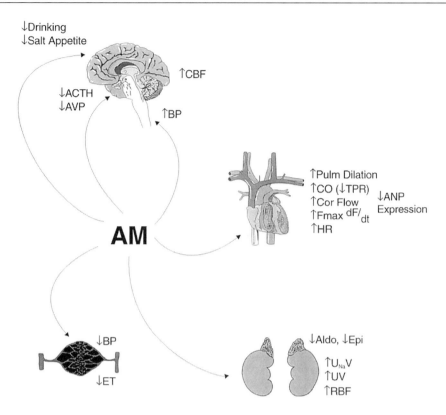

Fig. 3. Schematic representation of the multiple tissue sites of action of AM. ACTH, adrenocorticotropin; AVP, vasopressin; BP, mean arterial pressure; CO, cardiac output; TPR, total peripheral resistance; Cor Flow, coronary blood flow; Fmax, maximum coronary flow; HR, heart rate; ANP, atrial natriuretic peptide; Aldo, aldosterone; Epi, epinephrine; $U_{na}V$, urinary sodium excretion; UV, urine volume; RBF, renal blood flow; ET, endothelin.

REFERENCES

1. Kitamura K, Kangawa K, Kawamoto M, Ichiki Y, Nakamura S, Matsuo H, Eto T. Adrenomedullin: a novel hypotensive peptide isolated from human pheochromocytoma. Biochem Biophys Res Commun 1993;192:553–560.
2. Kitamura K, Sakata J, Kangawa K, Kojima H, Matsuo H, Eto T. Cloning and characterization of cDNA encoding a precursor for human adrenomedullin. Biochem Biophys Res Commun 1993;194:720–725.
3. Ishimitsu T, Kojima M, Hino J, Matsuoka H, Kitamura K, Eto T, Matsuo H. Genomic structure of human adrenomedullin gene. Biochem Biophys Res Commun 1994;203:631–639.
4. Sakata J, Shimokubo T, Kitamura K, Nakamura S, Kangawa K, Matsuo H, Eto T. Molecular cloning and biological activities of rat adrenomedullin, a hypotensive peptide. Biochem Biophys Res Commun 1993;195:921–927.
5. Ichiki Y, Kitamura K, Kangawa K, Kawamoto M, Matsuo H, Eto T. Distribution and characterization of immunoreactive adrenomedullin in human tissue and plasma. FEBS Lett 1994;338:6–10.
6. Satoh F, Takahashi K, Murakami O, Totsune K, Sone M, Ohneda M, Sasano H, Mouri T. Immunocytochemical localization of adrenomedullin-like immunoreactivity in the human hypothalamus and adrenal gland. Neurosci Lett 1996;203:207–210.
7. Washimine H, Asada Y, Kitamura K, Ichiki Y, Hara S, Yamamoto Y, et al. Immunohistochemical identification of adrenomedullin in human, rat, and porcine tissue. Histochem Cell Biol 1995;103:251–254.

8. Sakata J, Shimokubo T, Kitamura K, Nakamura S, Kangawa K, Matsuo H, Eto T. Distribution and characterization of immunoreactive rat adrenomedullin in tissue and plasma. FEBS Lett 1994;352: 105–108.

9. Ueta Y, Kitamura K, Isse T, Shibuya I, Kabashima N, Yamamoto S, et al. Adrenomedullin-immunoreactive neurons in the paraventricular and supraoptic nuclei of the rat. Neurosci Lett 1995;202:37–40.

10. Sugo S, Minamino N, Kangawa K, Miyamoto K, Kitamura K, Sakata J, Eto T, Matsuo H. Endothelial cells actively synthesize and secrete adrenomedullin. Biochem Biophys Res Commun 1994;201: 1160–1166.

11. Nishimori T, Tsujino M, Sato K, Imai T, Marumo F, Hirata Y. Dexamethasone-induced up-regulation of adrenomedullin and atrial natriuretic peptide genes in cultured rat ventricular myocytes. J Mol Cell Cardiol 1997;29:2125–2130.

12. Tsuruda T, Kato J, Kitamura K, Kuwasako K, Imamura T, Koiwaya Y, et al. Adrenomedullin: a possible autocrine or paracrine inhibitor of hypertrophy of cardiomyocytes. Hypertension 1998;31: 505–510.

13. Chun TH, Itoh H, Ogawa Y, Tamura N, Takaya K, Igaki T, et al. Shear stress augments expression of C-type natriuretic peptide and adrenomedullin. Hypertension 1997;29:1296–1302.

14. Jougasaki M, Wei CM, Mckinley LJ, Burnett JC. Elevation of circulating and ventricular adrenomedullin in human congestive heart failure. Circulation 1995;92:286–289.

15. Minamino N, Shoji H, Sugo S, Kangawa K, Matsuo H. Adrenocortical steroids, thyroid hormones and retinoic acid augment the production of adrenomedullin in vascular smooth muscle cells. Biochem Biophys Res Commun 1995;211:686–693.

16. Satoh F, Takahashi K, Murakami O, Totsune K, Sone M, Ohneda M, et al. Adrenomedullin in human brain, adrenal glands and tumor tissues of pheochromocytoma, ganglioneuroblastoma and neuroblastoma. J Clin Endocrinol Metab 1995;80:1750–1752.

17. Katoh F, Kitamura K, Niina H, Yamamoto R, Washimine H, Kangawa K, et al. Proadrenomedullin N-terminal 20 peptide (PAMP), an endogenous anticholinergic peptide: its exocytotic secretion and inhibition of catecholamine secretion in adrenal medulla. J Neurochem 1995;64:459–461.

18. Romppanen H, Marttila M, Magga J, Vuolteenaho O, Kinnunen P, Szokodi I, Ruskaoho H. Adrenomedullin gene expression in the rat heart is stimulated by acute pressure overload: blunted effect in experimental hypertension. Endocrinology 1997;138:2636–2639.

19. Samson WK. Cardiovascular hormones. In: Conn PM, Melmed S, eds. Endocrinology, Basic and Clinical Principles, Humana, Totowa, 1997, pp. 361–376.

20. Shimokubo T, Sakata J, Kitamura K, Kangawa K, Matsuo H, Eto T. Augmented adrenomedullin concentrations in right ventricle and plasma of experimental pulmonary hypertension. Life Sci 1995; 57:1771–1779.

21. Sugo S, Minamino N, Shoji H, Kangawa K, Kitamura K, Eto T, Matsuo H. Interleukin-1, tumor necrosis factor and lipopolysaccharide additively stimulate production of adrenomedullin in vascular smooth muscle cells. Biochem Biophys Res Commun 1995;207:25–32.

22. Kitamura K, Ichiki Y, Tanaka M, Kawamoto M, Emura J, Sakakibara S, et al. Immunoreactive adrenomedullin in human plasma. FEBS Lett 1994;341:288–290.

23. Sato K, Hirata Y, Imai T, Iwashina M, Marumo F. Characterization of immunoreactive adrenomedullin in human plasma and urine. Life Sci 1995;57:189–194.

24. Washimine H, Yamamoto Y, Kitamura K, Tanaka M, Ichiki Y, Kangawa K, Matsuo H, Eto T. Plasma concentrations of human adrenomedullin in patients on hemodialysis. Clin Nephrol 1995;44:389–393.

25. Meeran K, O'Shea D, Upton PD, Small CJ, Ghatei MA, Byfield PH, Bloom SR. Circulating adrenomedullin does not regulate systemic BP but increases plasma prolactin after intravenous infusion in humans: a pharmacokinetic study. J Clin Endocrinol Metab 1997;82:95–100.

26. Ishimitsu T, Nishikimi T, Saito Y, Kitamura K, Eto T, Kangawa K, et al. Plasma levels of adrenomedullin, a newly identified hypotensive peptide, in patients with hypertension and renal failure. J Clin Invest 1994;94:2158–2161.

27. Kohno M, Hanehira T, Kano H, Horio T, Yokokawa K, Ikeda M, et al. Plasma adrenomedullin concentrations in essential hypertension. Hypertension 1996;27:102–107.

28. Cheung B, Leung R. Elevated plasma levels of human adrenomedullin in cardiovascular, respiratory, hepatic and renal disorders. Clin Sci 1997;92:59–62.

29. Taniyama M, Kitamura K, Ban Y, Sigita E, Ito K, Katagiri T. Elevation of circulating proadrenomedullin N-20 terminal peptide in thyrotoxicosis. Clin Endocrinol 1997;46:271–274.

30. Kohno M, Hanehira T, Hirata K, Kawaguchi T, Okishio K, Kano H, Kanazawa H, Yoshikawa J. Accelerated increase of plasma adrenomedullin in acute asthma. Metabolism 1996;45:1323–1325.

31. Hirata Y, Mitaka C, Sato K, Nagura T, Tsunoda Y, Amaha K, Marumo F. Increased circulating adrenomedullin, a novel vasodilatory peptide, in sepsis. J Clin Endocrinol Metab 1996;81:1449–1453.
32. Nishio K, Akai Y, Murao Y, Doi N, Ueda S, Tabuse H, et al. Increased plasma concentration of adrenomedullin correlate with relaxation of vascular tone in patients with septic shock. Crit Care Med 1997;25:953–957.
33. Shoji H, Minamino N, Kangawa K, Matsuo H. Endotoxin markedly elevates plasma concentration and gene transcription of adrenomedullin in rat. Biochem Biophys Res Commun 1995;215:531–537.
34. Sugo S, Minamino N, Shoji H, Kangawa K, Matsuo H. Effects of vasoactive substance and cAMP related compounds on adrenomedullin production in cultured vascular smooth muscle cells. FEBS Lett 1995;369:311–314.
35. Kuchinke W, Hart RP, Jonakait GM. Identification of mRNAs regulated by interferon-gamma in cultured rat astrocytes by PCR differential display. Neuroimmunomodulation 1995;2:347–355.
36. Elhawary AM, Poon J, Pang CC. Effects of calcitonin gene related peptide antagonists on renal actions of adrenomedullin. Br J Pharmacol 1995;115:1133–1140.
37. Baskaya M, Suzuki Y, Anzai M, Seki Y, Saito K, Takayasu M, Shibuya M, Sigita K. Effects of adrenomedullin, calcitonin gene related peptide, and amylin on cerebral circulation in dogs. J Cereb Blood Flow Metab 1995;15:827–834.
38. Mori T, Takayasu M, Suzuki Y, Shibuya M, Yoshida J, Hidaka H. Effects of adrenomedullin on rat cerebral arterioles. Eur J Pharmacol 1997;330:195–198.
39. Berthiaume N, Claing A, Lippton H, Cadieux A, D'Orleans-Juste P. Rat adrenomedullin induces selective arterial vasodilation via CGRP1 receptors in the double perfused mesenteric bed of the rat. Can J Physiol Pharmacol 1995;73:1080–1083.
40. Nuki C, Kawasaki H, Kitamura K, Takenaga M, Kangawa K, Eto T, Wada A. Vasodilator effect of adrenomedullin and calcitonin gene related peptide receptors in rat mesenteric vascular beds. Biochem Biophys Res Commun 1993;96:245–251.
41. Lang MG, Paterno R, Faraci FM, Heistad DD. Mechanisms of adrenomedullin induced dilatation of cerebral arterioles. Stroke 1997;28:181–185.
42. Gardiner SM, Kemp PA, March JE, Bennett T. Regional hemodynamic effects of human and rat adrenomedullin in conscious rats. Br J Pharmacol 1995;114:584–591.
43. Haynes JM, Cooper ME. Adrenomedullin and calcitonin gene related peptide in the rat isolated kidney and the anesthetized rat: in vitro and in vivo effects. Eur J Pharmacol 1995;280:91–94.
44. Hjelmqvist H, Keil R, Mathai M, Hubschle T, Gertsberger R. Vasodilation and glomerular binding of adrenomedullin in rabbit kidney are not CGRP receptor mediated. Am J Physiol 1997;273:R716–R724.
45. Aiyar, H, Rand K, Elshourbagy NA, Zeng Z, Adamou JE, Bergsma DJ, Li Y. cDNA encoding the calcitonin gene-related peptide type 1 receptor. J Biol Chem 1996;271:11,325–11,329.
46. Owji AA, Smith DM, Coppock HA, Morgan DGA, Bhogal R, Ghatei MA, Bloom SR. Abundant and specific binding site for the novel vasodilator adrenomedullin in the rat. Endocrinology 1995;136:2127–2134.
47. Shimekake Y, Nagata K, Ohta S, Kambayashi Y, Teraoka H, Kitamura K, Eto T, Matsuo H. Adrenomedullin stimulates two signal transduction pathways, cAMP accumulation, and calcium mobilization, in bovine aortic endothelial cells. J Biol Chem 1995;270:4412–4417.
48. Samson WK, Murphy TC, Schell DA. Novel vasoactive peptide, adrenomedullin, inhibits pituitary adrenocorticotropin release. Endocrinology 1995;136:2349–2352.
49. Sabates BL, Pigott JD, Choe EU, Cruz MP, Lippton HL, Hyman AL, Flint LM, Ferrara JJ. Adrenomedullin mediates coronary vasodilation through adenosine receptors and KATP channels. J Surg Res 1997;67:163–168.
50. Iwasaki H, Hirata Y, Iwashina M, Sato K, Marumo F. Specific binding for proadrenomedullin N-terminal 20 peptide (PAMP) in the rat. Endocrinology 1996;137:3045–3050.
51. Feng CJ, Kang B, Kaye AD, Kadowitz PJ, Nossman BD. L-NAME modulates responses to adrenomedullin in the hindquarters vascular bed of the rat. Life Sci 1994;55:433–438.
52. Shimosawa T, Ito Y, Ando K, Kitamura K, Kangawa K, Fujita T. Proadrenomedullin NH_2-terminal 20 peptide, a new product of the adrenomedullin gene, inhibits norepinephrine overflow from nerve endings. J Clin Invest 1995;96:1672–1676.
53. Takano K, Yamashita N, Fujita T. Proadrenomedullin N-terminal 20 peptide inhibits the voltage-gated calcium channel current through a pertussis toxin-sensitive G protein in rat pheochromocytoma-derived PC12 cells. J Clin Invest 1996;98:14–17.
54. Lainchbury JG, Cooper GJ, Coy DH, Jiang NY, Lewis LK, Yandle TG, Richards AM, Nicholls MG. Adrenomedullin: a hypotensive hormone in man. Clin Sci 1997;92:467–472.

55. Nakamura M, Yoshida H, Makita S, Arakawa N, Niinuma H, Hiramori K. Potent and long-lasting vasodilatory effects of adrenomedullin in humans. Comparisons between normal subjects and patients with chronic heart failure. Circulation 1997;95:1214–1221.

56. Fukuhara M, Tsuchihashi T, Abe I, Fujishima M. Cardiovascular and neurohumoral effects of intravenous adrenomedullin in conscious rabbits. Am J Physiol 1995;269:R1289-R1293.

57. Kohno M, Yasunari Y, Yokokawa K, Horio T, Ikeda M, Minami M, Hanehira T, Yoshikawa J. Interaction of adrenomedullin and platelet derived growth factor on the production of endothelin. Hypertension 1996;27:663–667.

58. Nakamura K, Toda H, Terasako K, Nakuyama M, Hatano Y, Mori K, Kangawa K. Vasodilative effect of adrenomedullin in isolated arteries of the dog. Jpn J Pharmacol 1995;67:259–262.

59. Kato J, Kitamura K, Kangawa K, Eto T. Receptors for adrenomedullin in human vascular endothelial cells. Eur J Pharmacol 1995;289:383–385.

60. Eguchi S, Hirata Y, Kano H, Sato K, Watanabe Y, Watanabe TX, et al. Specific receptors for adrenomedullin in cultured rat vascular smooth muscle cells. FEBS Lett 1994;340:226–230.

61. Kureshi Y, Kobayashi S, Nishimura J, Nakano T, Kanaide H. Adrenomedullin decreases both cytosolic calcium concentration and calcium sensitivity in pig coronary arterial smooth muscle. Biochem Biophys Res Commun 1995;212:572–579.

62. Kano H, Kohno M, Yasunari K, Yokokawa K, Horio T, Ikeda M, et al. Adrenomedullin as a novel antiproliferative factor in vascular smooth muscle cells. J Hypertension 1996;14:209–213.

63. Kohno M, Yokokawa K, Kano H, Yasunari K, Minami M, Hanehira T, Yoshikawa J. Adrenomedullin is a potent inhibitor of angiotensin II induced migration of human coronary artery smooth muscle cells. Hypertension 1997;29:1309–1313.

64. Chini EN, Choi E, Grande JP, Burnett JC, Douse TP. Adrenomedullin suppresses mitogenesis in rat mesangial cells via cAMP pathway. Biochem Biophys Res Commun 1995;215:868–873.

65. Kato H, Shichiri M, Marumo F, Hirata Y. Adrenomedullin as an autocrine/paracrine survival factor for rat endothelial cells. Endocrinology 1997;138:2615–2620.

66. Ebara T, Mura K, Okumura M, Matsuura T, Kim S, Yukimura T, Iwao H. Effect of adrenomedullin on renal hemodynamics and functions in dogs. Eur J Pharmacol 1994;263:69–73.

67. Jougasaki M, Wei CM, Aarhus LL, Heublein DM, Sandberg SM, Burnett JC. Renal localization and actions of adrenomedullin: a natriuretic peptide. Am J Physiol 1995;268:F657-F663.

68. Hirata Y, Hayakawa H, Suzuki Y, Suzuki Y, Ikenouchi H, Kohmoto O, et al. Mechanisms of adrenomedullin-induced vasodilation in the rat kidney. Hypertension 1995;25:790–795.

69. Owada A, Nonoguchi H, Terada Y, Marumo F, Tomita K. Microlocalization and effects of adrenomedullin in nephron segments and in mesangial cells of the rat. Am J Physiol 1997;272:F691–F697.

70. Yokoi H, Arima T, Kondo K, Iwasaki Y, Oiso Y. Intracerebroventricular injection of adrenomedullin inhibits vasopressin release in conscious rats. Neurosci Lett 1996;216:65–67.

71. Andreis PG, Neri G, Prayer-Galetti T, Rossi GP, Gottardo G, Malendowicz LK, Nussdorfer GG. Effects of adrenomedullin on the human adrenal glands: an in vitro study. J Clin Endocrinol Metab 1997;82:1167–1170.

72. Yamaguchi T, Baba K, Doi Y, Yano K. Effect of adrenomedullin on aldosterone secretion by dispersed rat adrenal zona glomerulosa cells. Life Sci 1995;56:379–387.

73. Jougasaki M, Aarhus LL, Heublein DM, Sandberg SM, Burnett JC. Role of prostaglandins and renal nerves in the renal actions of adrenomedullin. Am J Physiol 1997;272:F260–F266.

74. Segawa K, Minami K, Sata T, Kuroiwa A, Shigematsu A. Inhibitory effect of adrenomedullin on rat mesangial cell mitogenesis. Nephron 1996;74:577–579.

75. Edwards RM, Trizna W, Stack E, Aiyar N. Effect of adrenomedullin on cAMP levels along the rat nephron: comparison with CGRP Am J Physiol 1996;271:F895–F899.

76. Jensen BL, Kramer BK, Kurtz A. Adrenomedullin stimulates renin release and renin mRNA in mouse juxtaglomerular granular cells. Hypertension 1997;29:1148–1155.

77. Andreis PG, Mazzocchi G, Rebuffat P, Nussdorfer GG. Effects of adrenomedullin and proadrenomedullin N-terminal 20 peptide on rat zona glomerulosa cells. Life Sci 1997;60:1693–1697.

78. Parkes DG, May CN. 1995; ACTH-suppressive and vasodilator actions of AM in conscious sheep. J Neuroendocrinology 7:923–929.

79. Grantham JA, Burnett JC. Natriuretic peptides in cardiovascular disease. In: Samson WK, Levin ER, eds. Contemporary Endocrinology, Natriuretic Peptides in Health and Disease Humana, Totowa, 1997, pp. 309–326.

80. Sumimoto T, Nishikimi T, Mukai M, Matsuzaki K, Murakami E, Takishita S, Miyata A, Matsuo H, Kangawa K. Plasma adrenomedullin concetrations and cardiac and arterial hypertrophy in hypertension. Hypertension 1997;30:741–745.

81. Inatsu H, Sakata J, Shimokubo T, Kitani M, Nishizoni M, Washimine H, et al. Distribution and characterization of rat immunoreactive proadrenomedullin N-terminal 20 peptide (PAMP) and the augmented cardiac PAMP in spontaneously hypertensive rat. Biochem Mol Biol Int 1996;38:365–372.

82. Sato A, Autelitano DJ. Adrenomedullin induces expression of c-fos and AP-1 activity in rat vascular smooth muscle cells and cardiomyocytes. Biochem Biophys Res Commun 1995;217:211–216.

83. Sato A, Canny BJ, Autelitano DJ. Adrenomedullin stimulates cAMP accumulation and inhibits atrial natriuretic peptide gene expression in cardiomyocyte. Biochem Biophys Res Commun 1997;230:311–314.

84. Szokodi I,, Kinnunen P,, Ruskoaho H. Inotropic effect of AM in the isolated perfused rat heart. Acta Physiol Scand 1996;156:151–152.

85. Parkes DG. Cardiovascular actions of adrenomedullin in conscious sheep. Am J Physiol 1995;268: H2574–H2578.

86. Charles CJ, Rademaker MT, Richards AM, Cooper CJ, Coy DH, Jing NY, Nicholls MG. Hemodynamic, hormonal, and renal effects of adrenomedullin in conscious sheep. Am J Physiol 1997;272: R2040–R2047.

87. Parkes DG, May CN. Direct cardiac and vascular actions of adrenomedullin in conscious sheep. Br J Pharmacol 1997;120:1179–1185.

88. Rademaker MT, Charles CJ, Lewis LK, Yandle TG, Cooper GJ, Coy DH, Richards AM, Nicholls MG. Beneficial hemodynamic and renal effects of adrenomedullin in an ovine model of heart failure. Circulation 1997;96:1983–1990.

89. DeWitt BJ, Cheng DY, Caminiti GN, Nossaman BD, Coy DH, Murphy WA, Kadowitz PA. Comparison of responses to adrenomedullin and calcitonin gene-related peptide in pulmonary vascular bed of the cat. Eur J Pharmacol 1994;257:303–306.

90. Shirai M, Shimouchi A, Ikeda S, Ninomiya I, Sunagawa K, Kangawa K, Matsuo H. Vasodilator effects of adrenomedullin on small pulmonary arteries and veins in anesthetized cats. Br J Pharmacol 1997; 121:679–686.

91. Yang BC, Lippton H, Gumusel B, Hyman A, Mehta JL. Adrenomedullin dilates rat pulmonary artery rings during hypoxia: role of nitric oxide and vasodilator prostaglandins, J Cardiovasc Pharmacol 1997;28:458–462.

92. Yoshibayashi M, Kamiya T, Kitamura K, Saito Y, Kangawa K, Nishikimi T, et al. Plasma levels of adrenomedullin in primary and secondary pulmonary hypertension in patients <20 years of age. Am J Cardiol 1997;79:1558–1558.

93. deVroomen M, Takahashi Y, Gournay V, Roman C, Rudolph AM, Heyman MA. Adrenomedullin increases pulmonary blood flow in fetal sheep. Pediatr Res 1997;41:493–497.

94. Kamoi H, Kanazawa K, Hirata K, Kurihara N, Yano Y, Otani S. Adrenomedullin inhibits the secretion of cytokine induced neutrophil chemoattractant, a member of the interleukin-8 family, from rat alveolar macrophages. Biochem Biophys Res Commun 1995;211:1031–1035.

95. Allen MA, Ferguson AV. In vitro recordings from area postrema neurons demonstrate responsiveness to adrenomedullin. Am J Physiol 1996;270:R920-R925.

96. Yeung VT, Ho SK, Nicholls MG, Cockram CS. Adrenomedullin, a novel vasoactive hormone, binds to mouse astrocytes and stimulates cyclic AMP production. J Neurosci Res 1996;46:330–335.

97. Dogan A, Suzuki Y, Koketsu N, Osuka K, Saito K, Takayasu M, Shibuya M, Yoshida J. Intravenous infusion of adrenomedullin and increase in regional cerebral blood flow and prevention of ischemic brain injury after middle cerebral artery occlusion in rats. J Cereb Blood Flow Metab 1997;17:19–25.

98. Zimmerman U, Fischer JA, Frei K, Fischer AH, Reinscheid RK, Muff R. Identification of adrenomedullin receptors in cultured rat astrocytes and in neuroblastoma x glioma hybrid cells (NG108-15). Brain Res 1996;724:238–245.

99. Levin ER. Natriuretic peptide C-receptor: more than a clearance receptor. Am J Physiol 1993;264: E484–E489.

100. Murphy TC, Samson WK. Novel vasoactive hormone, adrenomedullin, inhibits water drinking in the rat. Endocrinology 1995;136:2459–2463.

101. Samson WK, Murphy TC. Adrenomedullin inhibits salt appetite. Endocrinology 1996;138:613–616.

102. Krahn DD, Gosnell BA, Levine AS, Morley JE. Effects of calcitonin gene related peptide on food intake. Peptides 1984;5:861–864.

103. Taylor GM, Meeran K, O'Shea D, Smith DM, Ghatei MA, Bloom SR. Adrenomedullin inhibits feeding in the rat by a mechanism involving calcitonin gene related peptide receptors. Endocrinology 1996;137:3260–3264.
104. Samson WK, Murphy TC, Resch ZT. Central mechanisms for the hypertensive effects of preproAM derived peptides in conscious rats. Am J Physiol 1998;274:R1505–R1510.
105. Blackburn RE, Samson WK, Fulton RJ, Stricker EM, Verbalis JG. Central oxytocin inhibition of salt appetite in rats: evidence for differential sensing of plasma sodium and osmolality. Proc Natl Acad Sci USA 1993;90:10,380–10,384.
106. Blackburn RE, Samson WK, Fulton RJ, Stricker EM, Verbalis JG. Central oxytocin and ANP receptors mediate osmotic inhibition of salt appetite in rats. Am J Physiol 1995;269:R245-R251.
107. Martinez V, Cuttitta F, Tache Y. Central action of adrenomedullin to inhibit gastric emptying in rats. Endocrinology 1997;138:3749–3755.
108. Takahashi H, Watanabe T, Nishimura M, Nakanishi T, Sakamoto M, Yoshimura M, et al. Centrally induced vasopressor and sympathetic responses to a novel endogenous peptide, adrenomedullin, in anesthetized rats. Am J Hypertension 1994;7:478–482.
109. Allen MA, Smith PA, Ferguson AV. Adrenomedullin microinjection into the area postrema increases blood pressure. Am J Physiol 1997;272:R1698–1703.
110. Samson WK, Murphy TC, Resch ZT. Proadrenomedullin N-20 terminal peptide inhibits adrenocorticotropin secretion from cultured pituitary cells, possibly via activation of a potassium channel. Endocrine 1998;9:269–272.

3

Cardiac and Vascular Actions of Urocortin

David G. Parkes and Clive N. May

CONTENTS

BACKGROUND AND INTRODUCTION

Since 1981, when corticotropin-releasing factor (CRF) was isolated and characterized by Vale et al. at the Salk Institute *(1,2)*, peripheral cardiovascular actions of CRF have been observed across species ranging from rodents to humans *(3–8)*. However, researchers have been perplexed by the relevance of these hemodynamic actions, because very low levels of CRF actually circulate in normal peripheral blood, and relatively low levels of CRF gene expression are observed in the heart and vasculature *(9)*. It is well accepted that CRF is the primary hormone involved in the mammalian response to stress *(2,10,11)*, and produces central actions to increase blood pressure (BP) and stimulate pituitary adenocorticotrophic hormone (ACTH) and adrenal steroid release in all species studied. First isolated from ovine hypothalamus *(1)*, CRF belongs to a family of structurally related peptides, including fish urotensin 1 and amphibian sauvagine, which also possess bioactivity similar to CRF in several mammalian systems *(12,13)*. In 1993, the discovery of a specific and high-affinity receptor for CRF *(14)* added to the comprehension and acceptance of CRF as a physiologically relevant and important hormone present in the central nervous system (CNS) and pituitary blood supply. However, lack of any significant expression of this CRF type 1 receptor (CRF-R1) in peripheral tissues relevant to control of the cardiovascular system did not support the hypothesis that CRF may be controlling regional hemodynamics directly. CRF-R1 is expressed in high levels within the brain and the pituitary, with relatively low levels found in the periphery *(15)*. In 1994, a second type of CRF receptor was cloned and characterized *(16–19)*, and tissue expression of this type 2 receptor (CRF-R2) was reported soon thereafter. A splice variant of

From: *Contemporary Endocrinology: Hormones and the Heart in Health and Disease*
Edited by: L. Share © Humana Press Inc., Totowa, NJ

this type 2 receptor, CRF receptor type 2β (CRF-R2β), is present in both brain and peripheral tissues, including the heart, testis, and gastrointestinal tract *(16–19)*.

Two years later, Vaughan et al. *(20)* elegantly described the discovery of a CRF-related peptide expressed in rat brain, known as urocortin (Ucn), named after its peptide homology to both the teleost hormone, urotensin, and to mammalian CRF, and because it possesses biological activity exhibited by both these peptides *(20)*. In this same study, the authors also reported Ucn to have marked cardiovascular actions in conscious rats to lower BP and increase heart rate (HR) at a much greater potency and duration of action when compared to CRF. Preliminary results have shown that, in the rat heart, Ucn messenger RNA (mRNA) is expressed primarily within the vascular smooth muscle cells of the cardiac blood vessels (P. Sawchenko, personal communication). Whether this is the primary source of Ucn that may be acting on the heart is unclear. At present, plasma levels of Ucn are unknown, so it is difficult to determine to what extent Ucn may be circulating to the heart from local or distant sites of synthesis. However, the isolation of this peptide helped fill in the picture concerning potentially circulating CRF-like peptides being involved in physiological regulation of regional hemodynamics; subsequent studies in other species, such as sheep *(21)*, have confirmed potent actions of Ucn on the heart and vasculature. Although CRF-R2α mRNA expression lies exclusively within the CNS, high levels of CRF-R2β mRNA exist within the cardiac atria and ventricles (myocardium, epicardium, arterioles) *(18)*. Ucn has been shown to strongly bind and activate CRF-R2β receptors *(20)*, suggesting that there may now be an identified CRF-like peptide that binds to systemic receptors, and subsequently mediates cardiovascular effects in the periphery.

Since these two animal cardiovascular studies were published *(20,21)*, relatively few, if any, reports have appeared examining this specific biological action of Ucn. This chapter focuses on recent understanding of the cardiovascular actions of Ucn reported to date.

ISOLATION AND CHARACTERIZATION OF UROCORTIN

Rat Ucn is a 40-amino-acid peptide that exhibits 45% homology to rat/human CRF, 63% homology to teleost urotensin 1, and 35% homology to frog sauvagine (Fig. 1; *20*). The urotensin-like immunoreactivity possessed by Ucn enabled its initial identification within a discrete region of the rat midbrain known as the Edinger-Westphal nucleus, a region that lacks expression of CRF messenger RNA. Ucn cDNA was isolated from a library constructed with mRNA derived from rat midbrain, screened with a urotensin probe. The full-length cDNA clone contains a single open reading frame encoding a protein deduced to be 122 amino acids in length. The carboxy terminus contains Ucn, a putatively cleaved 40-amino-acid peptide, with a C-terminal amidation.

A detailed study on peripheral distribution of either Ucn gene expression or immunoreactivity by *in situ* hybridization/immunohistochemistry has yet to appear in the literature, although several studies have reported extensive distribution of Ucn within the rat CNS. Recently, Kozicz et al. *(22)* used a polyclonal antibody against rat Ucn to map Ucn-like immunoreactivity to areas including the supraoptic, paraventricular, and ventromedial nuclei within the rat hypothalamus, in addition to areas described previously using urotensin antisera, including the Edinger-Westphal nucleus, confirming the region containing the most abundant expression of urotensin-like immunoreactivity. Ucn distribution overlapped with gene expression of the CRF-R2 in several of these brain regions.

```
hUcn    - D D P P L S I D L T F H L L R T L L E L A R T Q S Q R E R A E Q N R I I F D S V *
r/oUcn  - D N P S L S I D L T F H L L R T L L E L A R T Q S Q R E R A E Q N R I I F D S V *
oCRF    S Q E P P I S L D L T F H L L R E V L E M T K A D Q L A Q Q A H S N R K L L D I A *
r/hCRF  S E E P P I S L D L T F H L L R E V L E M A R A E Q L A Q Q A H S N R K L M E I I *
cUro    N D D P P I S I D L T F H L L R N M I E M A R N E N Q R E Q A G L N R K Y L D E V *
Svg     - E G P P I S I D L S L E L L R K M I E I E K Q E K E K Q Q A A N N R L L L D T I *
```

Fig. 1. Comparison of amino acid sequences for human urocortin (hUcn), rat/ovine urocortin (r/oUcn), ovine CRF (oCRF), rat/human CRF (r/hCRF), carp urotensin (cUro), and frog sauvagine (Svg). Amino acid residues exhibiting identity to hUcn are shown in bold. *represents C-terminal amidation (20,26).

Other Ucn-like immunoreactive regions reported by Yamamoto et al. (23) include the substantia nigra pars compacta and ventral tegmental area, areas exhibiting immunoreactivity for tyrosine hydroxylase and possessing projections to the cervical spinal cord, which may potentially regulate the cardiovascular system. Oki et al. (24) have shown Ucn-like immunoreactivity to be present extensively throughout the digestive system, and Petraglia et al. (25) has elegantly shown expression of both mRNA and immunoreactivity for Ucn within human placenta and fetal membranes, suggesting that, like CRF, Ucn may be involved in regulation of placental endocrine function and uterine contractility. Co-expression of CRF-R2β within these peripheral tissues adds credence to the physiological relevance of CRF, Ucn, and related peptides outside the CNS.

Ucn possesses many characteristics of an endogenous ligand for the CRF-R2, and this peptide may mediate several of the peripheral physiological actions previously attributed to CRF. Ucn binds and activates CRF-R2 with much greater potency than does CRF itself (20,26), and may be a candidate for a peripherally circulating peptide, which can bind to type 2 receptors within the heart to modulate the cardiovascular system in mammals. Potential mechanisms of these hemodynamic effects are described in the following sections.

CARDIOVASCULAR ACTIONS

CRF and Related Peptides

CRF, sauvagine, and urotensin have been shown to produce potent actions on the cardiovascular system, effects that are dependent on whether the peptide is administered peripherally or directly into the CNS. Intravenous CRF is consistently seen to produce vasodilatation in rats, leading to a fall in BP and reflex increase in HR, although this action is not observed in species such as sheep (21), and is only observed at relatively high concentrations in man (6,7) and monkeys (27). The rat and dog are the most responsive species to this vasodilator action, and these are the two species from which much of the early hemodynamic data on CRF have been obtained. In rats, iv CRF produces a peripheral vasodilator action predominantly mediated by a reduction in mesenteric arterial resistance (3,28). In contrast, in all species studied, including sheep (29), icv administration of CRF increases BP, cardiac output, and HR. This effect is mediated by viscerotropic activation of sympathetic nervous outflow, to raise peripheral resistance and HR in rats (3,30,31), dogs (32), and rabbits (33); however, it is not blocked by peripheral concurrent administration of the CRF antagonist, α-helical CRF (9–41) (3). This contrasting action of CRF on BP, depending on the route of administration, has been observed with several other cardiovascular peptides, such as atrial natriuretic factor (or atrial natriuretic peptide [ANP]; 34,35) and, more recently, adrenomedullin (36,37). Samson et al. (38) have suggested that this may be an endogenous cardioprotective mechanism of peripheral peptides to counteract a large fall in arterial pressure/blood volume by a feedback or co-release mechanism in the brain to sustain BP. Several studies have provided evidence that these peptides may be signaling the brain via nuclei within the brain stem, such as the area postrema, which lack a blood–brain barrier, and allow communication of these hormones with central nuclei controlling cardiovascular function *(39)*.

In rats, evidence that CRF or a related peptide may produce direct cardiac actions to increase contractility now exists from several in vitro studies. Grunt et al. *(40)* have shown that CRF, perfused through isolated working rat hearts, can increase both coronary blood flow and maximal aortic pressure, suggesting direct effects of CRF on cardiac activity. These effects were not blocked by the β-adrenergic receptor antagonist, propranolol, nor by the nitric oxide synthesis inhibitor N^G-nitro-L-arginine. Saitoh et al. *(41)* have reported that CRF can directly increase the contractile force of isolated guinea pig ventricular myocardium independent of norepinephrine release or Na^+K^+-ATPase activity. More recently, Heldwein et al. *(42)* have demonstrated that CRF and related peptides can directly stimulate cyclic adenosine monophosphate (cAMP) accumulation in isolated neonatal rat cardiomyocytes.

Intravenous injection of CRF in conscious sheep promotes little change in mean arterial pressure (MAP), HR, or cardiac output (CO) (Fig. 2). Most notably, there is no change in cardiac contractility (Fig. 3; *21*). However, a robust increase in plasma ACTH and cortisol levels is observed. This lack of any significant peripheral hemodynamic action of CRF in sheep may be the result of species differences in binding of CRF to peripheral CRF-R2s. It is possible that ovine CRF is highly specific for type 1 receptors within the brain and pituitary, and lacks any significant binding and activation of ovine cardiac type 2 receptors.

Urocortin

Ucn has been shown to possess potent and long-lasting hypotensive actions in conscious Sprague-Dawley rats *(20)*, as reported by Vaughan et al. in 1995. Ucn produced a dose-dependent hypotension with the highest dose tested (19 µg/kg), lowering MAP by about 27 mmHg. CRF showed approx 30% of the hypotensive potency of Ucn, as did urotensin 1. The duration of hypotensive action of Ucn (3.8 µg/kg) in rats was approx 95 min, with those of CRF and urotensin being 50 and 79 min, respectively. Increases in HR were associated with these BP changes, although there was no change in arterial pulse pressure. The mechanism of this hypotension following Ucn injection would presumably be via a peripheral vasodilator action, possibly caused by a specific action on mesenteric vascular beds, as described for CRF, sauvagine, and urotensin *(43)*. The authors have recently observed, in isoflurane-anesthetized rats, that iv Ucn (6 µg/kg) can reduce arterial pressure, aortic flow, stroke volume, and aortic resistance, together with increasing HR and aortic conductance, suggesting that Ucn does indeed act to produce peripheral vasodilatation in rats (D. Parkes and C. May, unpublished observations). The authors also observed a 50% increase in maximum aortic flow, and a 90% increase in aortic *dF/dt*, two indicators of cardiac contractility; hence, Ucn does appear to have positive cardiac inotropic actions in anesthetized rats. Spina et al. *(44)* have reported that Ucn injected into the lateral cerebral ventricles in rats slightly increases BP, but they measured no change in myocardial contractility. This further supports the concept that the cardiac inotropic action of Ucn may be mediated by a peripheral action, probably directly on the heart.

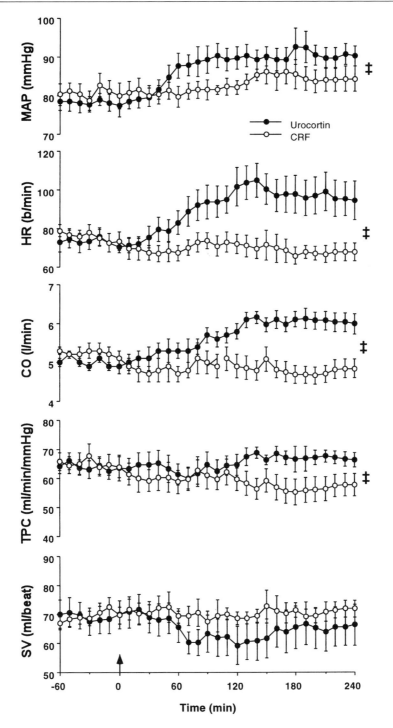

Fig. 2. Hemodynamic effects of iv rat Ucn (1–40) (●) or ovine CRF (1–41) (○) injected at 2 μg/ kg in five sheep. Mean arterial pressure (MAP), heart rate (HR), cardiac output (CO), total peripheral conductance (TPC), and stroke volume (SV) were measured every minute by a computer-based data collection system. Results are shown as the mean of 10-min grouped readings ± SE. ‡ represents significant difference between Ucn- and CRF-treated sheep. Reprinted with permission from ref. *21*.

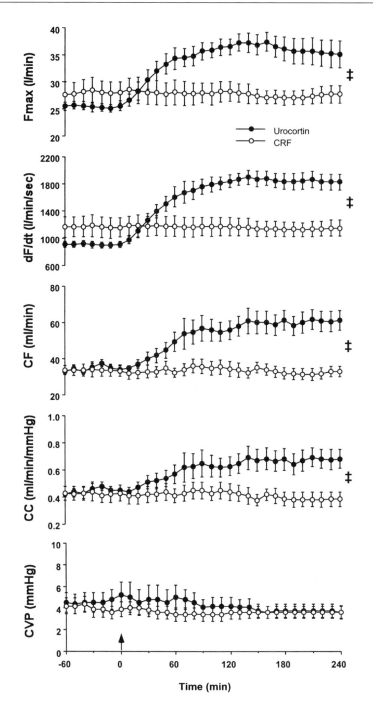

Fig. 3 Hemodynamic effects of iv rat Ucn (1–40) (●) or ovine CRF (1–41) (○) injected at 2 μg/kg in five sheep. Maximal aortic flow (F_{max}), aortic dF/dt, coronary blood flow (CF), and coronary conductance (CC) were measured every minute by a computer-based data collection system. Central venous pressure (CVP) was measured continuously by chart recorder. Results are shown as the mean of 10-min grouped readings ± SE. ‡ represents significant difference between Ucn and CRF treated sheep. Reprinted with permission from ref. *21*.

The authors' study in sheep investigated the detailed cardiovascular actions of rat Ucn (which has recently been shown to be identical in peptide sequence to ovine Ucn; W. Vale personal communication), and Figs. 2 and 3 show a summary of these effects when Ucn is injected intravenously at 2 μg/kg *(21)*. In conscious, chronically instrumented sheep, Ucn produced a slowly developing increase in MAP, which was first significant 60 min after injection. This was associated with a 40% rise in HR, and about a 16% rise in CO 120 min after injection. There was no change in total peripheral conductance or stroke volume at this dose, although, at a lower dose (1 μg/kg), stroke volume and total peripheral conductance decreased slightly.

The most striking cardiovascular change seen with iv Ucn in sheep was a rapid and extremely potent (twofold) increase in cardiac contractility within 30 min of injection, as reflected by the large increases in both maximum aortic flow and rate of change in aortic flow (*dF/dt*) (Fig. 3). Two hours following injection of Ucn at 2 μg/kg, coronary blood flow exhibited a significant increase from control, and this was associated with a rise in coronary conductance. The changes in arterial pressure, HR, CO, aortic F_{max}, *dF/dt*, coronary blood flow, and coronary conductance were all dose-dependent. The onset of the cardiac inotropic effect of Ucn, prior to any change in BP or central venous pressure, suggests that the primary action of Ucn in sheep is to increase cardiac contractility, and this effect is not a reflex response to changes in cardiac preload or afterload. The observed increase in HR indicates that Ucn has either a direct chronotropic action on the heart, or influences vagal or sympathetic reflexes acting on the heart. Because the onset of the inotropic action of Ucn in sheep is not immediate (within seconds to minutes), it is possible that Ucn may have a very slow "on rate" to cardiac CRF receptors, or may act indirectly to increase cardiac contractility via release of other endogenous inotropic factors. It is possible that Ucn may promote release of endogenous peptides, which can themselves influence cardiovascular function. CRF is known to stimulate release of ANP from isolated hearts, probably via its action on cardiac CRF receptors. However, the short-term hemodynamic actions of ANP in sheep are characterized by a large reduction in CO, stroke volume, and hypotension *(45)*, which are effects different from those seen following Ucn injection in sheep.

The increase in coronary arterial blood flow and conductance in sheep demonstrates that a coronary vasodilator action is associated with Ucn administration. Whether this is a direct action of Ucn to produce vascular relaxation, as suggested by several in vitro studies reported for CRF *(4,40,46)*, or a consequence of greater oxygen demand by the heart because of an increase in cardiac work, remains to be determined. As mentioned previously, specific receptors for Ucn (CRF-R2β) have been demonstrated by *in situ* hybridization to exist within arterioles/perivascular cells of the heart *(18)*, supporting the possibility of direct cardiac actions of Ucn.

The onset of cardiovascular actions following Ucn injection is intriguing. Cardiac contractility was seen to significantly increase prior to any other cardiovascular parameter measured. This suggests that Ucn can initially increase maximum aortic flow without affecting mean aortic flow (cardiac output) and BP. More detailed molecular studies are required to determine whether the effect on contractility is mediated solely via elevation of intracellular levels of cAMP, or whether other, perhaps as yet unidentified, signaling mechanisms are involved in this cardiac inotropic action.

The authors found that Ucn exhibits an extensive duration of action on cardiac contractility in sheep. The cardiac inotropic and coronary vasodilator actions of Ucn were still maximal 4 h following a bolus injection of Ucn. The peak response was reached approx 2 h after injection, and parameters plateaued after this time at maximal change. In three sheep monitored continuously for 3 days following injection, the authors observed that cardiac contractility remained significantly elevated for up to 24 h after injection; other hemodynamic variables had returned to control values within 14 h. There are no reports of such a long duration of inotropic action for any peptide, and the data suggest that once Ucn has bound to receptors mediating cardiovascular changes, it may maintain binding and signaling for extremely long periods, or persistently stimulate release of endogenous inotropic factors. Alternatively, clearance of Ucn from blood or local tissues may be slow, allowing prolonged exposure to CRF receptors in the heart. When comparing the inotropic activity of Ucn with another peptide known to increase cardiac contractility, the authors have shown that the vasodilator, adrenomedullin, produces a 15% increase in aortic dF/dt in sheep *(47)*. Ucn given at equimolar doses increased aortic dF/dt by almost 120%, providing evidence that Ucn is an extremely potent cardiac inotrope in conscious sheep.

The authors observed that the CRF antagonist, α-helical CRF (9–41), could abolish all cardiovascular changes produced by Ucn in sheep. This suggests that the effects are mediated via binding to CRF receptors accessed via the blood, because neither the antagonist nor Ucn are likely to cross the blood–brain barrier. However, it is possible that peripherally injected Ucn may reach areas of the brain that lack a blood–brain barrier, such as the area postrema, and stimulation of this brain nucleus is known to activate sympathetic afferents to increase BP and promote vagal withdrawal of HR control in rats *(48,49)*. The fact that the authors observed complete inhibition of the cardiovascular changes produced by Ucn, with a dose ratio of α-helical CRF (9–41): Ucn of 10:1, suggested that these changes are more likely to be mediated via CRF-R2s. Total blockade of CRF-R1-mediated effects, such as CRF-induced ACTH secretion, only occurs at antagonist: agonist ratios reaching 3000:1 in rats *(50)*. This lends further support to the hypothesis that this particular CRF antagonist is more effective at inhibiting agonist binding to CRF-R2s vs binding to CRF-R1s *(51)*.

CARDIAC ACTIONS OF UROCORTIN DURING TOTAL AUTONOMIC (GANGLION) BLOCKADE

The authors have recently assessed the ability of Ucn to produce a cardiac inotropic action in the absence of an intact autonomic nervous system (D. Parkes and C. May, unpublished observations). These experiments were designed to determine whether Ucn may be acting directly on the heart, or via a secondary mechanism, possibly via the brain or peripheral nervous system, to activate sympathetic outflow to the heart and periphery, in a similar fashion to how CRF acts when administered into the CNS.

Conscious sheep received iv Ucn (1 µg/kg/h) for 1 h in the absence or presence of iv hexamethonium chloride (2.5 mg/kg/h) started 3 h prior to, and continuing during, the Ucn infusion protocol (8 h total). The effectiveness of ganglion blockade with this dose of hexamethonium has been confirmed previously *(52,53)*. Intravenous infusion of Ucn (1 µg/kg/h for 1 h) alone caused quantitatively similar effects when compared to bolus administration of Ucn *(21)*. There was little hemodynamic change during Ucn infusion, but there were progressive and prolonged changes following the infusion. Results are presented in Fig. 4. In control animals, Ucn increased MAP from 78 ± 1 mmHg to 85 ± 1 mmHg. This was accompanied by increases in HR from 68 ± 1 to 90 ± 2 beats/min and CO from 4.54 ± 0.10 to 5.32 ± 0.13 L/min, but there was little effect on total

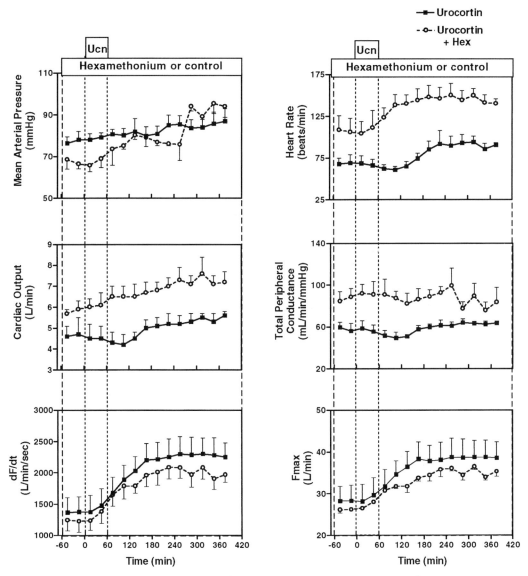

Fig. 4. Cardiovascular actions of Ucn (1 μg/kg/h for 60 min) in sheep with (○) and without (●) ganglion blockade (hexamethonium 2.5 mg/kg/h). Results are shown as the mean of 30-min grouped readings ± S.E. Abbreviations: dF/dt, maximum aortic rate of change of flow; Fmax, maximum aortic flow. No significant difference was seen in the Ucn-induced increase in cardiac contractility (dF/dt or F_{max}) in the absence or presence of ganglion blockade.

peripheral conductance (57.9 ± 1.3–62.7 ± 0.9 mL/min/mmHg), and central venous pressure was unchanged. There were large increases in two indices of cardiac contractility: *dF/dt* increased from 1352 ± 14 to 2278 ± 30 mL/min/s, and there was a parallel increase in peak aortic flow from 28.0 ± 0.3 to 38.6 ± 0.4 L/min.

In ganglion-blocked sheep, MAP was reduced, and there were increases in HR, CO, and total peripheral conductance, confirming the authors' previous findings *(52)*. Hence, ganglion blockade did not abolish the effects of Ucn. In sheep treated with hexamethonium, Ucn increased MAP from 68 ± 1 to 91 ± 2 mmHg, HR from 107 ± 1 to 146 ± 3 beats/

min, and CO from 5.71 ± 0.1 to 7.35 ± 0.25 L/min. In ganglion-blocked sheep the increases in dF/dt, from 1288 ± 16 to 1984 ± 74 L/min/s, and peak aortic flow, from 26.0 ± 0.2 to 35.0 ± 1.1 L/min, were similar to those in intact sheep. Central venous pressure was unchanged, and total peripheral conductance was 85 ± 1.8 during the control period, and 81.3 ± 5.9 mL/min/mmHg after Ucn.

The chief finding from this study is that ganglion blockade did not prevent any of the cardiovascular effects of Ucn. The Ucn-induced increases in CO and HR, and the striking increase in cardiac contractility, were similar in intact and ganglion-blocked sheep. These findings indicate that these actions of Ucn were not mediated by the autonomic nervous system, and it is likely that they are mediated by a direct action of Ucn on the heart, possibly via binding to CRF-R2β. This is supported by the demonstration that high levels of mRNA for CRF-R2βs are present within cardiac atria and ventricles (18), and by the authors' previous finding that all the effects of Ucn were blocked by low doses of α-helical CRF (9–41) (21), an antagonist that is thought to preferentially block CRF-R2βs, and does not cross the blood–brain barrier (11).

The effects of Ucn on MAP were enhanced in ganglion-blocked sheep, as a result of a greater increase in CO and a reduction in peripheral conductance, compared to an increase in conductance in intact sheep. Thus, the autonomic nervous system tends to offset the pressor response to Ucn. As mentioned previously, the authors have demonstrated that Ucn causes coronary vasodilatation, which is probably a response to the increase in cardiac work, but the effects of Ucn on other regional vascular beds are unknown.

OTHER BIOLOGICAL ACTIONS OF UROCORTIN

Synthetic Ucn can stimulate release of ACTH to a greater extent than CRF from isolated rat pituitary cells (20), and also in vivo in conscious rats (20). This is consistent with the peptide's ability to bind and activate CRF-R1s expressed by corticotropes within the anterior pituitary (20). In sheep, the authors observed that Ucn produced actions on the pituitary gland to increase secretion of ACTH and, subsequently, cortisol from the adrenal (21). This action was more potent than the effect of an equivalent dose of ovine CRF, consistent with the studies in conscious rats. Whether the effect on plasma ACTH secretion from the pituitary following iv Ucn is mediated via access from arterial blood supplying this gland, or subsequent transport via the hypophyseal portal circulation, remains unclear. It is also feasible that Ucn may promote release of peptides, such as arginine vasopressin, which may synergize with Ucn or CRF to enhance ACTH secretion, in addition to having cardiovascular actions to increase BP. It is unlikely that the rise in circulating ACTH levels would contribute to any cardiovascular changes during Ucn administration in normal sheep, because the earliest hemodynamic changes seen with infusion of ACTH in sheep occur after 4 h of infusion (54). Expression of both Ucn mRNA and immunoreactivity has recently been described in human pituitary, predominantly co-localizing with somatotropes (about 74% of Ucn-immunoreactive cells), and, to a lesser extent, with lactotropes and corticotropes (less than 1%) (55). Furthermore, Murakami et al. (56) has shown that Ucn can stimulate release of GH from pituitary tissue derived from pituitary adenoma patients, possibly via a CRF-R2-dependent mechanism.

It is well accepted that CRF can have marked effects on behavior to suppress appetite, stimulate arousal, and increase performance in various memory and learning exercises.

At higher doses, it can increase emotionality, leading to fear, anxiety, and depression-like effects in a variety of species *(57)*. Spina et al. *(44)* have demonstrated that Ucn, when given intracerbroventricularly to conscious rats, can dose-dependently suppress food and water intake in both food-deprived and freely feeding states. This appetite-suppressing action of Ucn was approximately equipotent to that of urotensin, but significantly more potent than CRF. Ucn did not produce any anxiogenic-like behavior when rats were tested in an emotionality test (elevated plus maze), a test in rats known to be sensitive to CRF. In contrast, another study by Moreau et al. *(58)* reported anxiogenic properties of Ucn in rats, using a similar elevated-plus maze, and also in mice when examining exploratory behavior in an open field. Significant behavioral actions were observed with iv Ucn administration in sheep, particularly at a higher dose of 2 µg/kg *(21)*. Ucn markedly suppressed appetite for food and water in sheep for at least 12 hours after the normal time of feeding, but the animals did not appear anxious or stressed. Significant levels of CRF-R2 expression are seen within the gastrointestinal tract of rats *(18)* and high levels of Ucn mRNA are also seen at several important junctions throughout this tract *(24*; J. Bittencourt, personal communication). Hence, Ucn may act directly on the gut to inhibit gastrointestinal motility, in combination with central actions to suppress feeding behavior.

Many of the other localized actions of CRF on inflammation, metabolism, respiration, and the immune system may be mimicked by Ucn, when examined in forthcoming studies, especially in regions or tissues in which there is a high level of expression of the CRF-R2.

CONCLUSIONS AND FUTURE DIRECTIONS

Ucn is now emerging as a potential hormone involved in cardiovascular control, and may be the piece of the puzzle missing for so long regarding peripheral actions of CRF. Increasing evidence, based on CRF/Ucn receptor expression, Ucn peptide expression, and Ucn physiology, indicates that this peptide may be present in significant concentrations and at relevant sites to control a number of local physiological systems, in addition to its marked actions within the CNS to regulate behavior, BP, and hormonal release from cells present within the anterior pituitary gland (Fig. 5). The marked and persistent cardiovascular, hormonal, and behavioral actions of Ucn following iv administration in sheep are intriguing. In particular, the cardiac inotropic action of Ucn is unique regarding its potency and duration of action when compared to other cardioactive peptides studied, and it appears to be the primary cardiovascular action of this peptide in conscious sheep. Whether this potent inotropic action of Ucn may prove useful in developing analogs/ therapeutics for treatment of diseases, such as congestive heart failure, will wait on confirmatory studies examining the cardiovascular actions of this peptide in primates or humans. However, preliminary studies for developing compounds that may free endogenous CRF and, potentially, Ucn, from the CRF binding protein *(59,60)* appear encouraging as a novel technique to raise endogenous levels of these peptides to concentrations that may be of clinical benefit. Of particular relevance, understanding the control of Ucn secretion within localized peripheral tissues should provide answers to the physiological and pathological significance of systemic Ucn, once a specific and reliable assay is developed. Overall, it is now evident that Ucn plays a significant role in the control of cardiac function and peripheral hemodynamics, and may be one of the primary factors involved in the cardiovascular response to a stressful stimulus.

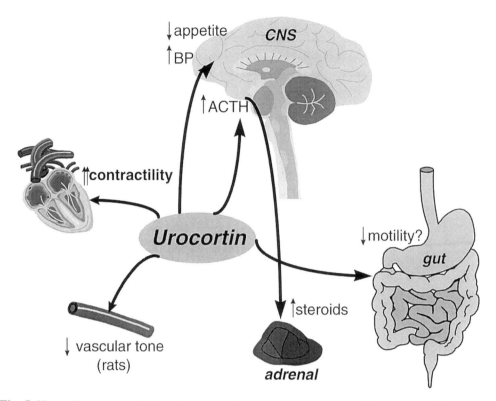

Fig. 5. Ucn actions on the CNS and peripheral physiological systems. The source of Ucn acting outside the CNS may be within the respective target tissue.

REFERENCES

1. Vale W, Spiess J, Rivier C, Rivier J. Characterization of a 41-residue ovine hypothalamic peptide that stimulates secretion of corticotropin and β-endorphin. Science 1981;213:1394–1397.
2. Vale W, Rivier C, Brown MR, Spiess J, Koob G, Swanson L, et al. Chemical and biological characterization of corticotropin releasing factor. Rec Prog Horm Res 1983;39:245–247.
3. Overton J, Fisher L. Differentiated hemodynamic responses to central versus peripheral administration of corticotropin-releasing factor in conscious rats. J Autonom Nerv Syst 1991;35:43–52.
4. Richter R, Mulvany M. Comparison of hCRF and oCRF effects on cardiovascular responses after central, peripheral, and in vitro application. Peptides 1995;16:843–849.
5. Udelsman R, Harwood JP, Millan MA, Chrousos GP, Goldstein DS, Zimlichman R, Catt KJ, Aguilera G. Functional corticotropin releasing factor receptors in the primate peripheral sympathetic nervous system. Nature 1986;319:147–145.
6. Hermus A, Pieters G, Willemsen J, Ross H, Smals A, Benrad T, Kloppenberg P. Hypotensive effects of ovine and human corticotrophin-releasing factor in man. Eur J Clin Pharmacol 1987;31:531–534.
7. Orth D, Jackson R, DeCherney G, DeBold C, Alexander A, Island D, et al. Effect of synthetic ovine corticotropin-releasing factor: dose response of plasma adrenocorticotropin and cortisol. J Clin Invest 1983;71:587–595.
8. Smith EM, Morrill AC, Meyer WJ 3rd, Blalock JE. Corticotropin releasing factor induction of leukocyte derived immunoreactive ACTH and endorphins. Nature 1986;321:881–882.
9. Muglia L, Jenkins N, Gilbert D, Copeland N, Majzoub J. Expression of the mouse corticotropin-releasing hormone gene in vivo and targeted inactivation in embryonic stem cells. J Clin Invest 1994; 93:2066–2072.
10. DeSouza E, Grigoriadis D. Corticotropin releasing factor: physiology, pharmacology, and role in central nervous system and immune disorders. In: Psychopharmacology: The 4th Generation of Progress. 1995, pp. 505–517.

11. Vale W, Vaughan J, Perrin M. Corticotropin-releasing factor (CRF) family of ligands and their receptors. Endocrinologist 1997;7:3S–9S.
12. Chadwick D, Marsh J, Ackryl J, eds. Corticotropin-Releasing Factor, John Wiley, Chichester, 1993.
13. Lederis K. Non-mammalian corticotropin-release-stimulating peptides. Ann NY Acad Sci 1987;512: 129–139.
14. Chen R, Lewis K, Perrin M, Vale W. Expression cloning of a human corticotropin-releasing-factor receptor. Proc Natl Acad Sci USA 1993;90:8967–8971.
15. Potter E, Sutton S, Donaldson C, Chen R, Perrin M, Lewis K, Sawchenko P, Vale W. Distribution of corticotropin-releasing factor receptor mRNA expression in the rat brain and pituitary. Proc Natl Acad Sci USA 1994;91:8777–8781.
16. Lovenberg T, Chalmers D, Liu C, DeSouza E. CRF2α and CRF2β receptor mRNAs are differentially distributed between the rat central nervous system and peripheral tissues. Endocrinology 1995;136: 4139–4142.
17. Kishimoto T, Pearse R, Lin C, Rosenfeld M. A sauvagine/corticotropin-releasing factor receptor expressed in heart and skeletal muscle. Proc Natl Acad Sci USA 1995;92:1108–1112.
18. Perrin M, Donaldson C, Chen R, Blount A, Berggren T, Bilezikjian L, Sawchecnko P, Vale W. Identification of a second corticotropin-releasing factor receptor gene and characterization of a cDNA expressed in heart. Proc Natl Acad Sci USA 1995;92:2969–2973.
19. Stenzel P, Kesterson R, Yeung W, Cone R, Rittenberg M, Stenzel-Poore M. Identification of a novel murine receptor for corticotropin-releasing hormone expressed in the heart. Mol Endocrinol 1995;9: 637–645.
20. Vaughan J, Donaldson C, Bittencourt J, Perrin M, Lewis K, Sutton S, et al. Urocortin, a mammalian neuropeptide related to fish urotensin 1 and corticotropin-releasing factor. Nature 1995;378:287–292.
21. Parkes D, Vaughan J, Rivier J, Vale W, May C. Cardiac inotropic actions of urocortin in conscious sheep. Am J Physiol 1997;272:H2115–H2122.
22. Kozicz, T, Yanaihara H, Arimura A. Distribution of urocortin-like immunoreactivity in the central nervous system of the rat. J Comp Neurol 1998;391:1–10.
23. Yamamoto H, Maeda T, Fujimura M, Fujimiya M. Urocortin-like immunoreactivity in the substantia nigra, ventral tegmental area and Edinger-Westphal nucleus of rat. Neurosci Lett 1998;243:21–24.
24. Oki Y, Iwabuchi M, Masuzawa M, Watanabe F, Ozawa M, Iino K, Tominaga T, Yoshimi T. Distribution and concentration of urocortin, and effect of adrenalectomy on its content in rat hypothalamus. Life Sci 1998;62:807–812.
25. Petraglia F, Florio P, Gallo R, Simoncini T, Saviozzi M, Blasio AD, Vaughan J, Vale W. Human placenta and fetal membranes express human urocortin mRNA and peptide. J Clin Endocrinol Metab 1996;81:3807–3810.
26. Donaldson C, Sutton S, Perrin M, Corrigan A, Lewis K, Rivier J, Vaughan J, Vale W. Cloning and characterization of human urocortin. Endocrinology 1996;137:2167–2170.
27. Udelsman R, Gallucci W, Bacher J, Lorriaux D, Chrousos G. Hemodynamic effects of corticotropin releasing hormone in the anesthetized cynomolgus monkey. Peptides 1986;7:465–471.
28. MacCannell K, Lederis K, Hamilton P, Rivier J. Amunine (ovineCRF), urotensin 1 and sauvagine, three structurally related peptides, produce selective dilation of the mesenteric circulation. Pharmacology 1982;25:116–120.
29. Scoggins B, Coghlan J, Denton D, Nelson M, Lambert P, Parkes D, et al. Effect of intracerebroventricular infusions of CRF, sauvagine, ACTH (1-24) and ACTH (4-10) on blood pressure in sheep. J Hypertens 1984;2(Suppl 3):67–68.
30. Fisher LA, Brown MR. Corticotropin-releasing factor and angiotensin II: comparison of CNS actions to influence neuroendocrine and cardiovascular function. Brain Res 1984;296:41–47.
31. Grosskreutz, C, Brody M. Regional hemodynamic responses to central administration of corticotropin-releasing factor (CRF). Brain Res 1988;442:363–367.
32. Brown M, Fisher L. Central nervous system effects of corticotropin-releasing factor in the dog. Brain Res 1983;280:75–79.
33. May C, Whitehead C, Mathias C. Effects of naloxone on the cardiovascular and respiratory effects of centrally administered corticotrophin releasing factor in conscious rabbits. Br J Pharmacol 1991;103: 1776–1780.
34. Parkes D, Coghlan J, Weisinger R, Scoggins B. Effects of intracerebroventriculat infusion fo atrial natriuretic peptide in conscious sheep. Peptides 1988;9:509–513.
35. Parkes D, Coghlan J, McDougall J, Scoggins B. Long-term hemodynamic actions of atrial natriuretic factor (99-126) in conscious sheep. Am J Physiol 1988;254:H811–H815.

36. Gardiner S, Kemp P, March J, Bennett T. Regional haemodynamic effects of human and rat adreno-medullin in conscious rats. Br J Pharmacol 1995;114:584–591.

37. Takahashi H, Watanabe, T, Nishimura M, Nakanishi T, Sakamoto M, Yoshimura M, et al. Centrally induced vasopressor and sympathetic responses to a novel endogenous peptide, adrenomedullin, in anesthetized rats. Am J Hypertens 1994;7:478–482.

38. Samson, WK, Murphy T, Resch Z. Central mechanisms for the hypertensive effects of preproadreno-medullin derived peptides in conscious rats. Am J Physiol 1998;274:R1505–R1509.

39. Allen M, Ferguson A. In vitro recordings from area postrema neurons demonstrate responsiveness to adrenomedullin. Am J Physiol 1996;270:R920–R925.

40. Grunt M, Glaser J, Schmidhuber H, Pauschinger P, Born J. Effects of corticotropin-releasing factor on isolated rat heart activity. Am J Physiol 1993;264:H1124–H1129.

41. Saitoh M, Hasegawa J, Mashiba H. Effect of corticotropin-releasing factor on the electrical and mechan-ical activities of the guinea-pig ventricular myocardium. Gen Pharmacol 1990;21:337–342.

42. Heldwein K, Redick D, Rittenberg M, Claycomb W, Stenzel-Poore M. Corticotorpin-releasing hormone receptor expression and functional coupling in neonatal cardiac myocytes and AT-1 cells. Endocrinology 1996;137:3631–3639.

43. Lenz, H, Fisher L, Vale W, Brown M. Corticotropin-releasing factor, sauvagine and urotensin I: effects on blood flow. Am J Physiol 1985;249:R85–R90.

44. Spina M, Merlo-Pich E, Chan R, Basso A, Rivier J, Vale W, Koob G. Appetite-suppressing effects of urocortin, a CRF-related neuropeptide. Science 1996;273:1561–1564.

45. Parkes D, Coghlan J, McDougall J, Scoggins B. Hemodynamic effects of atrial natriuretic peptide in conscious sheep. Clin Exp Hypertension 1987;A9:2143–2156.

46. Lei S, Richter R, Bienert M, Mulvaney M. Relaxing actions of corticotropin-releasing factor on rat resistance arteries. Br J Pharmacol 1993;108:941–947.

47. Parkes D. Cardiovascular actions of adrenomedullin in conscious sheep. Am J Physiol 1995;268:H2574–H2578.

48. Lowes V, Sun K, Li Z, Ferguson A. Vasopressin actions on area postrema neurons in vitro. Am J Physiol 1995;269:R463–R468.

49. Papas S, Smith P, Ferguson A. Electrophysiological evidence that systemic angiotensin influences rat area postrema neurons. Am J Physiol 1990;258:R70–R76.

50. Fisher L, Rivier C, Rivier J, Brown M. Differential antagonist activity of alpha-helical corticotropin-releasing factor antagonist 9-41 in three bioassay systems. Endocrinology 1991;129:1312–1316.

51. Turnbull A, Vale W, Rivier C. Urocortin, a corticotropin-releasing factor-related mammalian peptide, inhibits edema due to thermal injury in rats. Eur J Pharmacol, in press.

52. Parkes D, May C. Direct cardiac and vascular actions of adrenomedullin in conscious sheep. Br J Pharmacol 1997;120:1179–1185.

53. May C, McAllen R. Baroreceptor-independent renal nerve inhibition by intracerebroventricular angio-tensin II in conscious sheep. Am J Physiol 1997;273:R560–R567.

54. Bednarik J, May C. Differential regional hemodynamic effects of corticotropin in conscious sheep. Hypertension 1994;24:49–55.

55. Iino K, Sasano H, Oki Y, Andoh N, Shin R, Kitamoto T, et al. Urocortin expression in human pituitary gland and pituitary adenoma. J Clin Endocrinol Metab 1997;82:3842–3850.

56. Murakami Y, Mori T, Koshimura K, Kurosaki M, Hori T, Yanaihara N, Kato Y. Stimulation by urocortin of growth hormone (GH) secretion in GH-producing human pituitary adenoma cells. Endocr J 1997;4:627–629.

57. Koob G, Britton K. Behavioural effects of corticotropin-releasing factor. In DeSouza E, Nemeroff C, eds. Corticotropin-Releasing Factor: Basic and Clinical Studies of a Neuropeptide. CRC, Boca Raton, 1990, pp. 253–266.

58. Moreau J, Kilpatrick G, Jenck F. Urocortin, a novel neuropeptide with anxiogenic-like properties. Neuroreport 1997;8:1697–1701.

59. Behan D, Khongsaly O, Ling N, Souza ED. Urocortin interaction with corticotropin-releasing factor (CRF) binding protein (CRF-BP): a novel mechanism for elevating "free' CRF levels in human brain. Brain Res 1996;725:263–267.

60. Behan D, Heinrichs S, Troncoso J, Liu X, Kawas C, Ling N, DeSouza E. Displacement of corticotropin releasing factor from its binding protein as a possible treatment for Alzheimer's disease. Nature 1995;378:284–287.

4   The Renin-Angiotensin System and the Heart

Haralambos Gavras and Irene Gavras

INTRODUCTION

The discovery of the renin-angiotensin system (RAS) opened a new era in the research of the physiology and pathology of the cardiovascular system. Early studies relying on measurements of plasma renin levels had raised doubts about the participation of the RAS in the development and maintenance of hypertension (HT), but these doubts were laid to rest when antagonists or inhibitors of various components of the system were used to demonstrate its role. Use of these antagonists/inhibitors also permitted the elucidation of various aspects of the contribution of the RAS to the onset and progression of ischemic cardiac disease through the successive stages of ischemia, myocardial infarcts, diastolic and systolic dysfunction, and congestive heart failure (CHF). The corollary of this research was the introduction of angiotensin inhibition in the treatment of HT, ischemic heart disease, and heart failure (HF).

Angiotensin II (ANG II) is the effector hormone of the RAS. It is generated by a cascade of events starting with the secretion of the proteolytic enzyme, renin, mostly from the juxtaglomerular apparatus in the renal cortex, in response either to a fall of intrarenal perfusion pressure or to accumulation of sodium at the site of the adjacent macula densa. Renin acts on the polypeptide, angiotensinogen, an α_2-globulin of hepatic origin, to cleave off the biologically inactive decapeptide ANG I; the latter is the main substrate for the angiotensin-converting enzyme (ACE), which cleaves off two amino acids from the C terminal of ANG I to form the octapeptide ANG II, one of the most potent natural vasoconstricting substances. ANG II has a very short half-life, because it is rapidly degraded by angiotensinases into peptide fragments with little biologic activity.

From: *Contemporary Endocrinology: Hormones and the Heart in Health and Disease*
Edited by: L. Share © Humana Press Inc., Totowa, NJ

The remote vasoconstrictor and steroidogenic (i.e., aldosterone-stimulating) properties of circulating ANG II were the earliest to be recognized, and have been studied extensively since its discovery 60 yr ago. In the past two decades, intensive research into various aspects of the RAS has produced evidence suggesting additional properties of ANG II exerted via its capacity as a circulating hormone, as well as a locally acting autacoid.

The following is a brief review of the various effects of ANG II on the heart, including those exerted directly on myocardial cells and those resulting from the systemic hemodynamic and metabolic actions of the circulating or locally generated ANG II, acting on different parts of the coronary and peripheral vasculature.

CIRCULATING VS LOCALLY GENERATED ANG II

Renin of renal origin is the rate-limiting step in the production of circulating ANG II *(1)*. Hence, plasma renin activity (PRA), which is easily measured by radioimmunoassay of ANG I generated after incubation of plasma for a specified period of time, and is expressed as ng/mL/h, has been used as a substitute for actual levels of circulating ANG II in most clinical studies. The importance of circulating vs locally generated ANG II has been a matter of longstanding debate *(2,3)*. With the widespread use of molecular biology techniques in the 1980s, it was found that differentiated cells of various organs, including the cardiomyocytes and vascular smooth muscle cells (VSMCs), contain components of the RAS cascade, and may therefore possess the capability to generate ANG II. The functional significance of circulating vs locally produced (paracrine, autocrine, or intracrine) ANG II continues to be a matter of debate.

Although all components of the RAS have been identified in cardiac tissues by biochemical methods, it was not clear whether they were the product of genes for renin, angiotensinogen (ANGT), and ACE in cardiomyocytes, or whether they were the result of sequestration from plasma *(4)*. Presence of mRNA for ANGT and ACE *(5,6)* was convincingly demonstrated in cardiac cells, although at levels much lower than those of hepatic and endothelial cells (ECs). However, the presence of renin mRNA remained controversial for a long period: Some investigators reported evidence of renin mRNA produced by cardiac tissues *(7)*; others were unable to detect renin transcripts. A possible explanation for these discrepancies was that overestimates in the levels of mRNA could result from cross-hybridization of probes to transcripts of other proteases (e.g., cathepsin D), which have a high degree of sequence homology with renin *(4)*. It was also suggested that local synthesis of ANG I may be promoted by such proteases in cardiac tissue *(8)*, and that it may be converted to ANG II via alternative enzyme pathways (e.g., chymase) during inhibition of the ACE *(9)*. The bulk of the evidence suggests that intracardiac renin is constitutively produced by cardiomyocytes, as well as other cardiac cells (e.g., fibroblasts) in culture *(9)*. Therefore, all RAS components appear to be present and regulated at the molecular level in heart tissues, although the synthesis of ANG II in vivo may vary under different circumstances, such as species, age, and pathological condition of the heart. Nevertheless, the renal renin and the circulating components of the RAS are produced in amounts greater by several orders of magnitude, compared to those produced by extrarenal tissues, and are chiefly or solely responsible for the systemic hormonal and hemodynamic effects of ANG II. On the contrary, the minute amounts of ANG II produced locally may be responsible for its direct paracrine, autocrine, and, possibly, intracrine effects, (such as trophic, and so on) that persist even in the renoprival state.

Whether blood-borne or locally generated, ANG II exerts its effects on the heart via activation of its type 1 (AT_1) receptor, a G-protein-linked receptor identified on cardiac cell membranes *(10)*. This receptor activates protein kinase C (PKC) through formation of diacylglycerol and hydrolysis of phosphatidylinositol *(10,11)*. An AT_2 receptor has also been identified by radioligand binding studies, but has not been clearly linked to biologic responses; it is believed to play a role mostly in fetal growth and development, because its density declines sharply in the postnatal period *(12)*. Several subtypes of these receptors can be detected by pharmacological and molecular biological techniques. They seem to bind differentially to ANG II fragments (e.g., to the heptapeptide ANG III), but their possible biological functions remain unclear *(9)*.

Activation of the AT_1 receptors by ANG II elicits a variety of responses, depending on the cellular type. In cardiomyocytes and VSMCs, these responses alter the electrophysiologic milieu and the growth and proliferation of the cells. ECs respond by secreting various autocoids, such as nitric oxide (NO) and endothelin (ET), neural cells by modulating the release of neurotransmitters, fibroblasts and platelets by releasing growth factors, and so on. Accordingly, the effects of ANG II on the heart include those exerted directly via activation of AT_1 receptors and mobilization of intracellular messengers of myocardial cells, those mediated by locally released substances from other cells (endothelial, fibroblasts, and so on) as well as those resulting indirectly from the systemic and regional hemodynamic and metabolic actions of ANG II.

The AT_2 type receptor appears to be involved in the developmental effects of ANG II in the fetus, but its function postnatally remains elusive. About 30% of the ANG II receptors found in normal rat heart are AT_2 type, and their percentage increases to 60% in the hypertrophied heart *(13)*. The reports on their function seem to be contradictory: Some investigators have found evidence suggesting that AT_2 activation sets in motion intracellular events leading to apoptosis, i.e., programmed cell death *(14)*. On the contrary, others have attributed to these receptors a cardioprotective effect, possibly mediated via activation of kinins and other autocoids, similar to those participating in the actions of ACE inhibitors *(15)*. This is a field of active ongoing research, in which new data may soon reconcile seemingly conflicting pieces of evidence.

DIRECT EFFECTS OF ANG II ON THE HEART

Trophic/Mitogenic Properties of ANG II

Left ventricular hypertrophy (LVH) is the most common hypertensive complication, and is an independent coronary risk factor *(16)*, because it predisposes patients to myocardial ischemia and rhythm disturbances. The poor correlation between magnitude of LVH and severity or duration of hypertension, as well as the poor correlation between normalization of blood pressure (BP) and regression of LVH, indicates that the hemodynamic burden is only partly responsible for LVH. For this reason, neurohumoral factors, including ANG II, have been incriminated in this process. ANG II promotes LVH both directly and via pressure overload. AT_1 receptor activation stimulates release from cardiac and adjacent cells of numerous growth factors, which act in an autocrine fashion to activate enzymes and genes that induce proteins and DNA synthesis *(9)*. Such growth factors include the transforming growth factor beta (TGF-β_1) *(17)*, platelet-derived growth factor (PDGF) *(18)*, basic fibroblast growth factor (βFGF) *(19)*, insulin-like growth factor (IGF-1) *(20)*, and so on. ANG II per se can also act as a peptide growth factor, stimulating the expression of genes that regulate cell growth and proliferation, such as *c-fos, c-jun, c-myc, c-myb (18,21,22)*.

Furthermore, intracellular second messengers generated by activation of AT_1 receptors, such as phospholipases and phosphatidic acid, are now known to have trophic and mitogenic effects: They were shown to increase thymidine incorporation in various cells and to induce mRNA expression of proto-oncogenes *(23–25)*. Incubation of isolated cardiomyocytes with ANG II was shown long ago to produce increased turnover of DNA and RNA and increased protein synthesis *(26)*, thus proving that this is an intrinsic property of ANG II, and not the result of hemodynamic or mechanical conditions. By contrast, there is evidence suggesting that the AT_2 receptor may counteract the enhanced growth and proliferation triggered by the AT_1 receptor *(27,28)*, thus contributing to a constant equilibrium.

An additional mechanism by which ANG II promotes myocardial cell hypertrophy and proliferation is the permissive action on sympathetic nerve terminals to enhance the release of norepinephrine (NE), which possesses trophic and mitogenic properties of its own *(29)*. Likewise, ANG II has been shown to stimulate the expression of the ET-1 gene *(30,31)*, and to induce ET-mediated proliferation *(32)* and hypertrophy *(33)* of cardiac and vascular myocytes.

Mechanical conditions of pressure overload with increased ventricular wall stress, such as HT or CHF, produce stretching of myocardial and other cardiac cells. Stretching produces a humoral factor that activates a number of trophic and mitogenic factors, including protein kinases and proto-oncogenes *(34,35)*. There is evidence that the cardiac RAS is involved in this process, and the humoral factor may be locally produced ANG II acting in paracrine/autocrine manner, because LVH is associated with increased gene expression of some of the RAS components, such as ANGT *(36)* and ACE *(37)* in the hypertrophied myocardium (*see also* the following).

Contractile/Positive Inotropic Properties

Activation of the AT_1 receptor by ANG II triggers a series of intracellular responses, including calcium (Ca) mobilization, stimulation of Na^+/H^+ exchange, inositol phosphate metabolism, production of diacyl glycerol, activation of PKC and other kinases, activation of phosphorylation pathways, and alterations in cytoplasmic proteins *(9)*. It also triggers release of intracellular growth factors, as mentioned earlier, which, among other functions, control also the expression of contractile proteins *(38)*. The changes in electrolyte channels, especially in the Ca channels, along with the enhanced cardiac fiber shortening resulting from protein alterations, tend to increase contractility of cardiomyocytes and VSMCs, thus explaining the direct positive inotropic effect of ANG II that had been described many years ago *(39,40)*.

Facilitation of NE release by presynaptic sympathetic nerve endings *(41,42)* is an indirect mechanism contributing to the positive inotropic action of ANG II. In isolated perfused heart preparations, sympathetic nerve stimulation elicits a significantly lesser contractile response after pretreatment with an ACE inhibitor *(42,43)*, suggesting that this mechanism is physiologically important. In patients with CHF, ACE inhibition does induce a small negative inotropic effect *(44)*, probably attributable to both ANG II and sympathetic withdrawal, but this is by far outweighed by the hemodynamic improvement (reduced afterload, increased coronary blood flow) and its metabolic consequences (diminished myocardial oxygen consumption).

Chronotropic/Arrhythmogenic Effects of ANG II

High density of AT_1 receptors of ANG II has been demonstrated in the conduction system of the heart *(45)*. Stimulation of such receptors on the sinoatrial and atrioventricular nodes and the Purkinje fibers can generate spontaneous electrical activity or alter responses to electrical stimulation *(46)*. There is now evidence suggesting that ANG II decreases the intracellular resistance and increases significantly the conduction velocity *(47)*. Like the inotropic effect, this effect is believed to be mediated via activation of PKC *(48)* and increased Ca current resulting from altered conductance of Ca channels *(11)*. It has been demonstrated that ANG II shortens the refractory period in cardiac myocytes *(49)*. That this is a direct effect is best shown in cultured neonatal rat myocytes, in which ANG II increases the spontaneous contractile frequency, and ANG II antagonists can block this action *(10,11,50)*.

In addition to this direct mechanism, activation of AT_1 receptors of ANG II was also demonstrated to stimulate the release of ET-1 *(51)*, itself believed to be arrhythmogenic. Furthermore, ANG II exerts an indirect positive chronotropic and proarrhythmic effect by enhancing sympathetic activity and suppressing vagal activity. Facilitation of sympathetic neurotransmission in cardiac adrenergic nerve terminals *(52)* and sympathetic ganglia *(53)* is partly responsible for the previously mentioned positive inotropic, as well as the chronotropic and proarrhythmic properties of ANG II. Furthermore, an inhibitory action of ANG II on cardiac vagal afferents in the central nervous system has been reported *(54)*.

Disequilibrium between sympathetic and parasympathetic influences is one of the characteristics of decompensated CHF, which is associated with activation of several neurohormonal systems, including the sympathetic system and the RAS. This autonomic imbalance, with the attendant loss of parasympathetic restraint, is incriminated, in part, for the high rate of malignant ventricular arrhythmias and sudden death that are characteristic of CHF *(55)*. Experimental evidence indicates that enalapril increases the cardiac refractoriness *(56)*, and ACE inhibitors have long been known to diminish the rate of arrhythmias in myocardial ischemia, or during the reperfusion phase postmyocardial ischemia, as well as in CHF *(57,58)*. These findings had been attributed partly to ANG II withdrawal and partly to potentiation of bradykinin *(59)*, because they were attenuated in the presence of bradykinin antagonists. A surprising recent finding, however, was that selective AT_1 receptor blockade was significantly more efficacious than ACE inhibition in the treatment of elderly patients with chronic CHF, in whom mortality was decreased by 46% more with losartan than with captopril *(60)*. The authors attributed this finding to diminished propensity for arrhythmias. If these results are confirmed by further clinical trials, they will firmly establish the multifaceted cardioprotective role of ANG II blockade.

Thrombogenic Properties of ANG II

A constant equilibrium between forces that enhance intravascular coagulation and fibrinolytic/thrombolytic factors ensures normal blood rheology. The tissue-type plasminogen activator (tPA) is an important factor in the fibrinolytic process, and its inhibition has a prothrombotic effect *(61)*. Activation of the RAS has been shown to disturb this equilibrium by stimulating excess production of the plasminogen activator inhibitor type 1 (PAI-1), thus increasing the risk of thrombotic events *(62)*. In vitro, cultured VSMCs or ECs exposed to ANG II demonstrated induction of PAI-1 mRNA expression *(63,64)*. Infusion of ANG II in vivo resulted in a rapid increase in circulating levels of

PAI-1 in a dose-dependent manner, and this increase was observed in both normotensive and hypertensive individuals *(65)*. The role of elevated plasma level of PAI-1 as a risk factor for myocardial infarction (MI) has been recognized for some time *(66)*, and its suppression is now believed to be one of the mechanisms by which ACE inhibitors decrease the rate of reinfarction postmyocardial infarct *(67,68)*. Indeed, ACE inhibition was shown to suppress plasma PAI-1 activity levels *(69)*.

However, the exact mechanism by which ANG II induces expression of PAI-1 mRNA, and increases the production of this enzyme inhibitor, remains obscure. Recent evidence indicates that neither the AT_1 nor the AT_2 receptor is involved in this process, because selective ANG II receptor antagonists do not inhibit it *(70)*. Investigation of smaller ANG fragments suggested that the hexapeptide ANG IV (i.e., ANG II 3–8) may be the one responsible for this effect, acting via a novel-type receptor on endothelial and smooth muscle cells, designated as AT_4. If confirmed, these findings might mean that chronic ANG II inhibition by selective AT_1 receptor antagonists might turn out to be less effective than chronic ACE inhibition in terms of diminishing the rates of reinfarction. The cardio-protective potential of ACE inhibitors in this respect is firmly established *(71)*. The ability of ANG II blockade to prevent recurrence of myocardial infarcts may be diminished because of two important differences: The relatively lesser antithrombotic action, to the extent that such action is also exerted via potentiation of bradykinin, with its downstream effects on prostacyclin and nitric oxide (NO) *(72)*, and the inability to prevent conversion of ANG II into shorter active fragments, which may exert their own physiologic actions.

Oxidative Properties of ANG II

Increased oxidative stress is another theoretical mechanism by which ANG II may exert its direct and indirect deleterious effects on the heart *(73)*. It acts directly, by inflicting injury to myocardial and other cells, and, indirectly, by enhancing lipid peroxidation, which facilitates the atherosclerotic damage to the coronary vasculature.

ANG II has been found to cause increased activity of the nicotinamide adenine dinucle-otide and nicotinamide adenine dinucleotide phosphate oxidases, with production of large amounts of superoxide anions *(74)*. The data suggest that reactive oxygen intermedi-ates may be part of the normal intracellular signaling responses following stimulation of AT_1 receptors. Reactive oxygen species are known to cause oxidative damage to various cellular structures, including membranes, proteins such as intracellular enzymes, DNA sequences, and DNA repair enzymes *(75)*. Hypertension induced by ANG II was reported to be accompanied by marked increases in vascular production of superoxide radicals, associated with impairment of endothelial, NO-dependent vasodilation *(76,77)*, and inhibited by treatment with superoxide dismutase. The data suggest that, in addition to its own AT_1-mediated vasoconstriction, ANG II may raise BP by accelerating the degra-dation of endothelial NO via increased oxidation, as well as via a potential vasoconstric-tive effect of the superoxide anion itself *(78)*.

Acute MI is accompanied by activation of numerous systemic and local neurohumoral factors, including the RAS *(79,80)*. Furthermore, reperfusion of the acutely infarcted area (as obtained experimentally by removal of a coronary ligature, and clinically by thrombolytic agents) produces a surge in reactive oxygen species causing tissue damage beyond that inflicted by ischemia *(81)*, and attributed also in part to activation of local humoral factors, including ANG II. ACE inhibition was shown to minimize the extent of this damage *(82, 83)*, although it is unclear how much of this benefit should be attributed to ANG II suppression, and how much to potentiation of bradykinin.

Another type of oxidative damage relevant to coronary heart disease is lipid peroxidation, which is the auto-oxidation of polyunsaturated fatty acid chains of lipids *(84)*. Recent evidence indicates that low-density lipoprotein (LDL) cholesterol must be oxidized before it becomes atherogenic, and lipid peroxidation is the first step in this process. Oxidized LDL is taken up by macrophages, stimulates monocyte adhesion to the endothelium, and inhibits vasodilation, and is generally cytotoxic *(85)*. Recent clinical work suggests that LDL derived from hypertensive patients demonstrates increased susceptibility to lipid peroxidation, which the authors attributed to ANG II, because it could be reduced by ACE inhibition *(86)*. Reactive oxygen species may also act as an intracellular signal transduction pathway, by modulating the expression of cell-adhesion molecules on ECs *(87,88)*, and by activating proto-oncogenes *(89)*. All of these mechanisms would favor atheroma formation and neointimal proliferation, and would explain, in part, the increased tendency of hypertensive patients to develop atherosclerotic changes, leading to coronary obstruction, as well as peripheral arterial obstructive disease. Indeed, there is epidemiologic evidence to suggest that high-renin hypertensives are significantly more prone to heart attacks *(90,91)*, and to coronary disease in general. Moreover, successful treatment of HT by most conventional older medications (mostly diuretics, which are known to stimulate the RAS) was shown to significantly decrease the incidence of complications such as renal failure, HF, and stroke, but not of MIs *(92)*. Although no such studies are available for new antihypertensives, such as ACE inhibitors and ANG II blockers, it should be noted that ACE inhibitors have demonstrated antiatherogenic properties *(43)*. More importantly, in chronic trials on patients with preexisting ischemic heart disease or HF, such as the SAVE and SOLVD studies (*see* the following paragraphs), ACE inhibition was consistently found to reduce the rate of MIs by about 25%. This is probably partly the result of inhibition of the formation of ANG II, and partly because of the bradykinin-mediated release of prostacyclin and NO, whose oxidative degradation is retarded when ANG II is suppressed.

INDIRECT EFFECTS OF ANG II ON THE HEART

Coronary Vasoconstriction, Ischemia, and Myocardial Infarction

Acute vasoconstriction was the first effect observed in response to ANG II. Prolonged infusion of exogenous ANG II in rabbits was found to produce widespread areas of myocardial necrosis *(94)*, and surges of endogenous ANG II were shown to produce similar pathologic alterations in patients undergoing hemodialysis with ultrafiltration *(95)*. A series of experimental animal studies, using various ANG II antagonists or ACE inhibitors as pharmacologic tools, demonstrated that different vascular trees display different degrees of sensitivity to the vasoconstrictive action of ANG II; because the coronary vasculature is one of the most sensitive ones *(95,97)*, it would sustain far more pronounced vasospasm in response to excess ANG II. Subsequent experiments by other investigators have confirmed that ANG II produces myocardial necrosis *(98,99)*, and have suggested additional mechanisms by which it can be cardiotoxic, such as increased sarcolemmal permeability and death of cardiomyocytes, or increased permeability and destruction of coronary microvascular ECs. The particular sensitivity of the coronary arteries to the vasoconstrictive influence of ANG II explains also the preferential coronary vasodilation with ANG II antagonists *(100,101)* and ACE inhibitors *(102,103)*.

It is also known now that, in addition to AT_1-mediated direct vasoconstriction, ANG II stimulates or facilitates the release of other vasoconstricting forces, such as vasopressin *(104)*, NE *(29)*, and ET-1 *(51)*, which act both as systemic pressor hormones and as autocrine/paracrine factors, adding their own vascular effects to those of ANG II. Under conditions of neurohormonal activation, such as in decompensated CHF or after a MI, excessive release of these vasoconstrictors may have more than additive effects, because each may heighten the vascular responsiveness to the other. There is also evidence to suggest differences in responsiveness to ANG II among the coronary microvasculature of different regions within the myocardium: Selective AT_1 receptor inhibition in vivo, although increasing overall myocardial blood flow, seems to shunt blood away from the endocardium, as indicated by a decrease in the endocardial-to-epicardial ratio of blood flow *(105)*. This effect appears to be more pronounced in zones of experimentally induced coronary artery stenosis, where the normal endocardial dominance has been eliminated by the obstructive arterial lesion.

Acute myocardial ischemia is a potent stimulus for the local release of ANG II, as well as a host of vasoactive autacoids and local hormones *(80)*, including catecholamines, kinins, ET, and so on. Some of these tend to further accentuate cell damage; others, such as bradykinin and its tissue mediators, may have cardioprotective properties *(106)*. The multiple and complex interactions among these vasoactive substances are the subject of intensive ongoing basic research, with new aspects being constantly elucidated. However, the biological and clinical importance of the postinfarct activation of the RAS has been proven *ex juvantibus*: Chronic ACE inhibition after coronary ligation in rats was shown to attenuate the progressive LV dilation *(107)*, and to prolong survival. The first clinical trial in post-MI patients with some systolic dysfunction demonstrated that ACE inhibition could retard the progression of HF *(108)*. The mechanisms were retardation of the process of myocardial remodeling and attenuation of the progression of LV enlargement, with reduced cardiac filling and improved exercise tolerance *(67,109)*. A single study *(110)*, in which ACE inhibition was started within 24 h of a MI in patients unstable and prone to hypotension, did not benefit survival. Subsequent large controlled clinical trials, in which survivors of acute MI with various degrees of LV dysfunction were treated with ACE inhibition, showed reductions in overall mortality and reductions in risk for CHF, recurrence of infarct, or any major cardiovascular event. All of these events were consistently reduced by 20–30%, regardless of the particular ACE inhibiting agent tested. Such trials include the SAVE *(111)* with captopril, the AIRE *(112)* with ramipril, the TRACE *(113)* with trandolapril, the SMILE *(114)* with zofenopril, the GISSI-3 *(115)* with lisinopril, and others.

Systemic Vasoconstriction, Hypertension, and Congestive Heart Failure

The first immediately obvious result of renin-angiotensin excess is, of course, systemic vasoconstriction with acute BP elevation, as observed by Tigerstedt and Bergman *(116)* with administration of renal extracts to rabbits. The renal origin of the hypertensive principle was shown by Goldblatt et al. *(117)*, who induced immediate HT by clamping a renal artery, and reversal of HT by removing the clamp or the ischemic kidney, although the fact that this hypertensive principle was the RAS was not recognized until several years later *(118,119)*. Elevated peripheral vascular resistance as a result of sustained

ANG II-mediated systemic vasoconstriction is one pathogenic mechanism of HT; the steroidogenic effect of ANG II on the adrenal zona glomerulosa, with stimulation of aldosterone and retention of sodium and fluid, is a necessary component for the maintenance of chronic HT *(120)*.

Elevated systemic vascular resistance—the hallmark of HT—is a mechanical stimulus for LVH via increase in LV pressure and LV wall stretch. Although initially compensatory, LVH is now recognized to be an independent risk factor for cardiac morbidity and mortality *(16)*, because it predisposes to electrophysiological instability *(121)*, CHF *(122)*, myocardial ischemia *(123)*, and sudden death *(124)*. A vast body of literature has established that mechanical forces work in concert with locally prevailing neurohormonal influences to enhance, prevent, or reverse LVH. Vasopressor forces, such as ANG II, NE, and ET, tend to accentuate LVH; endogenous vasodilators, such as kinins *(125)*, tend to prevent or reverse it. It was even reported that an ACE inhibitor in low doses, insufficient to alter systemic BP in a renin-dependent HT, could reverse LVH *(126)*, which would suggest that the antihypertrophic effect was primarily caused by bradykinin, and that the pressor effect of ANG II was irrelevant to this action; however, this finding has been challenged by other investigators *(127)*. Most studies indicate that both the mechanical and biological effects of ANG II contribute to LVH. Although these effects can be dissociated, they are also interdependent, because stretching of cardiomyocytes induces them to release ANG II *(128)*, which then acts locally as a cellular growth factor. At the clinical level, reversal of LVH by chronic ACE inhibition is one of the recognized benefits of the treatment *(129)*.

Elevated systemic vascular resistance is also the hallmark of decompensated CHF. It is attributed to activation of pressor neurohormones *(130)*, such as ANG II, cathecholamines, vasopressin, and ET, in an effort to maintain circulatory homeostasis in the face of diminishing systolic force, but contributes to further deterioration of contractile capacity and decrease of cardiac output. The first attempt to treat CHF with ANG II blockade *(100)* demonstrated immediate hemodynamic amelioration of systemic and cardiac hemodynamics: fall in peripheral resistance, increase in cardiac output, improved left ventricular work index with increased coronary blood flow, despite decreased myocardial oxygen consumption. Acute treatment of HF first with the iv ACE inhibitor, teprotide, and later with captopril, produced virtually identical hemodynamic effects to those of ANG II blockade *(102,131,132)*, indicating that the systemic hemodynamic results were mostly attributable to inhibition of ANG II. Subsequent large controlled trials were designed to compare chronic ACE inhibition to placebo or to other vasodilators in patients with chronic cardiac insufficiency, ranging from subclinical LV dysfunction to advanced CHF. The first of those was the CONSENSUS trial *(133)* with enalapril, and was followed by the SOLVD *(134,135)*, V-HeFT II *(136)*, and so on. Along with the post-MI studies mentioned earlier, these trials demonstrated that hemodynamic amelioration can be chronically maintained, and leads to functional improvement. They also established the fact that ACE inhibition is the only treatment that consistently reduces morbidity and mortality in HF.

CONCLUSIONS

This has been a brief overview of the multifaceted properties of ANG II as they have emerged over the years. All of them lead to effects that are damaging for the heart. Some are now well established and universally accepted, because they have been demonstrated by rigorously controlled experiments, and are intuitively consistent with the long-known effects of the hormone: Acute myocardial necrosis and LVH fall in this category. Others are still conjectural, based on logical hypotheses or isolated observations whose actual clinical relevance remains to be proven: Examples are the putative oxidative and procoagulant properties of ANG II. Undoubtedly, continuing research will uncover additional, yet unsuspected mechanisms, that may explain and amplify new findings in this still-evolving field. It is noteworthy that the cardioprotective benefits of renin-angiotensin blockade were demonstrated first by pilot clinical studies, and then confirmed by large multicenter trials, long before basic research started uncovering the wide range of mechanisms contributing to these results.

REFERENCES

1. Lee MR. Kinetics of renin-substrate reaction. In: Renin and Hypertension. Williams & Wilkins, Baltimore, MD, 1969, pp.25–27.
2. Campbell DJ. Circulating and tissue angiotensin systems. J Clin Invest 1987;79:1–5.
3. Laragh JH. Extrarenal tissue prorenin systems do exist: are intrinsic vascular and cardiac tissue renins fact or fancy? Am J Hypertens 1989;2:262–265.
4. Dostal DE, Baker KM. Evidence for a role of an intracardiac renin-angiotensin. Trends Cardiovasc Med 1993;3:67–74.
5. Campbell DJ, Habener JF. Angiotensinogen gene is expressed and differentially regulated in multiple tissues of the rat. J Clin Invest 1986;78:31–39.
6. Schunkert H, Dzau VJ, Tang SS. Hirsch AT, Apstein CS, Lorell BH. Increased rat cardiac angiotensin converting enzyme activity and mRNA expression in pressure overload left ventricular hypertrophy: effects on coronary resistance, contractility, and relaxation. J Clin Invest 1990;86:1913–1920.
7. Dzau VJ, Ellison EK, Brody T, Ingelfinger J, Pratt R. Comparison study of the distribution of renin and angiotensinogen messenger ribonucleic acids in rat and mouse tissues. Endocrinology 1987;120: 2334–2338.
8. Hackenthal E, Paul M, Ganten D, Taugner R. Morphology, physiology, and molecular biology of renin secretion. Physiol Rev 1990;70:1067–1116.
9. Dostal DE, Baker KM. Biochemistry, molecular biology, and potential roles of the cardiac renin—angiotensin system. In: Dhalla NS, Takeda N, Nagano M, eds. The Failing Heart. Lippincott-Raven, Philadelphia, PA, 1995, pp. 275–294.
10. Rogers TB, Gaa ST, Allen IS. Identification and characterization of functional angiotensin II receptors on cultured heart myocytes. J Pharm Exp Ther 1986;236:438–444.
11. Allen IS, Cohen NM, Dhallan RS, Gaa ST, Lederer WJ, Rogers TB. Angiotensin II increases spontaneous contractile frequency and stimulates calcium current in cultured neonatal rat heart myocytes: insights into the underlying biochemical mechanisms. Circ Res 1988;62:524–534.
12. Urata H. Healy B, Stewart RW, Bumpus FM, Husain A. Angiotensin receptors in normal and failing human hearts. J Clin Endocrinol Metab 1989;69:54–66.
13. Lopez JJ, Lorell BH, Ingelfinger JR, Weinberg EO, Schunkert H, Diamant D, Tang S-S. Distribution and function of cardiac angiotensin AT_1 and AT_2 receptor subtypes in hypertrophied rat hearts. Am J Physiol 1994;267:H844–H852.
14. Yamada T, Horiuchi M, Dzau VJ. Angiotensin II type 2 receptor mediates programmed cell death. Proc Natl Acad Sci USA 1996;93:156–160.
15. Liu Y-H, Yang X-P, Sharov VG, Nass O, Sabbah HN, Peterson E, Carretero OA. Effects of angiotensin-converting enzyme inhibitors and angiotensin II type 1 receptor antagonists in rats with heart failure: role of kinins and angiotensin II Type 2 receptors. J Clin Invest 1997;99:1926–1935.
16. Levy D, Garrison RJ, Savage DD, Kannel WB, Castelli WP. Left ventricular mass and incidence of coronary heart disease in an elderly cohort; the Framingham Heart Study. Ann Intern Med 1989;110: 101–107.
17. Stouffer GA, Owens GK. Angiotensin II-induced mitogenesis of spontaneously hypertensive rat-derived cultured smooth muscle cells is dependent on autocrine production of transforming growth factor-beta. Circ Res 1992;70:820–828.

18. Naftilan AJ, Pratt RE, Dzau VJ. Induction of plaelet-derived growth factor A-chain and c-myc gene expression by angiotenin II in cultured rat vascular smooth muscle cells. J Clin Invest 1989;83: 1419–1424.
19. Schorb W, Singer HA, Dostal DE, Baker KM. Angiotensin II is a potent simulator of MAP-kinase activity in neonatal rat cardiac fibroblasts. J Mol Cell Cardiol 1995;27:1151–1160.
20. Delafontaine P, Lou H. Angiotensin II regulates insulin-like growth factor I gene expression in vascular smoth muscle cells. J Biol Chem 1993;268:16,866–16,870.
21. Naftilan AJ, Pratt RE, Eldrige CS, Lin HL, Dzau VJ. Angiotensin II induces c-fos expression in smooth muscle via transcriptional control. Hypertension 1989;13:706–711.
22. Pauet J-L, Baudouin-Legros M, Brunell G, Meyer P. Angiotensin II-induced proliferation of aortic myocytes in spontaneously hypertensive rats. J Hypertens 1990;8:565–572.
23. Yu C, Tsai M, Stacey DW. Cellular ras activity and phospholipid metabolism. Cell 1988;52:63–71.
24. Knauss TC, Jaffer FE, Abboud HE. Phosphatidic acid modulates DNA synthesis, phospholipase C, and platelet-derived growth factor mRNAs in cultured mesangial cells. J Biol Chem 1990;265:14,457–14,463.
25. Moolenaar WH, Kruijer W, Till BC, Verlaan I, Bierman AJ, deLaat SW. Growth factor-like action of phosphatidic acid. Nature 1991;323:171–173.
26. Khairallah PA, Robertson AL, Davila D. Effect of angiotensin II on DNA, RNA, and protein synthesis. In: Genest J, Koiw E, eds. Hypertension. Springer Verlag, New York, 1972, pp. 212–220.
27. Nakajima M, Hutchinson HG, Fujinaga W, Hayashida R, Morishita L, Zhang Horiuchi M, Pratt RE, Dzau VJ. Angiotensin II type 2 (AT_2) receptor antagonizes the growth effects of the AT_1 receptor: gain-of-function study using gene transfer. Proc Natl Acad Sci USA 1995;92:10,663–10,667.
28. Stoll M, Steckelings UM, Paul M, Bottari SP, Metzger R, Unger T. Angiotensin AT_2-receptor mediates inhibition of cell proliferation in coronary endothelial cells. J Clin Invest 1995;95:651–657.
29. Newling RP, Fletcher PJ, Coutis M, Shaw J. Noradrenaline and cardiac hypertrophy in the rat: changes in morphology, blood pressure and ventricular performance. J Hypertens 1989;7:561–567.
30. Imai T, Hirata Y, Emori T, Yanagisawa M, Masaki T, Marumo F. Induction of endothelin-1 gene by angiotensin and vasopressin in endothelial cells. Hypertension 1992;19:753–757.
31. Chua BH, Chua CC, Diglio CA, Siu BB. Regulation of endothelin-1 mRNA by angiotensin II in rat heart endothelial cells. Biochim Biophys Acta 1993;1178:201–206.
32. Sung CP, Arleth AJ, Storer BL, Ohlstein EH. Angiotensin type 1 receptors mediate smooth muscle proliferation and endothelin biosynthesis in rat vascular smooth muscle. J Pharmacol Exp Ther 1994; 271:429–437.
33. Ito H, Hirata Y, Adachi S, Tanaka M, Tsujino M, Koike A, et al. Endothelin-1 is an autocrine/paracrine factor in the mechanism of angiotensin II-induced hypertrophy in cultured rat cardiomyocytes. J Clin Invest 1993;92:398–403.
34. Yamazaki T, Tobe K, Hoh E, Maemura K, Kaida T, Komuro H. Mechanical loading activates mitogen-activated protein kinase and S6 peptide kinase in cultured rat cardiac myocytes. J Biol Chem 1993;268: 12,069–12,076.
35. Komuro I, Katoh Y, Kaida T, Shibazaki Y, Kurabayashi M. Mechanical loading stimulates cell hypertrophy and specific gene expression in cultured rat cardiac myocytes. J Biol Chem 1991;266: 1265–1268.
36. Lindpaintner K, Ganten D. The cardiac renin-angiotensin system. Circ Res 1991;68:905–921.
37. Fabris B, Jackson B, Kohzuki M, Perich R, Johnston CI. Increased cardiac angiotensin-converting enzyme in rats with chronic heart failure. Clin Exp Pharmacol Physiol 1990;17:309–314.
38. Scott-Burden T, Hahn AWA, Resink TJ, Buhler FR. Modulation of extracellular matrix by angiotensin II: stimulated glycoconjugate synthesis and growth in vascular smooth muscle cells. J Cardiovasc Pharmacol 1990;16(Suppl 4):36–41.
39. Vogin EE, Buckley JP. Cadiac effects of angiotensin II. J Pharmacol Sci 1964;53:1482–1486.
40. Kobayashi M, Furukawa Y, Chiba S. Positive chronotropic and inotropic effects of angiotensin II in the dog heart. Eur J Pharmacol 1978;50:17–25.
41. Malik KU, Nasjletti A. (1976) Facilitation of adrenergic transmission by locally generated angiotensin II in rat mesenteric arteries. Circ Res 38:26–30.
42. Carlsson L, Abrahamsson T. Ramiprilat attenuates the local release of noradrenaline in the ichemic myocardium. Eur J Pharmacol 1989;166:157–164.
43. Xiang JZ, Linz W, Becker H, Ganten D, Lang RE, Scholkens B, Unger T. Effects of converting enzyme inhibitors: ramipril and enalapril on peptide action and sympathetic neurotransmission in the isolated heart. Eur J Pharmacol 1985;113:215–223.

44. Foult JM, Travalaro O, Autony I, Nittenberg A. Direct myocardial and coronary effects of enalaprilat in patient with dilated cardiomyopathy: assessment by a bilateral intracoronary infusion technique. Circulation 1988;77:337–344.
45. Saito K, Gutkind JS, Saavedra JM. Angiotensin II binding sites in the conduction system of rat hearts. Am J Physiol 1987;253:H1618–H1622.
46. Kass RS, Blair ML. Effects of angiotensin II on membrane current in cardiac Purkinje fibers. J Mol Cell Cardiol 1981;13:797–809.
47. De Mello WC. Renin-angiotensin system and cell communication in the failing heart. Hypertension 1996;27:1267–1272.
48. De Mello WC. Is an intracellular renin-angiotensin system involved in control of cell communication in heart? J Cardiovasc Pharmacol 1994;23:640–646.
49. De Mello WC, Crespo MJ. Cardiac refractoriness in rats is reduced by angiotensin II. J Cardiovasc Pharmacol 1995;25:51–56.
50. Dosemeci A, Dhallan RS, Cohen NM, Lederer WJ, Rogers TB. Phorbol ester increases calcium current and stimulates the effects of angiotensin II on cultured neonatal rat heart myocytes. Circ Res 1988;62: 347–357.
51. Rajagopalan S, Laursen JB, Borthayre A, Kurz S, Keiser J, Haleen S, Giaid A, Harrison DG. Role for endothelin-1 in angiotensin II-mediated hypertension. Hypertension 1997;30(Part 1):29–34.
52. Starke K. Action of angiotensin on uptake, release, and metabolism of 14C NE by isolated rabbit hearts. Eur J Pharmacol 1971;14:112–123.
53. Aiken JW, Reit E. Stimulation of the cat stellate ganglion by angiotensin. J Pharmacol Exp Ther 1968; 159:107–114.
54. Lee WB, Ismay MJ, Lumbers ER. Mechanisms by which angiotensin affects the heart rate of the conscious sheep. Circ Res 1980;47:286–292.
55. Ponikowski P, Auker SD, Amadi A, Chua TP, Cerquetain D, Ondusova D, et al. Heart rhythms, ventricular arrhythmias and death in chronic heart failure. J Cardiac Failure 1996;2:1772–1783.
56. De Mello WC, Crespo MJ, Altieri PI. Enalapril increases cardiac refractoriness. J Cardiovasc Pharmacol 1992;20:820–825.
57. Kingma JH, De Graeff PA, Van Gilst WH, van Binsbergen E, de Langen CDJ, Wesseling H. Effects of intravenous captopril on inducible sustained ventricular tachycardia. Postgrad Med 1986;62:159–163.
58. Wesseling H, De Graeff PA, Van Gilst WH, Kingma JH, de Langen CDJ. Cardiac arrhythmias: a new indication for angiotensin converting enzyme inhibitors. J Hum Hypertens 1989;3:89–95.
59. Van Gilst WH, De Graeff PA, Wesseling H, de Langen CDJ. Reduction of reperfusion arrhythmias in the ischemic isolated rat heart by angiotensin converting enzyme inhibitors: a comparison of captopril, enalapril, and HOE498. J Cardiovasc Pharmacol 1986;8:722–728.
60. Pitt B, Segal R, Martinez FA, Meurers G, Cowley AJ, Thomas I. Randomized trial of losartan versus captopril in patients over 65 with heart failure (Evaluation of losartan in the Elderly Study, ELITE). Lancet 1997;349:747–752.
61. Ridker PM. Epidemiologic assessment of thrombotic risk factors for cardiovascular disease. Curr Opin Lipid 1992;3:285–290.
62. Olson JA Jr, Ogilvie S, Buhi WC, Raizata MK. Angiotensin II induces secretion of plasminogen activator inhibitor I and a tissue metallopeptidase inhibitor-related protein from rat brain astrocytes. Neurobiology 1991;88:1928–1932.
63. Van Leeuwen RT, Kol A, Andreotti F, Kluft C, Maseri A, Sperti G. Angiotensin II increases plasminogen activator inhibitor type 1 and tissue-type plasminogen activator messenger RNA in culture rat aortic smooth muscle cells. Circulation 1994;62:362–368.
64. Vaughn DE. Lazos SA, Tong K. Angiotensin II regulates the expression of plasminogen activator inhibitor-1 in cultured endothelial cells. A potential link between the renin-angiotensin system and thrombosis. J Clin Invest 1995;95:995–1001.
65. Ridker PM, Gaboury CL, Conlin PR, Seely EW, Williams GH, Vaughan DE. Stimulation of plasminogen activator inhibitor in vivo by infusion of angiotensin II. Evidence of a potential interaction between the renin-angiotensin system and fibrinolytic function. Circulation 1993;87:1969–1973.
66. Hamsten A, DeFaire U, Walldius G, Dahlen G, Szamosi A, Landou C, Blomback M, Wiman B. Plasminogen activator inhibitor in plasma: risk factor for recurrent myocardial infarction. Lancet 1987;2:3–9.
67. Pfeffer MA, Braunwald E, Moye LA, Basta L, Brown EJ, Cuddy TE, et al. Effect of captopril on mortality and morbidity in patients with left ventricular dysfunction after myocardial infarction. N Engl J Med 1992;327:669–677.

68. Yusuf S, Pepine FJ. Garces C, Pouleur H, Salem D, Kostis J, et al. Effect of enalapril on myocardial infarction and unstable angina in patients with low ejection fractions. Lancet 1992;340:1173–1178.

69. Wright RA, Flapan AD, Alberti GMM, Ludlam CA, Fox AAA. Effects of captopril therapy on endogenous fibrinolysis in men with recent, uncomplicated myocardial infarction. J Am Coll Cardiol 1994; 24:67–73.

70. Kerins DM, Hao Q, Vaughan DE. Angiotensin induction of PAI-1 expression in endothelial cells is mediated by the hexapeptide angiotensin IV. J Clin Invest 1995;96:2515–2520.

71. Gavras H. Angiotensin-converting enzyme inhibition and the heart. Hypertension 1994;23:813–818.

72. Gavras I. Bradykinin-mediated effects of ACE inhibition. Kidney Int 1992;42:1020–1029.

73. Oskarsson HJ, Heistad DD. Oxidative stress produced by angiotensin II: Implications for hypertension and vascular injury. Circulation 1997;95:557–559.

74. Griendling KK, Minieri CA, Ollerenshaw JD, Alexander RW. Angiotensin II stimulates NADH and NADPH oxidase activity in cultured vascular smooth muscle cells. Circ Res 1994;74:1141–1148.

75. Ames BN, Shigenaga MK, Hagen TM. Oxidants, antioxidants, and the degenerative disease of aging. Proc Natl Acad Sci USA 1993;90:7915–7922.

76. Rajagopalan S, Kurz S, Munzel T, Tarpey M, Freeman BA, Griendling KK, Harrison DG. Angiotensin II-mediated hypertension in the rat increases vascular superoxide production via membrane NADH/ NADPH oxidase activation: contribution to alterations of vasomotor tone. J Clin Invest 1996;97: 1916–1923.

77. Bech LJ, Rajagopalan S, Galis Z, Tarpey M, Freeman BA, Harrison DG. Role of superoxide in angiotensin II-induced but not catecholamine-induced hypertension. Circulation 1997;95:588–593.

78. Katusic ZS, Vanhoutte PM. Superoxide anion is an endothelium-derived contracting factor. Am J Physiol 1989;257:H33–H37.

79. McAlpine HM, Cobbe SM. Neuroendocrine changes in acute myocardial infarction. Am J Med 1988; 84(Suppl 3A):61–66.

80. Rouleau JL, Moye LA, de Champlain J, Klein M, Bichet D, Packer M, et al. Activation of neurohumoral systems following acute myocardial infarction. Am J Cardiol 1991;68:80D–86D.

81. Braunwald E, Kloner RA. Myocardial reperfusion: a double-edged sword? J Clin Invest 1986;76: 1713–1719.

82. Li K, Chen X. Protective effects of captopril and enalapril on myocardial ischemia and reperfusion damage of rat. J Mol Cell Cardiol 1987;19:909–915.

83. Tio RA, De Langen CDJ, De Graeff PA, Van Gilst WH, Bel KJ, Wolters KGTP, et al. The effects of oral pretreatment with zofenopril an angiotensin-converting enzyme inhibitor, on early reperfusion and subsequent electrophysiologic stability in the pig. Cardiovasc Drugs Ther 1990;4:695–704.

84. Frei B. Reactive oxygen species and antioxidant vitamins Mechanisms of action. Am J Med 1994; 97(Suppl 3A):5–13.

85. Keaney JF, Frei B. Antioxidant protection of low-density lipoprotein and its role in the prevention of atherosclerotic vascular disease. In: Frei B, ed. Natural Antioxidants in Human Health and Disease. Orlando, Academic, 1994, pp. 303–351.

86. Keidar S, Kaplan M, Shapira C, Brook JG, Avirom M. Low density lipoprotein isolated from patients with essential hypertension exhibits increased propensity for oxidation and enhanced uptake by macrophages: a possible role for angiotensin II. Atherosclerosis 1994;107:71–84.

87. Marui N, Offermann MK, Swerlick R, Kunsch C, Rosen CA, Ahmad M, Alexander RW, Medford RM. Vascular cell adhesion molecule-1 (VCAM-1) gene transcription and expression are regulated through an antioxidant-sensitive mechanism in human vascular endothelial cell. J Clin Invest 1993;92: 1866–1874.

88. Fraticelli A, Serrano CV Jr Bochner BS, Capogrossi MC, Zweier JL. Hydrogen peroxide and superoxide modulate leukocyte adhesion molecule expression and leukocyte endothelial adhesion. Biochim Biophys Acta 1996;1310:251–259.

89. Puri PL, Avantaggiati ML, Burgio VL. Chirillo P, Collepardo D, Natoli G, Balsano C, Levrero M. Reactive oxygen intermediates mediate angiotensin II-induced c-jun c-fos heterodimer DNA binding activity and proliferative hypertropic responses in myogenic cells. J Biol Chem 1995;270:22,129–22,134.

90. Brunner HR, Laragh JR, Baer L, Newton MA, Goodwin FT, Krakoff LR, Bard RM, Buhler FR. Essential hypertension: renin and aldosterone, heart attack and stroke. N Engl J Med 1972;286:441–449.

91. Alderman MH, Madhavan S, Ooi WL, Cohen H, Sealey JE, Laragh JH. Association of the renin-sodium profile with the risk of myocardial infarction in patients with hypertension. N Engl J Med 1991; 324:10,098–10104.

92. MacMahon SW, Cutler JA, Furberg CD, Payne GH. The effects of drug treatment for hypertension on morbidity and mortality from cardiovascular disease: a review of randomized controlled trials. Prog Cardiovasc Dis 1986;29(Suppl 1):99–118.

93. Chobanian AV, Haudenschild CC, Nickerson C, Drago R. Antiatherogenic effect of captopril in the Watanabe heritable hyperlipidemic rabbit. Hypertension 1990;15:327–333.

94. Gavras H, Brown JJ, Lever AF, MacAdam RF, Robertson JIS. Acute renal failure, tubular necrosis and myocardial infarction induced in the rabbit by intravenous angiotensin II. Lancet 1971;II:19–22.

95. Gavras H, Kremer D, Brown JJ, Gray V, Lever AF, Macadam RF, et al. Angiotensin and norepinephrine-induced myocardial lesions: experimental and clinical studies in rabbit and man. Am Heart J 1975; 89:321–332.

96. Gavras H, Liang C, Brunner HR. Redistribution of regional blood flow after inhibition of the angiotensin converting enzyme. Circ Res 1978;43(Suppl 1):59–63.

97. Liang C, Gavras H, Hood WB Jr. Renin-angiotensin system inhibition in conscious sodium-depleted dogs: effects on systemic and coronary hemodynamics. J Clin Invest 1978;61:874–883.

98. Tan LB, Jalil JE, Pick R, Janicki JS, Weber KT. Cardiac myocyte necrosis induced by angiotensin II. Circ Res 1991;69:1185–1195.

99. Weber KT, Brilla CG, Campbell SE, Reddy HK. Myocardial fibrosis and the concepts of cardioprotection and cardioreparation. J Hypertens 1992;10(Suppl 5):S87-S94.

100. Gavras H, Flessas A, Ryan TJ, Brunner HR, Faxon DP, Gavras I. Angiotensin II inhibition: treatment of congestive cardiac failure in a high-renin hypertension. JAMA 1977;238:880–882.

101. Wang Y-X, Gavras I, Wierzba T, Gavras H. Comparison of systemic and regional hemodynamic effects of a diuretic, an angiotensin-II receptor antagonist, and an angiotensin-converting enzyme inhibitor in conscious renovascular hypertensive rats. J Lab Clin Med 1992;119:267–272.

102. Faxon DP, Creager MA, Halperin JL, Sussman HA, Gavras H, Ryan TJ. The effect of angiotensin converting enzyme inhibition on coronary blood flow and hemodynamics in patients without coronary artery disease. Int J Cardiol 1982;2:251–262.

103. Magrini F, Shimizu M, Roberts N, Fouad F, Tarazi RC, Zanchetti A. Converting enzyme inhibition and coronary blood flow. Circulation 1987;75(Suppl 1):1168-1174.

104. Sladek CD. Regulation of vasopressin release by neurotransmitters, neuropeptides and osmotic stimuli. In: Gross BA, Leng C, eds. Neurophysics: Structure, Function and Control Progress in Brain Research. Elsevier, Amsterdam, 1983, pp. 71–90.

105. Ruocco NA Jr, Bergelson BA, Yu T-K, Gavras I, Gavras H. Augmentation of coronary blood flow by ACE inhibition: role of angiotensin and bradykinin. Clin Exper Hypertens 1995;17:1059–1072.

106. Gavras H. Brunner HR, Laragh JH, Sealey JE, Gavras I, Vukovich RA. An angiotensin converting enzyme inhibitor to identify and treat vasoconstrictor and volume factors in hypertensive patients. N Engl J Med 1974;291:817–821.

107. Pfeffer MA, Pfeffer JA, Steinberg C, Finn P. Survival after an experimental myocardial infarction: beneficial effects of long-term therapy with captopril. Circulation 1985;72:406–412.

108. Sharpe N, Murphy J, Smith H, Hannan S. Treatment of patients with symptomless left ventricular dysfunction after myocardial infarction. Lancet 1988;1:255–259.

109. Pfeffer MA, Lamas GA, Vaughan DE, Paris AF, Braunwald E. Effect of captopril on progressive ventricular dilation after anterior myocardial infarction. N Engl J Med 1988;319:80–86.

110. Swedberg K, Held P, Kjekshus J, Rasmussen K, Ryden L, Wedel H. Effects of early administration of enalapril on mortality in patients with acute myocardial infarction (CONSENSUS II). N Engl J Med 1992;327:678–684.

111. Pfeffer MA, Braunwald E, Moye LA, Basta L, Brown EJ Jr, Cuddy TE. Effect of captopril on mortality and morbidity in patients with left ventricular dysfunction after myocardial infarction. Results of the Survival and Ventricular Enlargement trial. The SAVE Investigators. N Engl J Med 1992;327:669–677.

112. The AIRE Study Investigators. Effect of ramipril on mortality and morbidity of survivors of acute myocardial infarction with clinical evidence of heart failure. Lancet 1993;342:821–828.

113. Kober L, Torp-Pedersen C, Clarsen JE, Carlsen JE, Bagger H, Eliasen P. A clinical trial of the angiotensin-converting enzyme inhibitor trandolapril in patients with left ventricular dysfunction after myocardial infarction. Trandolapril Cardiac Evaluation (TRACE) Study Group. N Engl J Med 1995; 333:1670–1676.

114. Ambrosioni E, Borghi C, Magnani B. The Effect of the angiotensin-converting enzyme inhibitor zofenopril on mortality and morbidity after anterior myocardial infarction. SMILE Study Investigators. N Engl J Med 1995;332:80–85.

115. GISSI. GISSI-3: Effect of lisinopril and transermal glyceryl trinitrate singly and together on 6-week mortality and ventricular function after acute myocardial infarction. Lancet 1994;343:1115–1122.
116. Tigerstedt R, Bergman PG. Niere und Kreislauf. Skand Arch Physiol 1898;8:223–271.
117. Goldblatt H, Lynch J, Hanzal RF, Summerville WW. Studies on experimental hypertension, I: the production of persistent elevation of systolic blood pressure by means of renal ischemia. J Exp Med 1934;59:347–379.
118. Page IH, Helmer OM. A crystalline pressor substance (angiotonin) resulting from the reaction between renin and renin activator. J Exp Med 1940;71:29–42.
119. Braun-Menendez E, Fasciolo JC, Leloir LF, Munoz JM. The substance causing renal hypertension. J Physiol 1940;98:283–298.
120. Laragh JH, Ames M, Kelly W, Lieberman S. Hypotensive agents and pressor substances. The effect of epinephrine, norepinephrine, angiotensin II, and others on the secretory rate of aldosterone in man. JAMA 1960;174:234–240.
121. TenEick RE, Houser SR, Bassett AL. Cardiac hypertrophy and altered cellular electrical activity of the myocardium: possible electrophysiological basis for myocardial contractility changes. In: Sperelakis N, ed. Physiology and Pathophysiology of the Heart, 2nd ed. Kluwer Academic, Boston, MA, 1989, pp. 57–94.
122. Katz AM. Cardiomyopathy of overload. A major determinant of prognosis in congestive heart failure. N Engl J Med 1990;322:100–110.
123. Manolis AJ, Beldekos D, Hatzissavas J, Foussas S, Cokkinos D, Bresnahan M, Gavras I, Gavras H. Hemodynamic and humoral correlates in essential hypertension. Relationship between patterns of LVH and myocardial ischemia. Hypertension 1997;30(Part 2):730–734.
124. Kannel WB, Doyle JT, McNamara PM, Puickenton P, Gordon T. Precursors of sudden death; Factors related to the incidence of sudden death. Circulation 1975;51:606–613.
125. Nolly H, Carbini LA, Scicli G, Carrertero OA, Scicli AG. A local kallikrein-kinin system is present in rat hearts. Hypertension 1994;23:919–923.
126. Ling W. Shaper J, Wiemer G, Albus U, Scholkens BA. Ramipril prevents left ventricular hypertrophy with myocardial fibrosis without blood pressure reduction: a one year study in rats. Br J Pharmacol 1992;107:970–975.
127. Rhaleb N-E, Yang X-P, Scicli AG, Carretero OA. Role of kinins and nitric oxide in the antihypertrophic effect of ramipril. Hypertension 1994;23:865–868.
128. Sadoshima J, Xu Y, Slayter HS, Izumo S. Autocrine release of angiotensin II mediates stretch-induced hypertrophy of cardiac myocytes in vitro. Cell 1993;75:977–984.
129. Pfeffer MA, Pfeffer JM. Reversing cardiac hypertrophy in hypertension. N Engl J Med 1990;329:1388–1390.
130. Francis GS, Goldsmith SR, Levine TB, Olivari MT, Cohn JN. The neurohumoral axis in congestive heart failure. Am J Med 1984;101:370–377.
131. Gavras H, Faxon DP, Berkoben J, Brunner HR, Ryan TJ. Angiotensin converting enzyme inhibition in patients with congestive heart failure. Circulation 1978;58:770–775.
132. Turini GA, Brunner HR, Ferguson RK, Rivier JL, Gavras H. Congestive heart failure in normotensive man: hemodynamics, renin and angiotensin II blockade. Brit Heart J 1978;40: 1134–1142.
133. The CONSENSUS Trial Study Group. Effects of enalapril on mortality in severe congestive heart failure: result of the Cooperative North Scandinavian Enalapril Survival Study (CONSENSUS). N Engl J Med 1987;316:1429–1435.
134. The SOLVD Investigators. Effect of enalapril on survival in patients with reduced left ventricular ejection fractions and congestive heart failure. N Engl J Med 1991;325:293–302.
135. The SOLVD Investigators. Effect of enalapril on mortality and the development of heart failure in asymptomatic patients with reduced left ventricular ejection fractions. N Engl J Med 1992;327:685–691.
136. Cohn JN, Johnson G, Ziesche S, Cobb F, Francis G, Tristawi F, et al. Comparison of enalapril with hydralazine-isosorbide dinitrate in the treament of chronic congestive heart failure. N Engl J Med 1991;325:303–310.

5

Adrenocortical Hormones and the Heart

A Steroidogenic Endocrine Organ as Well as Target Organ?

Celso E. Gomez-Sanchez

CONTENTS

EFFECTS OF ADRENAL STEROIDS ON THE HEART
THE HEART IS A STEROIDOGENIC ORGAN
ACKNOWLEDGMENTS
REFERENCES

Mineralocorticoid steroids, of which aldosterone is the most abundant and important, are produced in the zona glomerulosa of the adrenal gland in response to low sodium, high potassium, angiotensin II (ANG II) and adrenocorticotrophic hormone (ACTH). They act on the circulation indirectly by increasing the reabsorption of sodium and water by the kidney. leading to the expansion of the extracellular vascular space, resulting in an increase in cardiac output. Chronic administration of mineralocorticoids results in autoregulation by vascular smooth muscle cells (VSMCs) increase in peripheral vascular resistance, and elevation of blood pressure (BP). The increase in cardiac afterload produced by the elevation in BP was thought to cause a pressure-dependent cardiac hypertrophy *(1)*. Over the past two decades, it has become clear that mineralocorticoid action is far more global and diverse, and includes actions in nontransport epithelial tissues, notably specific organs of the brain and the cardiovascular system.

The heart is a target organ for mineralocorticoid and glucocorticoid steroids, which have direct effects on the heart, including cardiac hypertrophy and fibrosis. In addition, the heart is capable of synthesizing corticosteroids *de novo*. Although the physiological relevance of this synthesis is still not clear, cardiac corticosteroids may have paracrine and/or autocrine effects that produce the clinical and experimental phenomena described below.

Patients with Addison's disease, or primary adrenal insufficiency, have a tendency to low BP, and often complain of postural dizziness or syncope, and have postural hypotension *(2)*. Chest X-rays often show a small heart *(3)*. Conversely, hypertension (HT) is the primary risk factor associated with left ventricular hypertrophy (LVH), which has been assumed to represent a maladaptive response of the heart to increased afterload. The role of hemodynamic load is not as clear as previously assumed. It is not the only determinant

From: *Contemporary Endocrinology: Hormones and the Heart in Health and Disease*
Edited by: L. Share © Humana Press Inc., Totowa, NJ

of LVH, because similar elevations of BP result in a wide range of variations in the extent and type of hypertrophy; among these are genetic, demographic, and humoral factors *(4)*. Patients with primary aldosteronism have thicker interventricular septi and posterior walls and higher LV mass indexes, compared to patients with similar elevations in BP caused by essential HT or other forms of secondary HT *(5–7)*. Surgical removal of adrenal adenomas causing primary aldosteronism results in the reduction of LV mass in most patients *(6)*, but medical treatment with an aldosterone antagonist does not *(5)*. Thus, clinical observations demonstrate direct effects of aldosterone on the heart that are independent of HT.

EFFECTS OF ADRENAL STEROIDS ON THE HEART

Mineralocorticoids

Mineralocorticoids act through intracellular mineralocorticoid receptors (MRs), which act as transcription factors in the nucleus and mediate genomic effects, and by membrane receptors, which mediate rapid nongenomic effects *(8,9)*. The nongenomic actions of mineralocorticoids on the vasculature and the heart are slowly becoming more accepted, although membrane receptors remain poorly characterized, and have yet to be isolated or cloned.

The best-understood aldosterone actions are genomic effects through binding to the classical intracellular MR, or type I corticoid receptor, in transport epithelia responsible for the vectorial transfer of sodium and water. Occupation of the MR in these cells causes an increase in the expression of several proteins that promote the transfer of sodium from the lumen into the cells by increasing the activity of amiloride-sensitive sodium channels, and from the cells into the interstitial space, by increasing the activity of the sodium potassium ATPase. MRs are found in nonepithelial cells (ECs), including the heart, where MRs have been demonstrated in all four chambers of the heart, using cytosol binding studies in vitro *(10)* and in vivo *(11)*, and mRNA expression for MR has been shown by Northern blots and RNase protection assays *(12,13)*, as well as by immunohistochemistry using an anti-idiotypic monoclonal antibody *(14)*. Though genomic effects of mineralocorticoids are well accepted and have been extensively studied, nuclear events, particularly the effector mechanisms beyond DNA binding, remain unclear.

The intracellular MR is a member of the steroid receptor superfamily of ligand-induced transcription factors *(12)*. There are at least two splice variants with alternative 5' untranslated exons and a common exon 2 containing the translation start site *(15,16)*. The two transcriptional products are regulated by different promoters that exhibit a specific pattern of expression in different tissues *(15)*. In the heart, the two MR splice variants appear to occur in similar amounts. In addition, quantitative *in situ* hybridization studies have revealed evidence for the existence of a different isoform in the heart. In the kidney, the hybridization signal from an exon 2 probe is much stronger than the signal for an exon 1α or 1β probe, as would be expected, because the exon 2 is common to both $MR\alpha$ and $MR\beta$ isoforms. However, in the heart, the signals for the exon 1α and exon 1β isoforms are stronger than the exon 2 signal, suggesting the existence of a different, as yet undescribed, isoform of the MR in the heart *(13)*.

It was originally believed that the specificity of the MR for aldosterone was an inherent characteristic of the receptor, but most MRs in nonclassic, nonepithelial target organs, including the heart, exhibit poor ligand specificity. The affinity of corticosterone and cortisol for the isolated MR and recombinant MR protein is similar to that of aldosterone *(10,12,17)*. Because these glucocorticoids are present in concentrations 100–1000 times greater than the mineralocorticoids, without factors extrinsic to the MR to confer specificity to the receptor, all MRs must be occupied almost exclusively by glucocorticoids. Specificity of mineralocorticoid action in some tissues, notably transport epithelia, is mediated by the co-expression of the 11β-hydroxysteroid dehydrogenase enzymes in mineralocorticoid target organs. These enzymes interconvert corticosterone and cortisol and the inactive 11-dehydrocorticosterone and cortisone, but leave aldosterone intact *(18,19)*. Two different 11β-hydroxysteroid dehydrogenases have been described. Type 1 is a nicotinamide adenine dinucleotide phosphate ($NADP^+$)-dependent enzyme that is bidirectional, has an affininy for corticosterone and cortisol in the low micromolar range (too low to be an effective oxidase for physiologic circulating concentrations of glucocorticoids), and, in most organs, behaves primarily as a oxoreductase, converting the inactive 11-dehydrocorticosterone and cortisone into biologically active corticosterone and cortisol *(20)*. 11β-Hydroxysteroid dehydrogenase I is expressed in VSMCs and in rat heart, as well as in the liver, where it is most abundant *(21,22)*. Its role in the heart is as yet unclear, but it may be important in modulation of glucocorticoid binding to the MR, because it appears to be in the brain *(23,24)*. 11β-Hydroxysteroid dehydrogenase type II is nicotinamide adenine dinucleotide (NAD^+)-dependent, has very high affinity for corticosterone and cortisol in the nanomole range, functions exclusively as an oxidase with natural steroids under physiological conditions, and is co-expressed with MR in epithelial target organs. 11β-Hydroxysteroid dehydrogenase type II protects the MRs from occupancy by cortisol or corticosterone *(25)*. Its deficiency causes apparent mineralocorticoid excess with HT *(26)*. The human, but not rat, heart expresses the 11β-hydroxysteroid dehydrogenase type II *(22,27–29)*. The hippocampus has a greater concentration of MR than the kidney, yet, because these MRs are not protected, they are occupied primarily by glucocorticoids, and the hippocampus is considered a glucocorticoid target organ (30). A significant proportion of the MRs in the heart are bound by glucocorticoids, with only about 30% of the heart MR protected from glucocorticoids *(11,31,32)*; however, the expression of both the MR and the 11β-hydroxysteroid dehydrogenase enzyme type II in the heart suggests that the heart is a mineralocorticoid target organ. The specificity of aldosterone binding to the heart MR and the mediation of mineralocorticoid effects in the heart are not adequately explained by the relatively limited co-expression of the 11β-hydroxysteroid dehydrogenase type II enzyme. Other yet-unknown factors conferring specificity to the heart MR must exist *(31)*. The small proportion of protected MRs appear to mediate the fibrotic actions of chronic administration of aldosterone on the heart *(32,33)*.

Mineralocorticoids have both direct and indirect effects on the vessels and heart, via changes in neural influence. Rapid nongenomic effects were demonstrated in studies conducted many years ago, before the development of the concept of intracellular receptors acting as transcription factors, which take at least 30 min to produce a physiological effect. Administration of deoxycorticosterone acetate in bilaterally adrenalectomized dogs and rats increased BP, presumably by direct actions on the vasculature and/or the heart *(34)*. Administration of aldosterone to humans increased systemic peripheral resistance within 5 min of administration *(35)*. Both isolated rat heart and rat heart–lung preparations perfused with blood from adrenalectomized animals have a lower left ventricular work index than when perfused with blood from intact animals or adrenalectomized animals supplemented with physiological concentrations of corticosterone or aldosterone *(36,37)*. Aldosterone was also shown to have a direct inotropic effect on isolated cat papillary muscle and whole-heart preparations *(38)*. Spironolactone did not antagonize these inotropic effects of aldosterone *(38)*. Addition of aldosterone to the perfusate of an isolated working-heart preparation, using the Langendorff technique, increased coronary and aortic flow and cardiac output. The addition of spironolactone with aldosterone inhibited these effects; spironolactone by itself had a small negative inotropic effect *(39)*. The very short latency for these responses suggests that they are nongenomic effects, even though spironolactone does not appear to antagonize nongenomic effects of aldosterone in other systems *(38,40)*. The significance of rapid aldosterone effects in the heart is yet unclear.

Nongenomic effects have been studied at the cellular level in VSMCs and human mononuclear leukocytes. Incubation of human mononuclear cells with aldosterone results in the stimulation of the sodium-proton exchanger and inositol-1,4-5-phosphate production within 1–2 min *(41,42)*. These effects are not antagonized by canrenone, a spironolactone derivative *(43)*. Aldosterone also rapidly induces a decrease in intracellular pH, followed by activation of the sodium-proton exchanger and alkalinization in cultured VSMCs *(44,45)* and inositol-1,4-5-phosphate production and intracellular calcium increase in porcine ECs and myocardial fibroblasts within 2–3 min of incubation *(44)*.

Aldosterone increases the incorporation of tritiated leucine into neonatal cardiomyocytes, an effect that appears to be mediated by the stimulation of protein kinase C, and which is markedly enhanced by incubation with high glucose media *(32)*. This effect is blocked by co-incubation with spironolactone. A report that aldosterone directly stimulates collagen synthesis in cultured cardiac fibroblasts *(46)* has not been confirmed by others *(47,48)*.

The administration of aldosterone for 8 wk, in conjunction with a high salt intake, results in HT and marked interstitial fibrosis, with a lesser degree of perivascular collagen accumulation in the heart *(49)*. Desoxycorticosterone acetate (DOCA) produced a similar degree of HT and cardiac hypertrophy, though the interstitial fibrosis was less, but the perivascular collagen was greater with DOCA *(50)*. Co-administration of corticosterone had no significant effect on cardiac remodeling; administration of the antiglucocorticoid, RU486, significantly increased perivascular fibrosis *(50)*, suggesting that the glucocorticoid receptor (GR)- and MR-mediated effects in the heart, as in specific areas of the brain, may be in opposition *(30,51)*. Aldosterone-salt excess produced a significant increase in BP and left ventricular hypertrophy within 15 d, which was associated with an 83% increase in mRNA for procollagen III, but no increase in procollagen I and III by immunohistochemistry *(52)*. At 30 and 60 d of treatment, progressive cardiac fibrosis, with inflammatory cells, myocyte necrosis, and elevation of both type I and III procollagen mRNA and protein, was seen in both ventricles *(52)*.

The regression of left ventricular mass in patients with primary aldosteronism treated by surgical removal of the adrenal, but not in those treated with spironolactone, led to the proposal that cardiac remodeling is the result of a nongenomic effect of aldosterone, because the aldosterone membrane receptor has been reported to be insensitive to this antagonist *(5)*. However, spironolactone prevents myocardial scarring and reactive fibrosis in rats treated with aldosterone and high salt diets *(53)*. Amiloride, a sodium-channel blocker that antagonizes the MR-mediated influx of sodium into a mineralocorticoid target cell, prevents the hypokalemia and the reparative fibrosis, but not the reactive fibrosis, in these rats *(54)*. This suggests that the hypokalemia induced by mineralocorticoids resulted in the myocyte necrosis and a reparative fibrosis *(54)*. Patients with aldosterone-producing adenomas also have both a reactive and reparative fibrosis in the myocardium and other organs *(55)*.

There is experimental data to complement the clinical evidence cited in the introduction that mineralocorticoid excess produces cardiac hypertrophy and fibrosis independent of its effect on BP. The adrenal cortex, but not adrenal medulla, was necessary for the development of the cardiac hypertrophy associated with aortic coarctation in rats, even though the BP increases produced by aortic coarctation in the adrenalectomized, medullectomized, and sham adrenalectomized animals were similar *(56)*. The infusion of aldosterone into the lateral ventricle of the brain at concentrations too small to elevate the BP, when given systemically, produces HT in rats and dogs *(57,58)*. Increasing the BP by the same amount for the same duration with either the continuous intracerebroventricular or, at 100 times the dose, continuous sc infusion of aldosterone produces cardiac hypertrophy only in those animals receiving the systemic aldosterone excess *(59,60)*. The spironolactone derivative, RU28318, at a dose that is too small to have systemic effects, prevents the increase in BP produced by systemic excesses of aldosterone *(61)*. However, these rats still develop the same degree of hypertrophy and fibrosis as the group receiving the same dose of aldosterone subcutaneously, and is allowed to become hypertensive *(59)*. These experiments are definitive demonstrations that the effect of aldosterone on the myocardium is direct, and not mediated through an increase in BP or afterload.

Spironolactone treatment is beneficial in the treatment of congestive heart failure (CHF) and decreases myocardial collagen turnover in human patients *(62)*. The beneficial effects of angiotensin-converting enzyme inhibitors in the treatment of CHF are probably the result, at least in part, of their indirect inhibition of aldosterone production *(62)*. Adding a spironolactone to converting-enzyme inhibition in patients with congestive heart failure enhances this therapeutic effect *(63)*.

Glucocorticoids

The heart and vascular tissue express the corticosteroid receptor type II or GR, in addition to the MR *(64,65)*. Patients with Cushing syndrome, in which both glucocorticoids and mineralocorticoids are in excess, have a high incidence of HT and left ventricular hypertrophy *(66)*. Glucocorticoids modulate protein synthesis in cultured cardiomyocytes *(67,68)*. Glucocorticoid administration induces temporary cardiac hypertrophy in rats, which is reversed with prolonged treatment *(69)*. Although chronic administration of corticosterone does not produce cardiac hypertrophy or fibrosis *(59)*, glucocorticoids have several effects on the heart, including the inhibition of the cytokine-inducible isoform of nitric oxide synthase (NOS) in both myocytes and microvascular ECs *(70)*. Dexamethasone (DEX) appears to inhibit NOS expression by inducing osteopontin, a regulator of the location and extent of NOS induction in the heart *(70)*. DEX also induces the expression of the Kv1.5 potassium channel of the rat heart ventricle *(71)*. This channel is thought to be important in repolarization. Expression of the $AT_{1\alpha}$ and $AT_{1\beta}$ receptors for ANG II in rat hearts is significantly increased by DEX *(36)*. The increase in ANG II receptors in the heart might participate in the development of HT induced by glucocorticoids. Though multiple actions of glucocorticoids in the heart have been demonstrated, their role in health and disease is yet unclear.

THE HEART IS A STEROIDOGENIC ORGAN

Mineralocorticoid and glucocorticoid hormones are synthesized in the adrenal cortex. Aldosterone, the chief mineralocorticord, is synthesized in the zona glomerulosa, and corticosterone (rodents) and cortisol (many animals, including humans) are synthesized in the zona fasciculata. These hormones are secreted into the circulation and transported to their target organ, where they act. Recently, extra-adrenal synthesis of both classes of corticosteroids has been demonstrated in the aortic endothelium, vascular smooth muscle, heart, and brain (72–77). Studies in the 1960s and early 1970s by Mary F. Lockett and her collaborators (78–83), and confirmed by others (84,85), suggested that the heart was capable of secreting a heart factor, confirmed to be a steroid, that promoted sodium retention.

Isolated cat hearts released a factor into the perfusate, which, when infused into kidneys, promoted sodium retention (86). Its activity was similar to that of aldosterone when injected in the whole animal, but had a shorter latency. The release of the factor into the blood stream increased significantly when venous input into the heart was reduced (78). This heart factor was extracted by organic solvents, and resembled the steroid, aldosterone-18-monoacetate (aldo-18-MA), in solubility, chromatographic, and biological characteristics (81). Aldo-18-MA is several times more potent than aldosterone in promoting sodium retention by the kidney and releasing antidiuretic activity from the pituitary (78,80). High-discrimination chromatographic separation revealed that the heart factor could be differentiated from aldo-18-MA, but it was not identified (83). Hearts from adrenalectomized rats contain measurable, but significantly less amounts of the factor. Perfusion of isolated hearts that no longer secreted the measurable quantities of the heart factor with aldosterone caused a rapid increase in the factor in the output (83). Radioactively labeled aldosterone added to a perfused heart resulted in the incorporation of the radioactivity into the heart factor. The heart factor was isolated from cat, rat, and pig heart, and from sheep arterial blood, but was undetectable in venous blood (83,85,87), and was shown to be partially inactivated by a single passage through the lungs (88). These old studies elegantly demonstrated that the heart was capable of synthesizing a steroid derivative of aldosterone that was less polar than aldosterone, and was difficult to separate from aldo-18-MA. The presence of the heart factor in the hearts of adrenalectomized rats, albeit at reduced concentrations, suggested that the heart also aldosterone. These studies were mostly ignored until recently, in part because they challenged the conventional wisdom of the time, and because the steroid identification techniques used were crude even for that era.

In 1992, Brilla et al. (89), presented an abstract demonstrating that aortic ECs in culture secreted aldosterone when stimulated by ANG II, a finding met with profound skepticism. Using reverse transcription polymerase chain reaction and Southern blot analysis, human ECs and VSMCs in culture were shown to express the mRNA for the cytochrome P450 11β-hydroxylase and aldosterone synthase at a concentration estimated to be one-fiftieth that of the adrenal (74). Cultured ECs and VSMCs release aldosterone into the incubation media (74). Aldosterone synthase mRNA expression in human umbilical vein ECs in culture is increased by incubation with ANG II, and aldosterone release is stimulated by incubation with ANG II and ACTH (90). Aldosterone and corticosterone production can be shown to occur and to be stimulated by ANG II and ACTH in mesenteric artery perfusions in intact and adrenalectomized rats (72,73). These studies gave very convincing evidence that the vasculature was capable of synthesizing aldosterone and corticosterone. Similar evidence for corticosteroid synthesis by the brain has been presented *(75,76)*.

The rat heart expresses the cytochrome P-450 enzyme 21-hydroxylase, which is necessary to synthesize aldosterone, corticosterone, and cortisol; 11β-hydroxylase, corticosterone and cortisol; and aldosterone synthase *(77,91)*. The expression of the mRNAs for 11β-hydroxylase and aldosterone synthase are greater in the atria than ventricles, and the 11β-hydroxylase mRNA expression is sevenfold greater than that of the aldosterone synthase mRNA *(77)*.

Rat hearts perfused in a Langendorff-type preparation secrete aldosterone and corticosterone into the perfusion media. Addition of ANG II to the perfusate results in a dose-dependent stimulation of corticosteroid secretion, with an eightfold increase above the baseline for aldosterone, and 1.4-fold for corticosterone. ACTH also increased steroid secretion by the isolated heart in a dose-dependent manner, with a maximum of 4.9-fold increase for aldosterone, and lower increases for corticosterone.

New studies made possible by the advent of molecular biological techniques support these original studies, indicating that the heart can synthesize aldosterone from endogenous precursors. Long-term treatment with a low-sodium, high-potassium diet, and continuous infusion of ANG II or ACTH, also increased the production of aldosterone by isolated perfused rat hearts, even though the chronic ACTH treatment lowered the plasma concentration of aldosterone, as expected from other studies. Aldosterone synthase mRNA expression increased in rats fed a low-sodium, high-potassium diet, and in those chronically treated with ANG II, but not in those treated chronically with ACTH *(77)*. The production of aldosterone by the heart is minuscule in comparison to that of the adrenal, and probably does not contribute in any meaningful degree to circulating levels of the hormone. Aldosterone produced in the heart, if relevant, is likely to have paracrine or autocrine functions, and may mediate the trophic effects of chronic ANG II administration. The concentration of aldosterone in myocardium is approx 16 nM, a value that is clearly higher than the mean concentration in plasma (~0.93 nM) *(77)*. The author obtained similar values in myocardium and plasma, but found that over 70% of the aldosterone in fresh myocardium is in the fraction corresponding to the monoacetates (probably the aldosterone-20-monoacetate; C. E. Gomez-Sanchez, unpublished observation). The aldosterone monoacetates hydrolyze to aldosterone very rapidly; there is negligible monoacetate remaining in plasma left for 30 min at room temperature. Aldosterone monoacetates have been reported to be more potent and to act more rapidly at the MR than the parent compound, aldosterone *(78,80)*. Acetylation of aldosterone by the heart or other target tissues would amplify its actions at a specific site, with the rapid hydrolysis within the circulation quickly restoring aldosterone to its less potent form. It is tempting to speculate that the heart factor described by Mary Lockett is an aldosterone monoacetate.

The presence of mineralocorticoid and glucocorticoid receptors in the myocardium, the evidence for corticosteroid synthetic ability in the heart, and the evidence for a more active form of aldosterone within the heart, compared to the circulation, all suggest the possibility that these steroids are part of a cardiovascular system with paracrine or autocrine effects. Interaction of the cardiac renin angiotensin system and the cardiac steroidogenic system is likely. Because aldosterone is known to exert trophic effects both in vivo and in vitro, the angiotensin-induced cardiac remodeling may be primarily or entirely through stimulation of cardiac aldosterone synthesis and/or the acetylation of aldosterone within the heart.

ACKNOWLEDGMENTS

The expert editorial help of Elise P. Gomez-Sanchez is gratefully acknowledged. Work done in our laboratory has been supported by Medical Research Funds from the Department of Veterans Affairs and National Institutes of Health.

REFERENCES

1. Bohr DF. What makes the pressure go up? A hypothesis. Hypertension 1981;3:II-160–II-165.
2. Nerup J. Addison's disease. Clinical studies. A report of 108 cases. Acta Endocrinol 1974;76:127–141.
3. Jarvis JL, Jenkins D, Sosman MC. Roentgenologic observations in Addison's disease. A review of 120 cases. Radiology 1954;62:16–29.
4. Morgan HE, Baker KM. Cardiac hypertrophy: mechanical, neural and endocrine dependence. Circulation 1991;83:13–25.
5. Rossi GP, Sacchetto A, Pavan E, Palatini P, Graniero GR, Canali C, Pessina AC. Remodeling of the left ventricle in primary aldosteronism due to Conn's adenoma. Circulation 1997;95:1471–1478.
6. Denolle T, Chatellier G, Julien J, Battaglia C, Luo P, Plouin P-F. Left ventricular mass and geometry before and after etiologic treatment in renovascular hypertension, aldosterone-producing adenoma, and pheochromocytoma. Am J Hypertens 1993;6:907–913.
7. Tanabe A, Naruse M, Naruse K, Hase M, Yoshimoto T, Tanaka M, Seki T, Demura H. Left ventricular hypertrophy is more prominent in patients with primary aldosteronism than in patients with other types of secondary hypertension. Hypertension Res 1997;20:85–90.
8. Evans RM. Steroid and thyroid hormone receptor superfamily. Science 1988;240:889–895.
9. Wehling M. Nongenomic actions of steroid hormones. TEM 1994;5:347–353.
10. Pearce P, Funder JW. High affinity aldosterone binding sites (type I receptors) in rat heart. Clin Exp Pharmacol Physiol 1987;14:859–866.
11. Pearce PT, Funder JW. Steroid binding to cardiac type I receptors: in vivo studies. J Hypertension 1988; 6(Suppl 4):S131–S133.
12. Arriza JW, Weinberger C, Cerelli G, Glaser TM, Handelin BL, Housman DE, Evans RM. Cloning of human mineralocorticoid receptor complementary DNA: structural and functional kinship with the glucocorticoid receptor. Science 1987;237:268–275.
13. Zennaro MC, Farman N, Bonvalet JP, Lombes M. Tissue-specific expression of alpha and beta messenger ribonucleic acid isoforms of the human mineralocorticoid receptor in normal and pathological states. J Clin Endocrinol Metab 1997;82:1345–1352.
14. Lombes M, Oblin ME, Gasc JM, Baulieu EE, Farman N, Bonvalet JP. Immunohistochemical and biochemical evidence for a cardiovascular mineralocorticoid receptor. Circ Res 1992;71:503–510.
15. Zennaro MC, Lemenuet D, Lombes M. Characterization of the human mineralocorticoid receptor gene 5'-regulatory region—evidence for differential hormonal regulation of two alternative promoters via nonclassical mechanism. Mol Endocrinol 1996;10:1549–1560.
16. Kwak S, Patel PD, Thompson RC, Akil H, Watson SJ. 5'-Heterogeneity of the mineralocorticoid receptor messenger ribonucleic acid: differential expression and regulation of splice variants within the rat hippocampus. Endocrinology 1993;133:2344–2350.
17. Krozowski ZS, Funder JW. Renal mineralocorticoid receptors and hippocampal corticosterone binding species have identical intrinsic steroid specificity. Proc Natl Acad Sci USA 1983;80:6056–6060.
18. Funder JW, Pearce PT, Smith R, Smith AI. Mineralocorticoid action: target tissue specificity is enzyme, not receptor, mediated. Science 1988;242:583–585.
19. Edwards CRW, Burt D, McIntyre MA, De Kloet ER, Stewart PM, Brett L, Sutanto WS, Monder C. Localisation of 11β-hydroxysteroid dehydrogenase-tissue specific protector of the mineralocorticoid receptor. Lancet 1988;ii:986–989.
20. Monder C. Forms and functions of 11β-hydroxysteroid dehydrogenase. J Steroid Biochem Mol Biol 1993;45:161–165.
21. Brem AS, Bina RB, King T, Morris DJ. Bidirectional activity of 11β-hydroxysteroid dehydrogenase in vascular smooth muscle cells. Steroids 1995;60:406–410.
22. Smith RE, Krozowski ZS. The 11β-hydroxysteroid dehydrogenase type I enzyme in the hearts of normotensive and spontaneously hypertensive rats. Clin Exp Pharmacol Physiol 1996;23:642–647.
23. Teelucksingh S, Mackie ADR, Burt D, McIntyre MA, Brett L, Edwards CRW. Potentiation of hydrocortisone activity in skin by glycyrrhetinic acid. Lancet 1990;1:1060–1063.

24. Seckl JR, Dow RC, Low SC, Edwards CRW, Fink G. 11β-hydroxysteroid dehydrogenase inhibitor glycyrrhetinic acid affects corticosteroid feedback regulation of hypothalamic corticotrophin-releasing petides in rats. J Endocrinol 1993;136:471–477.

25. Mune T, White PC. Apparent mineralocorticoid excess: genotype is correlated with biochemical phenotype. Hypertension 1996;27:1193–1199.

26. Mune T, Rogerson FM, Nikkilä H, Agarwal AK, White PC. Human hypertension caused by mutations in the kidney isozyme of 11β-hydroxysteroid dehydrogenase. Nature Genet 1995;10:394–399.

27. Slight S, Ganjam VK, Nonneman DJ, Weber KT. Glucocorticoid metabolism in the cardiac interstitium: 11β-hydroxysteroid dehydrogenase activity in cardiac fibroblasts. J Lab Clin Med 1993;122:180–187.

28. Slight SH, Ganjam VK, Gomez-Sanchez CE, Weber KT. High affinity NAD$^+$-dependent 11β-hydroxysteroid dehydrogenase in the human heart. J Mol Cell Cardiol 1996;28:781–787.

29. Lombes M, Alfaidy N, Eugene E, Lessana A, Farman N, Bonvalet J-P. Prerequisite for cardiac aldosterone action. Mineralocorticoid receptor and 11β-hydroxysteroid dehydrogenase in the human heart. Circ Res 1995;92:175–182.

30. De Kloet ER. Brain corticosteroid receptor balance and homeostatic control. Frontiers Neuroendocrinol 1991;12:95–164.

31. Funder J, Myles K. Exclusion of corticosterone from epithelial mineralocorticoid receptors is insufficient for selectivity of aldosterone action: in vivo binding studies. Endocrinology 1996;137:5264–5268.

32. Sate A, Funder JW. High glucose stimulates aldosterone-induced hypertrophy via type I mineralocorticoid receptors in neonatal rat cardiomyocytes. Endocrinology 1996;137:4145–4153.

33. Young MJ, Funder JW. Mineralocorticoids, salt, hypertension: effects on the heart. Steroids 1996; 61:233–235.

34. Langford HG, Snavely JR. Effect of DCA on development of renoprival hypertension. Am J Physiol 1959;196:449–450.

35. Klein K, Henk W. Klinisch-experimentelle untersuchungen über den einfluss von aldosteron auf haemodynamik und gerinnung. Z Kreisl Forsch 1964;52:40–53.

36. Solomon N, Sayers G. Work performance of the isolated rat heart preparation: standarization and influence of corticosteroids. In: Currie AR, Symington T, Grant JK, eds. Human Adrenal Cortex. William and Wilkins, Baltimore, 1962, pp. 314–324.

37. Ballard K, Lefer A, Sayers G. Effect of aldosterone and plasma extracts on a rat heart-lung preparation. Am J Physiol 1960;199:221–225.

38. Tanz RD. Studies on the inotropic action of aldosterone on isolated cardiac tissue preparations: including the effect of pH, ouabain and SC-8109. J Pharmacol Exp Ther 1962;135:71–78.

39. Moreau D, Chardigny JM, Rochette L. Effects of aldosterone and spironolactone on the isolated perfused rat heart. Pharmacol 1996;53:28–36.

40. Wehling M, Eisen C, Christ M. Aldosterone-specific membrane receptors and rapid non-genomic actions of mineralocorticoids. Mol Cell Endocrinol 1992;90:C5–C9.

41. Christ M, Eisen C, Aktas J, Theisen K, Wehling M. Inositol-1,4,5-trisphosphate system is involved in rapid effects of aldosterone in human mononuclear leukocytes. J Clin Endocrinol Metab 1993;77:1452–1457.

42. Wehling, M, Käsmayr J, Theisen K. Fast effects of aldosterone on electrolytes in human lymphocytes are mediated by the sodium-proton-exchanger of the cell membrane. Biochem Biophys Res Commun 1989;164:961–967.

43. Wehling M, Christ M, Gerzer R. Aldosterone-specific membrane receptors and related rapid, non-genomic effects. Trends Pharmacol Sci 1993;14:1–4.

44. Wehling M, Ulsenheimer A, Schneider M, Neylon C, Christ M. Rapid effects of aldosterone on free intracellular calcium in vascular smooth muscle and endothelial cells: subcellular localization of calcium elevations by single cell imaging. Biochem Biophys Res Commun 1994;204:475–481.

45. Wehling M, Neylon CB, Fullerton M, Bobik A, Funder JW. Nongenomic effects of aldosterone on intracellular Ca^{2+} in vascular smooth muscle cells. Circ Res 1995;76:973–979.

46. Brilla CG, Zhou G, Matsubara L, Weber KT. Collagen metabolism in cultured adult rat cardiac fibroblasts: response to angiotensin II and aldosterone. J Mol Cell Card 1994;26:809–820.

47. Fullerton MJ, Funder JW. Aldosterone and cardiac fibrosis: in vitro studies. Cardiovasc Res 1994;128: 1863–1867.

48. Köhler, E, Bertschin S, Woodtli T, Resink T, Erne P. Does aldosterone-induced cardiac fibrosis involve direct effects on cardiac fibroblasts? J Vascular Res 1996;33:315–326.

49. Brilla CG, Weber KT. Mineralocorticoid excess, dietary sodium and myocardial fibrosis. J Lab Clin Med 1992;120:893–901.

50. Young M, Fullerton M, Dilley R, Funder J. Mineralocorticoids, hypertension, and cardiac fibrosis. J Clin Invest 1994;93:2578–2583.

51. Gomez-Sanchez EP. Central hypertensive effects of aldosterone. Frontiers Neuroendocrinol 1997;18: 440–462.

52. Robert V, Silvestre JS, Charlemagne D, Sabri A, Trouve P, Wassef M, Delcayre C. Biological determinants of aldosterone-induced cardiac fibrosis in rats. Hypertension 1995;26:971–978.

53. Brilla CG, Matsubara LS, Weber KT. Antifibrotic effects of spironolactone in preventing myocardial fibrosis in systemic arterial hypertension. Am J Cardiol 1993;71:12A–16A.

54. Campbell SE, Janicki JS, Matsubara BB, Weber KT. Myocardial fibrosis in the rat with mineralocorticoid excess, prevention of scarring by amiloride. Am J Hypertens 1993;6:487–495.

55. Campbell SE, Diaz-Ariaz AA, Weber KT. Fibrosis of the human heart and systemic organs in adrenal adenoma. Blood Pressure 1992;1:149–156.

56. Nichols JR, Clancy RL, Gonzales NC. Role of adrenals on development of pressure-induced myocardial hypertrophy. Am J Physiol 1983;244:H234–H238.

57. Gomez-Sanchez EP. Intracerebroventricular infusion of aldosterone induces hypertension in rats. Endocrinology 1986;118:819–823.

58. Kageyama Y, Bravo EL. Hypertensive mechanisms associated with centrally administered aldosterone in dogs. Hypertension 1988;11:750–753.

59. Young M, Head G, Funder JW. Determinants of cardiac fibrosis in experimental hypermineralocorticoid states. Am J Physiol 1995;269:E657–E662.

60. Gomez-Sanchez EP. Mineralocorticoid modulation of central control of blood pressure. Steroids 1995; 60:69–72.

61. Gomez-Sanchez EP, Fort CM, Gomez-Sanchez CE. Intracerebroventricular infusions of RU28318 blocks aldosterone-salt hypertension. Am J Physiol 1990;258:E482–E484.

62. MacFadyen RJ, Barr CS, Struthers AD. Aldosterone blockade reduces vascular collagen turnover, improves heart rate variability and reduces early morning rise in heart rate in heart failure patients. Cardiovasc Res 1997;35:30–34.

63. Barr CS, Lang CC, Hanson J, Arnott M, Kennedy N, Struthers AD. Effects of adding spironolactone to an angiotensin-converting enzyme inhibitor in chronic congestive heart failure secondary to coronary artery disease. Am J Cardiol 1995;76:1259–1265.

64. Duval D, Funder JW, Devynck M, Meyer P. Arterial glucocorticoid receptors: the binding of tritiated dexamethasone in rabbit aorta. Cardiovasc Res 1977;11:529–535.

65. Funder JW, Duval D, Meyer P. Cardiac glucocorticoid receptors: the binding of tritiated dexamethasone in rat and dog heart. Endocrinology 1973;93:1300–1308.

66. Tsuda K, Saikawa T, Yonemochi H, Maeda T, Shimoyama N, Hara M, Ito Y, Sakata T. Electrocardiographic abnormalities in patients with Cushing's syndrome. Jpn Heart J 1995;36:333–339.

67. Sato A, Sheppard KE, Fullerton MJ, Funder JW. cAMP modulates glucocorticoid-induced protein accumulation and glucocorticoid receptor in cardiomyocytes. Am J Physiol 1996;271:E827–E833.

68. Nichols NR, McNally M, Campbell JH, Funder JW. Overlapping but not identical protein synthetic domains in cardiovascular cells in response to glucocorticoid hormones. J Hypertension 1984;2:663–669.

69. Kuroski TT, Czerwinski SM. Glucocorticoid modulation of cardiac mass and protein. Med Sci Sports Exerc 1990;22:312–315.

70. Singh K, Balligand JL, Fischer TA, Smith TW, Kelly RA. Glucocorticoids increase osteopontin expression in cardiac myocytes and microvascular endothelial cells. Role in regulation of inducible nitric oxide synthase. J Biol Chem 1995;270:28,471–28,478.

71. Takimoto K, Levitan ES. Glucocorticoid induction of Kv1.5 K+ channel gene expression in ventricle of rat heart. Circ Res 1994;75:1006–1013.

72. Takeda Y, Miyamori I, Yoneda T, Iki K, Hatakeyama H, Blair IA, Hsieh FY, Takeda R. Production of aldosterone in isolated rat blood vessels. Hypertension 1995;25:170–173.

73. Takeda Y, Miyamori I, Yoneda T, Iki K, Hatakeyama H, Blair IA, Hsieh FY, Takeda R. Synthesis of corticosterone in the vascular wall. Endocrinology 1994;135:2283–2286.

74. Hatakeyama H, Miyamori I, Fujita T, Takeda Y, Takeda R, Yamamoto H. Vascular aldosterone. Biosynthesis and a link to angiotensin II-induced hypertrophy of vascular smooth muscle cells. J Biol Chem 1994;269:24,316–24,320.

75. Gomez-Sanchez CE, Zhou MY, Cozza EN, Morita H, Eddleman FC, Gomez-Sanchez EP. Corticosteroid synthesis in the central nervous system. Endocr Res 1996;22:463–470.

76. Gomez-Sanchez CE, Zhou MY, Cozza EN, Morita H, Foecking MF, Gomez-Sanchez EP. Aldosterone biosynthesis in the rat brain. Endocrinology 1997;138:3369–3373.
77. Silvestre J-S, Robert V, Heymes C, Aupetit-Faisant B, Moalic J-M, Swynghedauw B, Delcayre C. Myocardial production of aldosterrone and corticosterone in the rat. Physiological regulation. J Biol Chem 1998;273:4883–4891.
78. Ilett KF, Lockett MF. Renally active substance from heart muscle and from blood. J Physiol 1968;196: 101–109.
79. Lockett, MF, Retallack RW. Isolation of a substance very closely resembling the 18-monoacetate of d-aldosterone from the venous blood of activated muscle and from contracting muscle. J Physiol 1969; 204:435–442.
80. Lockett MF. Factors affecting the antidiuretic actions of the 18-monoacetate of (+)-aldosterone and of a substance secreted by heart muscle, in rats. J Pharm Pharmac 1973;25:690–699.
81. Knox JR, Lockett MF. Similarity between a substance produced by the heart in vitro and the 18-monoacetyl derivative of d-aldosterone. J Endocr 1969;43:315–316.
82. Escubet B, Coureau C, Blot-Chabaud M, Bonvalet J-P, Farman N. Corticosteroid receptor mRNA expression is unaffected by corticosteroids in the rat kidney, heart and colon. Am J Physiol 1996;270: C1343–C1353.
83. Lockett MF, Retallack RW. Release of a renally active substance by perfused rat hearts. J Physiol 1971; 212:733–738.
84. Arora RB, Siddiqui HH. Role of sodium-retaining hormones in cardiac control. Indian J Med Res 1970; 8:275–277.
85. Arora RB, Gupta SK, Sharma RC, Siddiqui HH. Isolation and characterization of a sodium retaining substance from pig heart muscle and its role in myocardial infarction. Indian J Med Res 1971;59:483–493.
86. Locket MF. Hormonal actions of the heart and of lungs on the isolated kidney. J Physiol 1967;193: 661–679.
87. Locket MF, Retallack RW. Isolation of a renally active substance from arterial blood. J Physiol 1972;225: 477–484.
88. Lockett MF, Retallack RW, Sayers L. Extent of the destruction, during passage through the lungs of a substance secreted by the heart. J Physiol 1972;225:477–484.
89. Brilla CG, Guarda E, Zhou G, Myers PR, Weber KT. Angiotensin II-mediated aldosterone synthesis in aortic endothelial cells. Circulation 1992;86(Suppl 4):1–90 (abstract).
90. Takeda Y, Miyamori I, Yoneda T, Hatakeyama H, Inaba S, Mabuchi H, Takeda R. Regulation of aldosterone synthase in human vascular endothelial cells by angiotensin II and adrenocorticotropin. J Clin Endocrinol Metab 1996;81:2797–2800.
91. Zhou MY, Vila MC, Gomez-Sanchez EP, Gomez-Sanchez CE. Cloning of two alternatively spliced 21-hydroxylase cDNAs from rat adrenal. J Steroid Biochem 1997;62:277–286.

6

Catecholamines and the Heart

Matthew N. Levy

INTRODUCTION

Under ordinary conditions, the principal catecholamine that regulates cardiac function is the norepinephrine (NE) liberated from the sympathetic nerve endings in the heart. In this chapter, initially, the factors that regulate the release of NE and its concentration in the cardiac interstitium are discussed. The various factors that govern the rate at which the cardiac responses develop in response to the initiation of sympathetic neural activity, and that govern the rate at which those responses decay when that activity ceases, are then considered. Because the neural control of the heart depends on the antagonistic influence of the two divisions of the autonomic nervous system (ANS), the powerful influence of the sympathetic and parasympathetic interactions on cardiac performance are then described in detail.

SOURCES OF CATECHOLAMINES IN THE HEART

The naturally occurring catecholamines that are physiologically important in mammals are epinephrine, NE, and dopamine. Epinephrine is the principal hormone secreted by the adrenal medulla. NE is the major transmitter released from postganglionic neurons of the sympathetic nervous system (SNS) and also from certain neurons in the central nervous system. Dopamine is a precursor of epinephrine and NE, and it is the chief neurotransmitter released by neurons in the extrapyramidal system, and in certain other centers in the central nervous system. NE is by far the most important of these catecholamines in the regulation of cardiac function, because it is the principal mediator of the sympathetic neural influence on the heart *(1–4)*.

From: *Contemporary Endocrinology: Hormones and the Heart in Health and Disease*
Edited by: L. Share © Humana Press Inc., Totowa, NJ

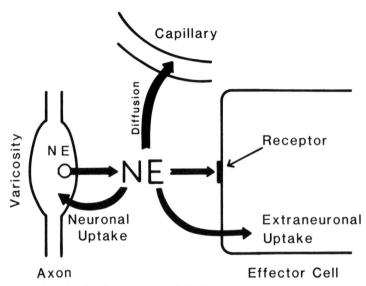

Fig. 1. Mechanisms involved in the removal of NE from the neuroeffector gaps between the post-ganglionic sympathetic nerve endings and the myocytes in cardiac tissues. Reproduced with permission from ref. *13*.

Most of the NE in blood plasma is derived from the sympathetic nerve endings throughout the body; most of the epinephrine in plasma is derived from the adrenal medulla *(2–6)*. The source of the dopamine in plasma is uncertain. The sympathetic postganglionic neurons in the lungs and skeletal muscles are the major sources of the NE that spills over into the circulating blood stream; these structures account for about 40 and 25%, respectively *(2,7)*. The sympathetic neurons in the heart account only for about 3% of the NE that appears in the peripheral blood *(7)*.

In the heart and other structures innervated by sympathetic nerves, the precursor for the adrenergic neurotransmitter, NE, is the amino acid, tyrosine, which is generally present throughout the extracellular fluid compartment of the body *(8)*. In the vicinity of a sympathetic nerve ending (varicosity), tyrosine is transported from the interstitial fluid into the neuronal axoplasm, where it is converted to dihydroxyphenylalanine (DOPA) by the enzyme, tyrosine hydroxylase. This hydroxylation of tyrosine is the rate-limiting step in the synthesis of NE. The enzyme, dopa decarboxylase, converts dopa into dopamine, which is then transported into vesicles in the axonal varicosities. In these vesicles, the dopamine is converted to NE by dopamine β-hydroxylase. Each varicosity contains about 200–400 vesicles, which serve as storage granules for the NE.

During neural activity, the vesicles tend to migrate toward the plasma membrane of the varicosity. As the vesicles reach the membrane, their content of NE and of other transmitters and modulators is extruded into the neuroeffector gap from the axon by the process of exocytosis; the neuroeffector gap is the zone of interstitium that lies between the neuronal varicosity and the effector cell (Fig. 1).

NOREPINEPHRINE EXCHANGE IN CARDIAC INTERSTITIUM

The NE that is released into the neuroeffector gap has various alternative fates (Fig. 1): The NE may temporarily occupy the α- or β-adrenoceptors on the surface of the cardiac effector cell; much of the NE in the neuroeffector gap can be taken up again by the sympathetic nerve endings (neuronal uptake); some of the NE that is released into the neuroeffector gap is taken up by nonneuronal tissues, including the effector cells themselves (extraneuronal uptake); and the NE that escapes either neuronal or extraneuronal uptake ultimately diffuses out of the neuroeffector gap and into the myocardial capillary network, which constitutes the NE spillover.

Norepinephrine Removal

The neuronal uptake of NE is an active transport process that can be inhibited by a large number of humoral substances and drugs *(2,8–10)*, the prototype of which is cocaine. The NE that is taken up by the varicosities is mostly recycled to the storage granules, although some of it is degraded by the monoamine oxidase in the mitochondria. The NE that is taken up by extraneuronal cells is degraded in these cells to several metabolites by monoamine oxidase and catechol-*O*-methyl transferase *(2,8,11,12)*, and these metabolites are excreted, ultimately, by the kidneys, or they are degraded elsewhere in the body.

Neuronal Release of Norepinephrine

The cardiac spillover of NE into the bloodstream (Fig. 1) essentially represents the difference between the rate at which NE is released from the nerve endings in the cardiac tissues and the rate at which it is taken up by neuronal and extraneuronal tissues in the heart *(9,13)*, as will be described shortly. Many factors regulate the rate at which NE is released from the sympathetic nerve endings in the heart. The major determinant of NE release is the activity level within the SNS. The general level of neural activity in this system is very sensitive to a host of psychological, environmental, pathophysiological, and exertional factors. Furthermore, for any given level of neural activity, the release of neurotransmitter from the nerve endings is influenced by many locally released humoral factors.

The rate at which NE spills over into the myocardial venous drainage varies with the frequency of the neural activity in the cardiac sympathetic nerves *(2,10,14)*. These changes in NE efflux elicited by alterations in stimulation frequency are paralleled by changes in cardiac performance, such as changes in heart rate (HR) and in left ventricular pressure *(10,14)*. In healthy human subjects, the spillover of NE into the coronary sinus blood increased about 30-fold, when the subjects exercised for 10 min at about 50% of their maximum exercise capacity *(15)*. The increased levels of catecholamines in the arterial blood during exercise are responsible for only a small fraction of the exercise-induced changes in cardiac function, however. When NE was infused at rates sufficient to raise the arterial concentrations of this catecholamine in conscious dogs to those that prevail during strenuous exercise, the increase in cardiac contractility (Fig. 2) was only a small fraction of the increment in contractility that prevailed during exercise *(16,17)*.

The amount of NE released from the sympathetic nerve endings per neuronal action potential is regulated by a number of humoral substances *(18–20)*. Notably, the presence of NE itself within the neuroeffector gap tends to inhibit its own neuronal release by interacting with presynaptic α_2-adrenoceptors in the plasma membrane of the varicosity. This constitutes an effective negative feedback system by which the neurally released NE inhibits the subsequent release of this transmitter. Drugs that block α_2-adrenoceptors augment the release of NE and its co-transmitters from the nerve endings *(18–20)*. Various substances that act on other specific presynaptic receptors may also affect the release of NE. For example, histamine, dopamine, enkephalins, acetylcholine, and prostaglandins inhibit the release of NE, but angiotensin II enhances its release *(18,19)*.

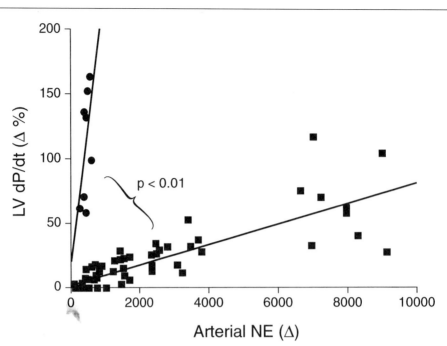

Fig. 2. Relationships between the per cent changes in left ventricular dP/dt and the arterial blood concentrations of NE produced by iv infusions of NE (squares) and by treadmill exercise (circles) in conscious, chronically instrumented dogs. Reproduced with permission from ref. *17*.

CARDIAC RESPONSES TO SYMPATHETIC NEURAL ACTIVITY

The sympathetic nerve endings are distributed extensively throughout virtually all regions of the heart. The innervation is the most dense in the atrial myocardium and in the sinoatrial and atrioventricular nodes *(4)*. The effects almost exclusively facilitate the important functions of the heart, notably myocardial contraction, HR, and atrioventricular conduction *(1,4,17)*. In general, the rates at which the facilitatory effects on the heart develop and decay at the beginning and end, respectively, of sympathetic neural activity are very slow compared with the development and decay of the inhibitory responses to parasympathetic neural activity. When the cervical vagus nerves (which include parasympathetic nerve fibers to the heart) of an anesthetized dog are stimulated for about 20 s *(21,22)*, for example, a steady-state reduction in HR is achieved within one or two cardiac cycles (Fig. 3A). When the stimulation is discontinued, the HR returns to the basal level within a few cardiac cycles. By contrast, when the cardiac sympathetic nerves are tonically stimulated (Fig. 3B), the increase in HR requires more than 30 s to achieve a steady state level, and, when the stimulation is discontinued, about 2–3 min are required for the HR to return to the basal level.

Kinetics of the Onset of Response

The heart responds so quickly to vagal stimulation because many of the muscarinic receptors are coupled directly via G proteins to acetylcholine (ACh)-regulated K^+ channels in the automatic cell membranes; a slow second messenger system is not interposed *(23,24)*. The prompt response enables beat-by-beat control of the cardiac rhythm *(22)*.

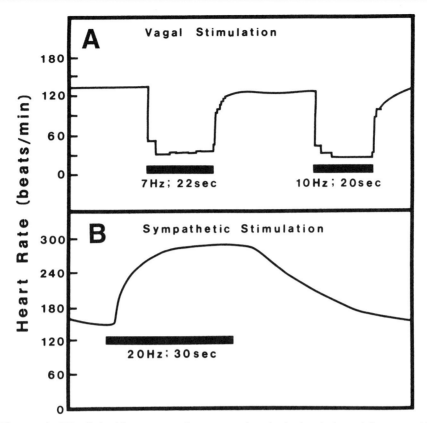

Fig. 3. Changes in HR elicited by constant frequency electrical stimulation of the vagus (**A**) and sympathetic (**B**) nerves in anesthetized dogs. Reproduced with permission from ref. *21*.

Furthermore, when vagal activity ceases, the response decays promptly *(21,22)*. The ACh released into the cardiac tissues is quickly hydrolyzed, because the enzyme, acetylcholinesterase, is so abundant in the nodal regions of the heart *(25,26)*.

The HR increases gradually in response to sympathetic stimulation (Fig. 3B), in contrast to the more abrupt change that characterizes the vagal response (Fig. 3A). The latency of the response to sympathetic stimulation is long and its rise to a plateau is gradual, partly because the process that transduces the signal from the β-adrenergic receptors to certain ion channels in the cardiac cell membranes involves a slow second messenger system, notably the adenylyl cyclase system *(4,27–29)*. Certain evidence suggests that some of the β-adrenergic receptors are coupled to the ion channels directly via G proteins *(30,31)*, but this evidence is controversial *(22,32)*. Such direct coupling would permit a rapid cardiac response to sympathetic stimulation.

The characteristically sluggish cardiac response to sympathetic stimulation (e.g., Fig. 3B) probably depends primarily on the slow rate at which NE is released from the sympathetic nerve endings in the heart *(22)*. The amount of NE ordinarily released from the sympathetic nerve endings in the heart during one heart beat is probably too small to alter cardiac performance substantially within one beat. When the sympathetic nerves are stimulated supramaximally at a frequency of 4 Hz, which would ordinarily induce a cardiac response that exceeds the half-maximal steady-state response, the fraction of the

NE released per impulse has been estimated to be only 10^{-5} of the quantity of NE stored in the nerve terminals *(33)*. This slow rate of transmitter release may have evolved as a protective mechanism that would counter the potentially damaging influence of the slow removal of NE from the cardiac interstitium *(22)*. If NE were released copiously from the cardiac sympathetic nerves, but removed slowly from the cardiac interstitium, the concentration of NE in the cardiac tissues would quickly rise to noxious levels *(4,22)*.

Toxic Effects of High Concentrations of Norepinephrine

That high concentrations of NE in the cardiac tissues are toxic has been well established *(1,3,4,34)*, but the mechanisms remain to be elucidated. In human subjects with head trauma, strokes, or pheochromocytoma, intense sympathoadrenal activation is accompanied by depression of myocardial function *(35,36)*. Intense activation of the SNS also impairs myocardial performance in experimental animals *(37–39)*. The principal mechanisms that have been implicated in the sympathetically mediated myocardial dysfunction are calcium overload in the myocytes *(40,41)*, generation of free radicals in the myocardial tissues *(42,43)*, and an imbalance between the supply and demand for oxygen and metabolic substrates *(39,44)*.

Kinetics of Response Decay

After sympathetic neural activity to the heart ceases, the chronotropic response gradually decays back to the control level (Fig. 3B). The principal mechanisms that remove the neuronally released NE in the heart (Fig. 1) are uptake by the sympathetic nerve endings (neuronal uptake), uptake by the cardiac cells (extraneuronal uptake), and diffusion away from the neuroeffector gap and into the coronary bloodstream *(2,4,7–9,11–13,22)*. These processes are much slower than those that remove ACh from the cardiac interstitium. For example, the time constant for the neuronal reuptake of NE is about 20 s *(45)*, in contrast to about 0.2 s for the hydrolysis of ACh by acetylcholinesterase *(26)*.

Regarding the two uptake processes, the neuronal mechanisms are much more potent than are the extraneuronal processes *(2,13,46)*. Neuronal uptake is especially effective in tissues that have relatively narrow neuroeffector gaps *(2)*, and cardiac tissues generally do have narrow neuroeffector gaps *(47)*. The relative effects of the two uptake processes on the kinetics of the decay of the cardiac inotropic responses to 30 s iv infusions of NE have been determined in anesthetized dogs *(46)*. The effects of cocaine on the response decay were compared with those of metanephrine; cocaine and metanephrine are potent inhibitors of neuronal and extraneuronal uptake, respectively *(48)*.

The animals were subdivided into five experimental groups, as shown in Table 1; five animals were included in each group *(46)*. In each animal, the experiment was divided into three observation periods, during each of which an infusion of NE was given. The U group was the untreated, control group, in which the animals received no uptake antagonist prior to the NE infusion during any of the observation periods. Period 1, served as the control period for all of the groups; that is, an uptake antagonist was not administered during this period. In the CC group, cocaine (COC) was administered throughout periods 2 and 3. In the CM group, cocaine was administered throughout periods 2 and 3, and metanephrine (MET) was infused throughout period 3. In the MM group, MET was administered throughout periods 2 and 3. Finally, in the MC group, MET was administered throughout periods 2 and 3, and COC was infused throughout period 3.

Table 1
Experimental Protocol Used to Determine Effects
of Cocaine, Metanephrine, or the Combination of These Two Drugs,
on the Half-Life for Decay of the Responses to Three Sequential Periods

	Experimental Groups				
Periods	*U*	*CC*	*CM*	*MM*	*MC*
1	No drug	No drug	No drug	No drug	No drug
2	No drug	COC	COC	MET	MET
3	No drug	COC	COC, MET	MET	MET, COC

NE was infused intravenously for 30 s in five groups of anesthetized dogs; there were five animals in each group. Reproduced with permission from ref. *46*.

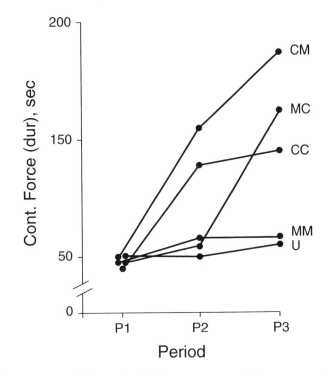

Fig. 4. Half-lives for recovery of the contractile force responses to three consecutive iv infusions (P1, P2, and P3) of NE, each for 30 s, in the five groups of anesthetized dogs listed in Table 1. Reproduced with permission from ref. *46*.

The effects of COC and MET on the half-lives for the decay of the inotropic responses to infusions of NE are shown in Fig. 4. In the U group, the 50% recovery time remained at about 50–60 s throughout the three observation periods. Neuronal blockade by cocaine during periods 2 and 3 (group CC) prolonged the recovery time substantially, to about 130–140 s. In the group (MM) that received metanephrine during the second and third periods, the recovery times did not differ materially from those in the untreated group. Thus, extraneuronal blockade, by itself, did not alter the kinetics of NE removal substantially. However, in group MC, when metanephrine was given together with cocaine during the third period, the increase in recovery time was significantly greater than was the

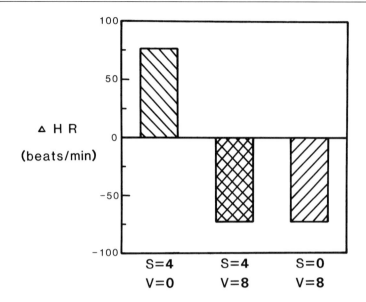

Fig. 5. Changes in heart rate (ΔHR) evoked by stimulation of (**A**) the cardiac sympathetic nerves alone at 4 Hz (S = 4, V = 0), (**B**) of the vagus nerves alone at 8 Hz (S = 0, V = 8), and (**C**) of the sympathetic and vagus nerves together (S = 4, V = 8) in an anesthetized dog. Adapted with permission from ref. *49*.

increase when cocaine alone was given in that same period (group CC). Furthermore, when metanephrine was given along with cocaine during period 3 in group CM, the effect was significantly greater than when cocaine alone was given during period 2. Thus, although extraneuronal blockade alone does not affect the kinetics of the response decay appreciably, it does potentiate substantially the effects of concomitant neuronal blockade *(46)*.

SYMPATHETIC–PARASYMPATHETIC INTERACTIONS

The regulation of cardiac function by the sympathetic division of the ANS does not operate in isolation. Instead, it usually operates in close association with the parasympathetic division of that system, most often in a reciprocal fashion. The parasympathetic nerve fibers to the heart are carried by the vagus nerves. The sympathetic effects are usually facilitatory on most aspects of cardiac function; the parasympathetic effects are usually inhibitory. Furthermore, these reciprocal effects do not antagonize each other in a simple algebraic fashion, but, in general, these reciprocal effects are highly nonlinear; that is, profound interactions prevail.

Sympathetic–vagal interactions are evident in most aspects of cardiac regulation, but they are especially pronounced in the neural control of HR. In the experiment *(49)* illustrated in Fig. 5, stimulation of the cardiac sympathetic nerves alone, at a frequency of 4 Hz (S = 4; V = 0), increased the HR by 75 beats/min. Vagal stimulation alone, at a frequency of 8 Hz (S = 0; V = 8), decreased the HR by the same amount (75 beats/min). However, when both nerves were stimulated simultaneously at these respective frequencies (i.e., S = 4 Hz, V = 8 Hz), the steady-state change in HR did not differ appreciably from that evoked by vagal stimulation alone. Hence, the facilitatory effect of the sympathetic stimulation was virtually abolished by the vagal activity, that is, the vagal effects clearly exceeded the sympathetic effects. This profound autonomic interaction has been

Cardiac Cell

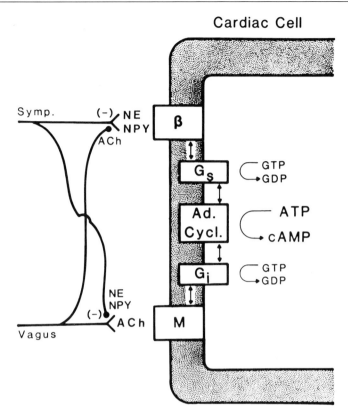

Fig. 6. Prejunctional and postjunctional mechanisms that contribute to the cardiac sympathetic–parasympathetic interactions. Abbreviations: ACh, acetylcholine; Ad. Cycl, adenylyl cyclase; β, β-adrenergic receptor; cAMP, cyclic AMP; G_i and G_s, inhibitory and stimulatory G proteins; M, muscarinic receptors; NE, norepinephrine; NPY, neuropeptide Y. Adapted with permission from ref. *51*.

termed accentuated antagonism *(50)*. Note that, in these experiments, stimulations of the two autonomic divisions were begun simultaneously. However, when the two divisions are not activated synchronously, the interactions may be entirely different, as described below.

Interaction Mechanisms

Accentuated antagonism is mediated at postjunctional and prejunctional levels of the neuroeffector junction (Fig. 6). Postjunctionally, the adrenergic and cholinergic transmitters interact at the level of the cardiac effector cell itself. Prejunctionally, transmitters and modulators released from the nerve terminals of one autonomic division inhibit the release of transmitters and modulators released from the nerve endings of the other division.

POSTJUNCTIONAL MECHANISMS

Autonomic interactions in the heart have been evinced not only by neural stimulation, but also by infusions of adrenergic and cholinergic agonists *(25,32,50,51)*. Therefore, such interactions must occur both at prejunctional and postjunctional levels of the cardiac neuroeffector junction.

The postjunctional interactions (Fig. 6) in the heart are mediated principally by the adenylyl cyclase system *(25,32,50–53)*. The adrenergic neurotransmitter, NE, occupies β-adrenergic receptors in the cardiac cell membrane. This process stimulates the membrane-bound enzyme, adenylyl cyclase, which catalyzes the intracellular production of cyclic adenosine monophosphate (cAMP) from adenosine triphosphate. The coupling of the β-adrenergic receptors to the adenylyl cyclase is mediated by a stimulatory protein, G_s. This coupling involves the hydrolysis of guanosine triphosphate (GTP) to guanosine diphosphate (GDP). The ACh released from vagal nerve endings antagonizes these adrenergic effects by occupying muscarinic receptors on the effector cell surface (Fig. 6). The muscarinic receptors inhibit adenylyl cyclase through an inhibitory protein, G_i, which also facilitates the hydrolysis of GTP to GDP.

The principal postjunctional interaction thus operates through adenylyl cyclase. The facilitatory effects of sympathetic activity are mediated by raising the intracellular levels of cAMP. Concomitant vagal activity antagonizes this process by inhibiting adenylyl cyclase, and thereby attenuates the adrenergically induced rise in the cAMP concentration.

PREJUNCTIONAL MECHANISMS

As stated, various receptors on the postganglionic autonomic nerve endings in the heart regulate the release of neurotransmitters and neuromodulators (18–20,50,51). Muscarinic receptors located on postganglionic sympathetic endings (Fig. 6) serve to inhibit the release of NE, and probably also of neuropeptide Y (NPY) from those endings; NE and NPY receptors act to inhibit the release of ACh from parasympathetic endings.

The prejunctional inhibition of NE release by vagally released ACh is well established (17,19,25,50,51,54,55). The release of NE from the cardiac sympathetic terminals has been estimated by measuring the NE overflow into the coronary sinus blood in anesthetized dogs (55). As explained, the overflow of NE represents the difference between the rate of NE release from the cardiac nerve endings and the rate at which it is taken up again by the nerve endings and extraneuronal tissues (Fig. 1). The NE not removed by these uptake processes overflows into the coronary venous blood. If the uptake processes are not affected appreciably by the experimental procedures, the changes in NE overflow during an experiment reflect the changes in transmitter release.

In the experiment (55) shown in Fig. 7, the rate of NE overflow into the coronary sinus blood of anesthetized dogs was measured under control conditions (C), during cardiac sympathetic stimulation alone (S), and during combined sympathetic and vagal stimulation (S + V). The NE overflows were 30 and 55 ng/min during sympathetic stimulations at 2 and 4 Hz, respectively (Fig. 7). During combined stimulation, the NE overflows decreased by 33%. Atropine abolished this inhibitory effect of vagal stimulation.

Changes in the neuronal release of NE are accompanied by parallel changes in NPY release. NPY is co-localized, along with NE, in a substantial fraction of the storage vesicles in the sympathetic nerve terminals (56,57), and the overflows of NE and NPY into the coronary sinus blood both increase as the frequency of sympathetic nerve stimulation is raised (58). Experiments conducted by Revington and McCloskey (59) strongly suggest that neurally released ACh can effectively suppress the release of NPY, as well as of NE, from sympathetic varicosities, as described below.

Another prejunctional autonomic interaction involves the inhibition of ACh release from vagal nerve endings by the NE and NPY released from neighboring sympathetic nerve endings (Fig. 6). Vagal neurotransmission is suppressed by neurally released NE while the sympathetic nerves are being stimulated, but the inhibition wanes quickly after the sympathetic stimulation ceases. The inhibitory effects of NE on the release of ACh

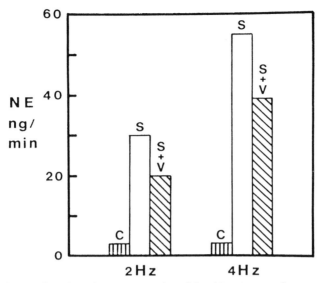

Fig. 7. Mean overflows of NE into the coronary sinus blood in a group of seven anesthetized dogs under control conditions (C), during sympathetic stimulation (S) alone at 2 and 4 Hz, and during combined stimulation (S + V) of the sympathetic (2 and 4 Hz) and vagus (15 Hz) nerves. Adapted from ref. *55*, with permission from the American Heart Association.

from the vagus nerve endings appear to be mediated by prejunctional α_1-receptors. In experiments on isolated atria, the suppression of ACh release was prevented by α_1-adrenergic receptor antagonists, such as prazosin, but not by β-adrenergic receptor antagnists, such as propranolol *(60,61)*.

The NPY released from the sympathetic nerve endings induces a much more sustained inhibition of ACh release from vagus nerve fibers than does the NE that is co-released with this neuropeptide *(NP; 56–58,62)*. Potter *(62)* was the first to demonstrate the pronounced effect of this NP on vagal neurotransmission (Fig. 8). She showed that a brief train of intense sympathetic stimulation could substantially attenuate the cardiac chronotropic responses to periodic vagal test stimulations in anesthetized dogs (Fig. 8A), presumably by inhibiting the release of ACh from vagal endings in the heart. The attenuation of the chronotropic response to vagal stimulation persisted for as long as 1 h. This inhibitory effect of sympathetic stimulation was mimicked by an iv injection of NPY (Fig. 8B). Furthermore, neither neurally released nor exogenous NPY altered the chronotropic responses to muscarinic agonists. By exclusion, therefore, the most likely explanation is that NPY suppresses vagal neurotransmission by diminishing the release of ACh from the vagal nerve endings. Confirmatory results have been reported by other investigators *(58,59)*. Certain species differences exist, however. For example, many of the actions of NPY in cardiovascular control in dogs are carried out by a different NP (namely, galanin) in cats *(63)* and possums *(64)*.

Sᴇǫᴜᴇɴᴄᴇ ᴏꜰ Aᴜᴛᴏɴᴏᴍɪᴄ Exᴄɪᴛᴀᴛɪᴏɴ

The experiments described above indicate that the NPY released by antecedent sympathetic activity may profoundly inhibit the responses to subsequent vagal activity. These findings strongly suggest that antecedent sympathetic activity of sufficient intensity and duration will attenuate or abolish the vagal preponderance that would otherwise

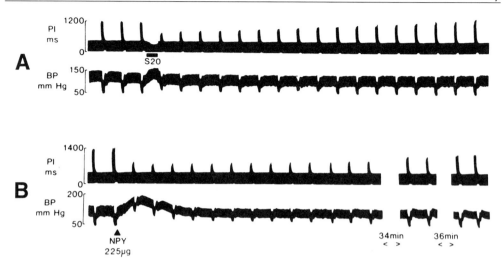

Fig. 8. Effects of stimulation (**A**) of the cardiac sympathetic nerves at a frequency of 20 Hz (S20) for 1 min, or of an iv injection (**B**) of NPY, on the PI and arterial blood pressure (BP) responses to repetitive 15 s trains of vagal stimulation, delivered once every 2 min, in an anesthetized dog. Reproduced with permission from ref. *62*.

prevail when activity in the two autonomic divisions is initiated simultaneously (as illustrated by the data in Fig. 5).

This contention has been supported by the experiments of Revington and McCloskey *(59)*. When these investigators stimulated the cardiac sympathetic nerves alone at 16 Hz for 1 min (at S16 in Fig. 9A), the pulse interval (PI) responses to periodic vagal stimuli were suppressed for about 45 min. This reaction was almost identical to that (Fig. 8A) obtained previously by Potter *(62)* under similar experimental conditions. The persistent attenuation of the responses to the periodic vagal test stimulations in Figs. 8A and 9A was presumably mediated by the NPY released during the brief, but intense, sympathetic stimulation.

Revington and McCloskey *(59)* found, however, that if the identical sympathetic stimulation was accompanied by vagal stimulation, also at 16 Hz for 1 min (V16 + S16), and, if the two stimulations were initiated simultaneously, the responses to the subsequent vagal test stimulations were not attenuated (Fig. 9C). In fact, they were somewhat facilitated, much as they were when the vagus nerves alone were stimulated at 16 Hz (V16) for 1 min (Fig. 9B). The absence of an enduring attenuation of the responses to the subsequent vagal test stimulations indicates that the ACh released during the combined sympathetic and vagal stimulations at 16 Hz (Fig. 9C) must have inhibited the release of NE and NPY from the sympathetic nerve endings. Furthermore, the PIs were markedly prolonged during the simultaneous vagal and sympathetic stimulations (Fig. 9C), just as they were during the period of intense vagal stimulation alone (Fig. 9B). This response demonstrates clearly that the vagal effects predominated over the sympathetic effects during the course of the combined stimulation, and thereby confirms the data shown in Fig. 5.

The finding *(59)* that concomitant sympathetic and vagal stimulation did not suppress subsequent vagal neurotransmission (Fig. 9C) suggests that the ACh released from the vagus nerve endings during the initial period of combined stimulation must have acted very quickly and powerfully to suppress the release of NE and NPY from the sympathetic nerve endings during the same period of combined stimulation. Furthermore, the diminished release of NE and NPY during the period of combined stimulation must account

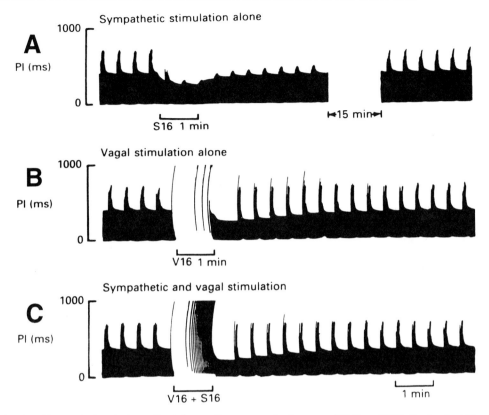

Fig. 9. Effects of stimulation of a right cardiac sympathetic nerve (S16) at 16 Hz for 1 min (**A**), of the right vagus nerve (V16) at 16 Hz for 1 min (**B**), and of both nerves simultaneously (V16 + S16), both at 16 Hz for 1 min (**C**) on the responses to supramaximal test stimulations of the right vagus nerve for 5 s every 30 s in an anesthetized dog. Reproduced with permission from ref. *59.*

for the observed attenuation of the responses to the subsequent vagal test stimulations. The principal inhibitor of the responses to the vagal test stimulations is probably NPY rather than NE, because NPY does act slowly but persistently (as do most NPs). Therefore, when the two autonomic divisions are stimulated simultaneously, one can postulate that the rapidly acting ACh quickly suppresses the release of NE and NPY, and hence the vagal effects predominate. However, when the sympathetic nerves are stimulated alone for a sufficient time before the beginning of vagal stimulation, one can postulate that appreciable amounts of NPY can be released from the sympathetic nerve endings. Thus, the NPY would have enough time to effectively suppress the release of ACh during subsequent vagal test stimulations (Fig. 9A).

The experiments heretofore described *(59)* strongly suggest that the NPY released by antecedent sympathetic activity may profoundly inhibit the responses to subsequent vagal activity. These findings would support the hypothesis that antecedent sympathetic activity of sufficient intensity and duration will attenuate or abolish the vagal preponderance that would otherwise prevail when activity in the two autonomic divisions is initiated simultaneously, or when the vagal activity begins prior to the sympathetic activity.

This hypothesis was subsequently tested by Yang and Levy *(65)*, who compared the changes in HR elicited by two neural stimulation patterns in anesthetized dogs. In one pattern (SV), the sympathetic stimulation preceded the vagal stimulation, and the order was reversed in the other pattern (VS). Each animal was assigned randomly to one of the two stimulation patterns; eight animals were included in each group. Regardless of the pattern of excitation, the nerves of each autonomic division were stimulated supramaximally at a constant frequency of 10 Hz.

With either pattern type, the durations of the stimulations of the sympathetic (S) and vagus (V) nerves varied from 0 to 11 min, and the two types of nerves were stimulated simultaneously during the last minute of stimulation *(65)*. For pattern SV, for example, the following stimulation combinations were used (subscripts denote the stimulation duration, in min): S_0V_1, S_1V_1, $S_{3.5}V_1$, S_6V_1, and $S_{11}V_1$. In each animal, the sequence of the various stimulation combinations was randomized. The steady state responses were measured near the end of that last minute, and both stimulations were terminated simultaneously.

The mean changes in HR in the animals subjected to pattern SV stimulations are shown in Fig. 10. Curve S_tV_1 shows that vagal stimulation alone for 1 min (S_0V_1) decreased HR by 64 beats/min; curve S_tV_0 shows that sympathetic stimulation alone (S_1V_0) for 1 min increased HR by 100 beats/min (subscript t in S_tV_0 and S_tV_1 represents the different durations of sympathetic stimulation). Thus, combined sympathetic and vagal stimulation (S_1V_1) for 1 min would be expected to increase HR by 36 beats/min, if the combined effects did sum algebraically. However, curve S_tV_1 shows that S_1V_1 stimulation actually decreased HR by 31 beats/min. The experimental data demonstrate, therefore, that the vagal effects predominated substantially over the sympathetic effects *(65)*.

Comparison of the S_1V_0 and S_1V_1 responses in Fig. 10A indicates that, during sympathetic stimulation (S_1) for 1 min, concomitant vagal stimulation decreases HR by 131 beats/min. This difference is represented by the height of bar S_1 in Fig. 10B. Similarly, the other bars in Fig. 10B denote the differences between the corresponding ordinate values for curves S_tV_1 and S_tV_0. The height of each bar above the horizontal dashed line in Fig. 10B reflects the vagal preponderance. Note that the vagal preponderance diminished significantly as the elapsed time between the beginnings of sympathetic and vagal stimulation was progressively increased.

Activation pattern VS in these experiments *(65)* was similar to pattern SV, except that, when the durations of V and S were not equal, V preceded S. The mean responses to this pattern of combined stimulations are shown in Fig. 11. Curve V_tS_1 shows that sympathetic stimulation alone for 1 min (V_0S_1) increased HR by 83 beats/min; curve V_tS_0 shows that vagal stimulation alone for 1 min (V_1S_0) decreased HR by 70 beats/min. Thus, although the sympathetically induced increment in HR exceeded the vagally induced decrement by 13 beats/min, simultaneous stimulation of the two autonomic divisions for 1 min (V_1S_1) actually decreased the HR by 39 beats/min (curve V_tS_1). Thus, the vagal effects on HR predominated over the sympathetic effects, just as it did in the preceding group of experiments (Fig. 10).

The differences between the ordinate values for curves V_tS_1 and V_tS_0 are reflected by the heights of the bars in Fig. 10B. In this figure, therefore, vagal preponderance is denoted by the extent to which the tops of the bars fall below the horizontal dashed line in panel B. Note that when the two autonomic divisions were activated simultaneously for 1 min (V_1S_1), vagal preponderance was most pronounced; i.e., the shortest bar in Fig. 11B was bar V_1. When the elapsed times between the beginnings of vagal and sympathetic stimulation were increased, the vagal preponderance was slightly attenuated, but this change was not significant statistically.

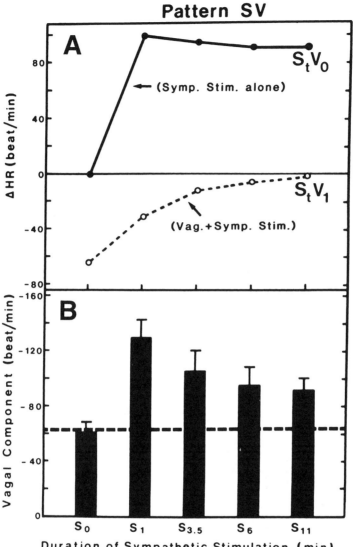

Fig. 10. Mean changes in heart rate (ΔHR) induced by sympathetic and vagal stimulation in a group of eight anesthetized dogs. (**A**) Curve S_tV_0 represents the changes in HR induced by sympathetic stimulation alone for durations (t) of 0, 1, 3.5, 6, and 11 min; curve S_tV_1 represents the changes in HR induced by the same durations of sympathetic stimulation, but vagal stimulation was also given during the last 1 min of the sympathetic stimulation. (**B**) Bars represent the differences between curves S_tV_0 and S_tV_1 for each value of t. The height of each bar above the horizontal dashed line is an index of vagal predominance. Adapted from ref. *65*, with permission from the American Heart Association.

The diminution of vagal preponderance induced by antecedent sympathetic stimulation (Fig. 10) is compatible with previous findings *(57–59,62)*, which show that intense sympathetic stimulation alone attenuates subsequent vagal neurotransmission. The attenuation is probably chiefly mediated by an inhibition of ACh release from vagal nerve endings by the NE or NPY released from the sympathetic varicosities (Fig. 6). The sustained inhibition of ACh release elicited by an antecedent period of sympathetic

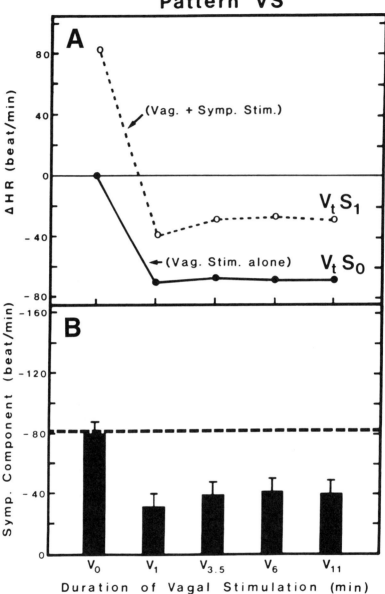

Fig. 11. Mean changes in heart rate (ΔHR) induced by sympathetic and vagal stimulation in a group of eight anesthetized dogs. (**A**) Curve V_tS_0 represents the changes in HR induced by vagal stimulation alone for durations (t) of 0, 1, 3.5, 6, and 11 min; curve V_tS_1 represents the changes in HR induced by the same durations of vagal stimulation, but sympathetic stimulation was also given during the last 1 min of the sympathetic stimulation. (**B**) Bars represent the differences between curves V_tS_1 and V_tS_0 for each of the above values of t. The distance from the top of each bar to the horizontal dashed line is an index of vagal predominance. Adapted from ref. *65,* with permission from the American Heart Association.

stimulation suggests that the principal inhibitor of vagal neurotransmission is the NPY that is co-released with NE from the sympathetic nerve endings *(57–59,62)*.

In the experiments shown in Figs. 10 and 11, attention was directed toward the steady state chronotropic responses that were attained during concomitant sympathetic and

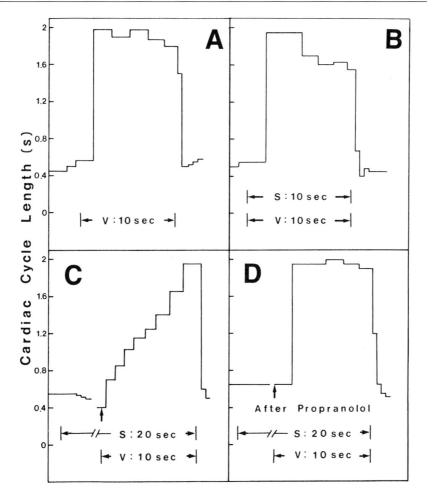

Fig. 12. Changes in cardiac cycle length induced by sympathetic (S) and vagal (V) stimulation in an anesthetized dog. (**A**) Vagus nerve alone was stimulated for 10 s. (**B**) Sympathetic and vagal nerves were stimulated simultaneously. (**C**) Sympathetic stimulation was initiated 10 s before vagal stimulation. (**D**) Propranolol (1 mg/kg) was given intravenously, and then sympathetic stimulation was again initiated 10 s before vagal stimulation. Reproduced with permission from ref. *66*.

vagal activity. In those experiments, it was incidentally observed that the temporal relation between the beginnings of sympathetic and vagal stimulation also appeared to affect the kinetics of the chronotropic responses to vagal stimulation. When vagal stimulation either preceded or began simultaneously with sympathetic stimulation, the chronotropic response to the vagal stimulation was abrupt; i.e., the beginning of the response resembled the initial response to vagal stimulation alone (as in Fig. 3A). However, when sympathetic stimulation preceded vagal stimulation, the chronotropic response to the vagal stimulation usually developed much more gradually; that is, the response was often blunted.

Experiments were conducted subsequently on anesthetized dogs to determine the mechanism responsible for the observed effects of antecedent sympathetic stimulation on the kinetics of the initiation of the response to vagal stimulation *(66)*. The representative effects of antecedent sympathetic stimulation on the time-course of the initial response to vagal stimulation are shown in Fig. 12. When a vagus nerve alone was stimulated in this experiment, the cardiac cycle length (CCL) increased abruptly to its steady-state value, and the response decayed very rapidly, as well (Fig. 12A); this constitutes the characteristic vagal response (similar to that shown in Fig. 3A). Similarly, when sympathetic and vagal stimulation were initiated simultaneously, CCL increased to its maximum value within one cardiac cycle (Fig. 12B).

However, when vagal stimulation was started 10 s after the beginning of sympathetic stimulation, CCL responded to the vagal excitation in a stepwise fashion (Fig. 12C), rather than abruptly. Propranolol abolished this blunting effect of antecedent sympathetic stimulation on the chronotropic response to subsequent vagal stimulation (Fig. 12D), but phentolamine did not abolish the blunting effect (not shown). Hence, the blunting effect appears to involve β-adrenergic, rather than α-adrenergic, mechanisms. Also, NE infusions were found to blunt the responses to vagal stimulation in a manner similar to that evoked by sympathetic stimulation (66). Therefore, the mechanism responsible for the blunting is probably postjunctional (at the level of the cardiac effector cells), rather than prejunctional (at the level of the postganglionic autonomic nerve endings). Finally, the blunting effect of sympathetic stimulation disappeared almost entirely within 30 s (66). Because the blunting becomes evident within a few seconds after the initiation of sympathoadrenal activity and the effect disappears soon after sympathoadrenal activity ceases, one may conclude that the blunting effect is mediated by a classical transmitter (NE), rather than by a NP (such as NPY), because NP effects are typically much more persistent than are the effects of classical transmitters, such as NE (56,57,62).

CONCLUSIONS

The catecholamines released from the sympathetic nerve endings in the heart, and from the adrenal medulla, exert profound facilitatory effects on most of the important aspects of cardiac function. The NE released from the sympathetic nerve endings generally has a much greater influence on cardiac function than does the epinephrine released from the adrenal medulla. The neuronal release of NE is regulated very tightly. The concentration of NE in the neuroeffector junction inhibits the release of NE from the sympathetic nerve endings via α-adrenergic autoreceptors in those terminals. The ACh released from the vagal nerve endings in the heart and the NPY released from the sympathetic nerve endings also inhibit the neuronal release of NE. These inhibitory effects of ACh, NPY, and of NE itself have a protective effect, in that they tend to prevent the concentration of NE from rising to noxious levels in the cardiac interstitium. The neurotransmitters and neuromodulators released from the sympathetic and vagal nerve endings exert strong antagonistic effects at the prejunctional and postjunctional levels of the cardiac neuroeffector junctions. Consequently, the antagonistic effects of spontaneous activity in the two divisions of the ANS are not additive in an algebraic sense, but, instead, strong interactions prevail. Hence, the temporal sequence of the changes in activity of those two divisions of the ANS greatly influence the magnitude and direction of the ultimate cardiac response.

REFERENCES

1. Riemersma RA, Oliver MF, eds. Catecholamines in the Non-Ischaemic and Ischaemic Myocardium. Elsevier, Amsterdam, 1982.
2. Esler M, Jennings G, Lambert G, Meredith I, Horne M, Eisenhofer G. Overflow of catecholamine neurotransmitters to the circulation: source, fate, and functions. Physiol Rev 1990;70:963–985.

3. Ganguli PK, ed. Catecholamines and Heart Disease. CRC, Boca Raton, FL, 1991.
4. Goldstein DS. Stress, Catecholamines, and Cardiovascular Disease. Oxford University Press, New York, 1995.
5. Cryer PE. Physiology and pathophysiology of the human sympathoadrenal neuroendocrine system. N Engl J Med 1980;303:436–444.
6. Shah S, Tse TF, Clutter WE, Cryer PE. Human sympathochromaffin system. Am J Physiol 1984;247: E380–E384.
7. Esler M, Jennings G, Korner P, Blombery P, Sacharias N, Leonard P. Measurement of total and organ-specific norepinephrine kinetics in humans. Am J Physiol 1984;247:E21–E28.
8. Levy MN. Neural and reflex control of the circulation. In: Garfein OB, ed. Current Concepts in Cardio-vascular Physiology. Academic, San Diego, 1990, pp. 133–207.
9. Goldstein DS, Eisenhofer G. Plasma catechols—What do they mean? News Physiol Sci 1988;3:138–144.
10. Yamaguchi N, de Champlain J, Nadeau R. Noradrenaline liberation from the dog heart. Can J Physiol Pharmacol 1973;51:297–305.
11. Lindmar R, Löffelholz K. Neuronal and extraneuronal uptake and efflux of catecholamines in the isolated rabbit heart. Naunyn-Schmiedeberg's Arch Pharmacol 1974;284:63–92.
12. Trendelenburg U. Metabolizing systems involved in the inactivation of catecholamines. Naunyn-Schmiedeberg's Arch Pharmacol 1986;332:201–207.
13. Levy MN, Masuda Y. Effects of heart rate on the myocardial disposition of norepinephrine. In: Zipes DP, Jalife J, eds. Cardiac Electrophysiology and Arrhythmias. Grune & Stratton, Orlando, FL, 1985, pp. 145–150.
14. Blombery PA, Heinzow BGJ. Cardiac and pulmonary norepinephrine release and removal in the dog. Circ Res 1983;53:688–694.
15. Esler M, Jennings G, Korner P. Willett I, Dudley F, Hasking G, Anderson W, Lambert G. Assessment of human sympathetic nervous system activity from measurements of norepinephrine turnover. Hyper-tension 1988;11:3–20.
16. Young MA, Hintze TH, Vatner SF. Correlation between cardiac performance and plasma catecholamine levels in conscious dogs. Am J Physiol 1985;248:H82–H88.
17. Vatner SF, Hittinger L. Sympathetic mechanisms regulating myocardial contractility in conscious animals. In: Shepherd JT, Vatner SF, eds. Nervous Control of the Heart. Harwood, Amsterdam, 1996, pp. 1–28.
18. Langer SZ. Presynaptic regulation of the release of catecholamines. Pharmacol Rev 1981;32:337–362.
19. Vanhoutte PM, Verbeuren TJ, Webb RC. Local modulation of adrenergic neuroeffector interaction in the blood vessel wall. Physiol Rev 1981;61:151–247.
20. Starke K, Göthert M, Kilbinger H. Modulation of neurotransmitter release by presynaptic autoreceptors. Physiol Rev 1989;69:864–989.
21. Warner HR, Cox A. Mathematical model of heart rate control by sympathetic and vagus efferent information. J Appl Physiol 1962;17:349–355.
22. Levy MN, Yang T, Wallick DW. Assessment of beat-by-beat control of heart rate by the autonomic nervous system: molecular biology technics are necessary, but not sufficient. J Cardiovasc Electrophysiol 1993;4:183–193.
23. Pfaffinger PJ, Martin JM, Hunter DD, Nathanson NM, Hille B. GTP-binding proteins couple cardiac muscarinic receptors to a K channel. Nature 1985;317:536–538.
24. Holmer SR, Homcy CJ. G proteins in the heart. Circulation 1991;84:1891–1902.
25. Löffelholz K, Pappano AJ. Parasympathetic neuroeffector junction of the heart. Pharmacol Rev 1985; 37:1–24.
26. Dexter F, Levy MN, Rudy Y. Mathematical model of the changes in heart rate elicited by vagal stimu-lation. Circ Res 1989;65:1330–1339.
27. Hartzell HC. Regulation of cardiac ion channels by catecholamines, acetylcholine and second messen-ger systems. Prog Biophys Mol Biol 1988;52:165–247.
28. Reiter M. Calcium mobilization and cardiac inotropic mechanisms. Pharmacol Rev 1988;40:189–217.
29. Clapham D. Control of intracellular calcium. In: Zipes DP, Jalife J, eds. Cardiac Electrophysiology: From Cell to Bedside 2nd ed. W. B. Saunders, Philadelphia, 1995, pp. 127–136.
30. Yatani A, Brown AM. Rapid β-adrenergic modulation of cardiac calcium channel currents by a fast G protein pathway. Science 1989;245:71–74.
31. Brown AM. Ion channels as G protein effectors. News Physiol Sci 1991;6:158–161.
32. Hartzell HC, Mery P-F, Fischmeister R, Szabo G. Sympathetic regulation of cardiac calcium current is due exclusively to cAMP-dependent phosphorylation. Nature 1991;351:573–576.

33. Folkow B, Nilsson H. Transmitter release at adrenergic nerve endings: total exocytosis or fractional release. News Physiol Sci 1997;12:32–36.

34. Haft JI. Cardiovascular injury induced by sympathetic catecholamines. Prog Cardiovasc Dis 1974;17: 73–86.

35. Hammermeister KE, Reichenbach DD. QRS changes, pulmonary edema, and myocardial necrosis associated with subarachnoid hemorrhage. Am Heart J 1969;78:94–100.

36. Quezado ZN, Keiser HR, Parker MM. Reversible myocardial depression after massive catecholamine release from a pheochromocytoma. Crit Care Med 1992;20:549–551.

37. Downing SE, Chen V. Myocardial injury following endogenous catecholamine release in rabbits. J Mol Cell Cardiol 1985;17:377–387.

38. Shanlin RJ, Sole MJ, Rahimifar M, Tator CH, Factor SM. Increased intracranial pressure elicits hypertension, increased sympathetic activity, electrocardiographic abnormalities and myocardial damage in rats. J Am Coll Cardiol 1988;12:727–736.

39. Lang SA, Maron MB, Bosso FJ, Pilati CF. Temporal changes in left ventricular function after massive sympathetic nervous system activation. Can J Physiol Pharmacol 1994;72:693–700.

40. Novitzky D, Cooper DKC, Rose AG, Reichart B. Prevention of myocardial injury by pretreatment with verapamil hydrochloride prior to experimental brain death. Am J Emerg Med 1987;5:11–18.

41. Todd GL, Eliot RS. Cardioprotective effects of diltiazem when given before, during or delayed after infusion of norepinephrine in anesthetized dogs. Am J Cardiol 1988;62:25G–29G.

42. Singal PK, Kapur N, Dhillon KS, Beamish RE, Dhalla NS. Role of free radicals in catecholamine-induced cardiomyopathy. Can J Physiol Pharmacol 1982;60:1390–1397.

43. Haggendal J, Jonsson L, Johansson G, Bjurstrom S, Carlsten J, Thoren-Tolling K. Catecholamine-induced free radicals in myocardial cell necrosis on experimental stress in pigs. Acta Physiol Scand 1987;131:447–452.

44. Pilati CF, Bosso FJ, Maron MB. Factors involved in left bentricular dysfunction after massive sympathetic activation. Am J Physiol 1992;263:H784–H791.

45. Cousineau D, Goresky CA, Bach GG, Rose CP. Effect of β-adrenergic blockade on in vivo norepinephrine release in canine heart. Am J Physiol 1984;246:H283–H292.

46. Masuda Y, Matsuda Y, Levy MN. Effects of cocaine and metanephrine on the cardiac responses to norepinephrine infusions. J Pharmacol Exp Ther 1980;215:20–27.

47. Novi A. Electron microscopic study of the innervation of the papillary muscle of the rat. Anat Rec 1968; 160:123–142.

48. Iversen LL. Catecholamine uptake processes. Brit Med Bull 1973;29:130–135.

49. Levy MN, Zieske H. Autonomic control of cardiac pacemaker activity and atrioventricular transmission. J Appl Physiol 1969;27:465–470.

50. Levy MN. Sympathetic-parasympathetic interactions in the heart. Circ Res 1971;29:437–445.

51. Levy MN. Sympathetic-parasympathetic interactions in the heart. In: Kulbertus HE, Franck G, eds. Neurocardiology. Futura, Mount Kisco, New York, 1988, pp. 85–98.

52. Stiles GL, Caron MG, Lefkowitz RJ. β-Adrenergic receptors: biochemical mechanisms of physiological regulation. Physiol Rev 1984;64:661–743.

53. Fleming JW, Strawbridge RA, Watanabe AM. Muscarinic receptor regulation of cardiac adenylate cyclase activity. J Mol Cell Cardiol 1987;19:47–61.

54. Löffelholz K, Muscholl E. Inhibition by parasympathetic nerve stimulation of the release of the adrenergic transmitter. Naunyn-Schmiedebergs Arch Pharmakol 1970;267:181–184.

55. Levy MN, Blattberg B. Effect of vagal stimulation on the overflow of norepinephrine into the coronary sinus during cardiac sympathetic nerve stimulation in the dog. Circ Res 1976;38:81–85.

56. Potter EK. Neuropeptide Y as an autonomic neurotransmitter. Pharmacol Ther 1988;37:251–273.

57. Warner MR, Levy MN. Role of neuropeptide Y in neural control of the heart. J Cardiovasc Electrophysiol 1990;1:80–91.

58. Warner MR, Senanayake P, Ferrario CM, Levy MN. Sympathetic stimulation-evoked overflow of norepinephrine and neuropeptide Y from the heart. Circ Res 1991;69:455–465.

59. Revington ML, McCloskey DI. Sympathetic-parasympathetic interactions at the heart, possibly involving neuropeptide Y, in anaesthetized dogs. J Physiol (London) 1990;428:359–370.

60. Wetzel GT, Brown JH. Presynaptic modulation of acetylcholine release from cardiac parasympathetic neurons. Am J Physiol 1985;248:H33–H39.

61. Wetzel GT, Goldstein D, Brown JH. Acetylcholine release from rat atria can be regulated through an a_1-adrenergic receptor. Circ Res 1985;56:763–766.

62. Potter EK. Prolonged non-adrenergic inhibition of cardiac vagal action following sympathetic stimulation: neuromodulation by neuropeptide Y? Neurosci Lett 1985;54:117–121.

63. Revington M, Potter EK, McCloskey DI. Prolonged inhibition of cardiac vagal action following sympathetic stimulation and galanin in anaesthetized cats. J Physiol (London) 1990;431:495–503.

64. Courtice GP, Potter EK, McCloskey DI. Inhibition of cardiac vagal action by galanin but not neuropeptide Y in the brush-tailed possum trichosurus vulpecula. J Physiol (London) 1993;461:379–386.

65. Yang T, Levy MN. Sequence of excitation as a factor in sympathetic-parasympathetic interactions in the heart. Circ Res 1992;71:898–905.

66. Yang T, Senturia JB, Levy MN. Antecedent sympathetic stimulation alters the time course of the chronotropic response to vagal stimulation in dogs. Am J Physiol 1994;266:H1339–H1347.

7

Vasopressin and the Heart

Vernon S. Bishop and Max G. Sanderford

Arginine vasopressin (AVP) is an important hormone in the regulation of H_2O excretion *(1–3)*. Increases in AVP result in a rapid modification of renal excretion of H_2O, resulting in a concentrated urine and a retention of H_2O. In addition to playing a central role in the regulation of H_2O, AVP has additional actions that contribute to the regulation of the cardiovascular system *(4,5)*. AVP is a potent vasoconstrictor and, as such, has the potential to play an important role in the maintenance of blood pressure (BP) in both physiological and pathophysiological states *(4,5)*.

The secretion of AVP from the neurohypophysis is influenced by plasma osmolality, as well as by cardiopulmonary and arterial baroreflexes (ABRs) *(1–3,5–9)*. In most conditions, plasma osmolality is the principle regulator of plasma AVP concentration *(1–3,6,10–12)*. Osmoreceptors located in the anterior hypothalamus and in the peripheral circulation (hepatoportal region) are sensitive to small changes in plasma osmolality *(6,10,11)*. Increases in AVP release are also initiated by cardiac and arterial baroreflexes in response to decreases in cardiac filling and/or arterial pressure *(6–9)*. These reflexes can also influence the osmotic-stimulated release of AVP *(3,6)*. In general, small changes in blood volume or arterial pressure do not influence AVP release. However, substantial decreases in arterial pressure or cardiac filling can result in large increases in plasma AVP, which are important in the restoration of arterial pressure during hemorrhage *(6,13)*.

Even though AVP has potent vasoconstrictor activities, circulating levels of AVP must exceed those required for maximal antidiuretic activity, before BP is increased *(4,13–15)*. The modest pressor action to acute increases in AVP is caused by an interaction of AVP with specific regions of the brain involved in regulation of sympathetic outflow to the systemic circulation *(13,14,16)*. This interaction results in an enhanced sympathoinhibitory response when pressure is increased with AVP, which is far greater than observed with other pressor agents *(13,14,16–21)*. Studies in conscious rabbits indicate that the enhanced sympathoinhibition involves a resetting of the ABR to lower pressures *(20)*.

From: *Contemporary Endocrinology: Hormones and the Heart in Health and Disease*
Edited by: L. Share © Humana Press Inc., Totowa, NJ

VASOPRESSIN CONTRIBUTION TO BASAL BLOOD PRESSURE

Resting BP is maintained by three primary pressor systems *(22–24)*: the sympathetic nervous system (SNS), the renin-angiotensin system (RAS), and AVP. Each of these systems has been shown to contribute to the maintenance of normal BP in physiological states, in addition to changes that may occur in pathophysiological states, such as hypertension (HT) and congestive heart failure.

In general, the SNS is known to be the principle determinant of resting BP, but, depending on the conditions, both angiotensin II (ANG II) and AVP contribute to BP. Arterial and cardiopulmonary reflexes modulate the relative activities of the three systems *(23)*. Both refluxes exert a tonic inhibitory influence on sympathetic outflow, renin release, and the secretion of AVP *(23)*. Also, the reflexes are important determinants of neural and hormonal responses when one or more of the systems is blocked *(22–24)*. Using linear control system analysis, the contribution of each of the three pressor systems in maintaining BP has been quantitated in the dog *(23)*. As expected, studies in dogs showed that, when ABRs are intact, the gain of the SNS was significantly greater than that of either AVP or ANG II. This indicates that, without these two systems, the SNS was able to maintain BP near the control level. Compared to the SNS, the gain for ANG II and AVP is substantially smaller, indicating that either of these systems is less able to maintain BP when they are the sole remaining pressor systems. In the absence of ABR as demonstrated, in sinoaortic denervated dogs (SAD), the SNS and ANG II were the major contributors to BP. AVP contributed to BP in the SAD state only when the SNS and ANG II were blocked. The important finding in these studies was that, although the SNS is the principle contributor to BP, the contribution of AVP and ANG II is increased in the absence of the SNS *(22,25–27)*.

The potential contribution of humoral pressor systems in BP regulation was evaluated following 48 h of H_2O deprivation. Such stress increases plasma osmolality and sodium concentration, resulting in increases in plasma levels of AVP, plasma renin activity (PRA), and catecholamines *(22)*. In studies in conscious rats and rabbits, the contribution of AVP and PRA to the maintenance of BP was increased following 48 h of H_2O deprivation. The important observation in these studies is that the stress of dehydration increased the relative importance of AVP and ANG II in BP regulation.

In a similar study, endogenous levels of AVP were increased by an iv infusion of hypertonic NaCl *(24)*. In awake dogs with intact ABRs, the infusion of hypertonic saline resulted in an increase in plasma AVP and peripheral vascular resistance (PVR), and a decrease in cardiac output (CO). When the experiments were repeated in dogs following denervation of the ABRs, iv infusion of hypertonic NaCl resulted in an increase in mean arterial pressure (MAP) and PVR. The assumption that these changes were related to the direct action of AVP was subsequently tested in awake dogs, in which, when ganglionic blockade was initiated, infusion of NaCl increased MAP to a significantly greater extent than that observed with the autonomic nervous system intact *(24)*. Also, in SAD dogs, the increase in MAP, caused by an osmotic stimuli, was greater than in the intact dog, but similar to that in the intact dog with ganglionic blockade. Administration of the AVP V_1 receptor antagonist abolished the pressor response.

Several important points should be mentioned. First, the pressor response to hypertonic NaCl is opposed by the ABR, as indicated by the greater pressor response in SAD dogs, or during ganglionic blockade. Ganglionic blockade in SAD animals does not enhance the pressor response. Finally, the pressor responses in each condition is prevented by V_1 receptor blockade, indicating that AVP, and not the SNS, is involved.

HEART RATE, CORONARY BLOOD FLOW, AND CARDIAC FUNCTION

In addition to its direct action on the peripheral vascular system to increase resistance, AVP also alters CO. Two mechanisms are thought to contribute to the decrease in CO observed in response to large increases in systemic AVP concentrations. In dogs, rabbits, and rats, the depression in CO is primarily caused by a baroreflex decrease in heart rate (HR) *(13,15,17)*. In the dog, rabbit, and sheep, the decrease in HR involves the parasympathetic limb of the baroreflex *(16,28,29)*. In the rat, the decrease in HR is thought to involve a baroreflex-initiated decrease in sympathetic outflow to the sinoatrial (SA) node *(17)*, and is mediated via AVP V_2 receptors *(30)*. The reflex slowing of HR in the rabbit and dog during AVP administration is enhanced relative to the slowing observed with other pressor agents, suggesting that AVP may enhance the cardiac inhibitory influence of the ABR. In contrast to the rat, the reflex slowing of HR in the dog and rabbit appears to be blocked by AVP V_1 receptor antagonists *(31,32)*. There is little data to suggest that AVP has a direct effect on the SA nodes. In fact, in isolated myocardial cells, application of AVP does not alter the automaticity *(33)*.

In the isolated perfused rat heart, the addition of AVP to the perfusate results in a dose-dependent decrease in coronary blood flow. At high coronary vascular resistance, cardiac function is depressed *(34,35)*. These effects of AVP on coronary vascular resistance and cardiac function are prevented by pretreatment with the AVP V_1 receptor antagonist, $d(Ch_2)_5Tyr(Me)VAVP$ *(34)*. To determine whether AVP had an effect on cardiac function independent of its effects to reduce coronary blood flow, Walker et al. *(34)* evaluated the effects of AVP on cardiac contractile function when coronary blood flow was constantly maintained. At doses of AVP encountered in pathophysiological conditions, AVP caused a mild increase in cardiac contractility. Both the vasoconstrictor and contractility responses were blocked by the AVP V_1 receptor antagonists.

HYPERTENSION

Investigating endogenous factors that could initiate the development and maintenance of HT, ANG II and AVP are logical choices. Both hormones are involved in volume and electrolyte regulations *(4,5)*, and both have central and vascular actions that could contribute to chronic increases in BP *(36,37)*. However, less is known about the potential role of AVP in HT, which is certainly more controversial than ANG II. AVP is one of the more powerful vasoconstrictor agents, and, in experimental conditions, increases in circulating levels of AVP within the physiological range can cause marked increases in vascular resistances in rats, dogs, and humans *(4,5,14,17,18)*. The antidiuretic action of AVP, which involves renal tubular V_2 receptors, can result in significant expansion of body fluid volume *(38,39)*. Extended administration of AVP, together with constant H_2O intake, leads to substantial blood volume expansion.

In the normal conscious dog, increasing levels of AVP, with constant H_2O intake, results in an increase in MAP *(38,39)*. Under these conditions, the increase in MAP is not maintained, because the antidiuretic actions of AVP are opposed by pressure diuresis, resulting in renal escape *(38,40)*. However, if renal perfusion pressure is clamped at the control pressure, no escape occurs, and the elevated BP is maintained. When fluid balance is maintained, no HT develops, even though the level of circulating AVP is above levels required to increase arterial pressure.

AVP has also been shown to reduce medullary blood flow, an effect that may contribute to the development of HT *(41)*. There is also evidence suggesting AVP may increase systemic pressure via an action in the central nervous system *(36,42)*. In addition to these actions of AVP, which suggest the likelihood that AVP is involved in HT, there are studies suggesting that endogenous AVP is a contributing factor in certain models of HT. For example, the development of HT in spontaneously hypertensive rats (SHR) is attenuated by treatment with the AVP V_1 receptor antagonist *(43,44)*.

In studies involving both SHRs and stroke prone (SP) SHRs, administration of AVP antiserum, or chronic infusion of an AVP V_1V_2 receptor antagonist, $d(CH_2)_5$-D-Tyr(Me) VAVP, lowered BP *(45,46)*. In these studies, plasma AVP was elevated. However, it has also been reported *(47)* that plasma levels of AVP are unaltered in young SPSHRs and SHR, and that BP is unchanged in young SHRs in response to acute or chronic administration of the V_1 antagonist *(47)*. In SPSHRs, AVP V_1 vascular receptors contribute to BP in the malignant HT phase. Evidence that AVP may not be a major contributor to the elevation of BP in this model of HT is the lack of an apparent role of AVP in HT rats crossbred from SHRs and diabetes insipidus rats. These rats developed HT, even though they lacked measurable quantities of AVP *(48)*.

AVP may also contribute to the elevated pressure in other types of HT, including certain models of renal HT, in which plasma levels of AVP are elevated. In deoxycorticosterone acetate (DOCA)-salt models *(44)*, the HT is related to the plasma level of AVP, and can be attenuated with blockade of AVP. The role of AVP is underscored by the fact that Brattleboro rats, which are unable to secrete AVP, do not develop HT when treated with DOCA salt. However, when AVP is replaced, HT develops *(49)*. The involvement of AVP in this type of HT includes vascular (V_1 receptors) and renal (V_2 receptors) actions *(15)*. There is also indication that DOCA-salt HT involves a central action of AVP *(50)*.

Intravenous or intrarenal (medullary) administration of an AVP V_1 agonist (Phe^2, Ile^3, Orn^8) vasopressin V_1 agonist results in a sustained HT uninephrectomized rats. The HT to iv administration of V_1 agonist could be blocked by intrarenal injection of the V_1 antagonist into the renal medulla *(41,57)*. Moreover, intrarenal infusion of the V_1 agonist, at a rate that showed no evidence of spillover into the systemic circulation, also caused HT. In this situation, iv administration of a V_1 antagonist had no effect on lowering BP. The HT, resulting from administration of the V_1 agonist, occurred without evidence of sodium or volume retention. The authors suggest that the HT may depend on a reduction in renal medullary blood flow. Indeed, previous studies show that the injection of N_ω-nitro-L-arginine methyl ester (L-NAME), a nitric oxide synthase inhibitor, into the renal medulla decreased medullary blood flow and increased BP *(58)*. One theory is that the HT resulting from the administration of V_1 agonists into the renal medulla involves the release of a potent vasoconstrictor or the release of a vasodilator inhibitor into the circulation. In any case, the sustained HT appears to be nonadapting. An important point is that sustained increases in plasma levels of AVP, under circumstances in which V_2 receptors are downregulated, may lead to an increase in BP, especially if renal function is compromised. Thus, even though increases in circulating AVP do not seem to result in a sustained increase in MAP, it may be a contributing factor to an elevation in BP under certain circumstances.

Studies by Liard *(51,52)* have indicated that vascular smooth muscle expresses two types of AVP receptors. The V_1 receptor, when activated, causes vasocontriction and an increase in BP. The V_2 receptor initiates vasorelaxation and a fall in BP. Data suggest a time-dependent interaction between V_1 and V_2 receptors. Short exposures to AVP or AVP V_1 agonist attenuates the expression of V_2 agonism-dependent hemodynamic responses (increase in HR and CO); prolonged exposure to V_1 agonism appeared to sensitize the system to V_2 agonists. These observations suggest that acute increases in plasma AVP can produce vasoconstriction and an increase in BP, with little opposition from V_2 receptor activation, and that chronic elevation of AVP levels could lead to modulation of the initial vasoconstrictor actions of V_1 receptors by the V_2-mediated countereffect.

A recent study using isolated vascular smooth muscle cells (VSMC) showed that AVP, acting via V_2 receptors, enhanced agonist-stimulated increases in cyclic adenosine monophosphate (cAMP) formation by a Ca^{2+} calmodulin-dependent mechanism *(53)*. Thus, it seems likely that this or similar mechanisms may explain the time-dependent differences in the vascular response to acute vs chronic exposure to elevated AVP *(52)*. It should also be mentioned that prior exposure to AVP enhances the vasodilation to isoproterenol. Other studies have shown that AVP actions at the VSMC increases prostaglandin I2 *(54)*, and the action in the kidney releases prostaglandin E_2 *(55)*. There is also a report suggesting that hemodynamic responses to selective AVP V_2 agonists involved endothelial nitric oxide (NO) *(56)*. Because the study only showed that the vascular response to V_2 agonism was blocked by prior treatment with L-NAME, the effect may have been a permissive interaction, rather than a release of NO by activation of V_2 receptors on endothelial cells.

In another laboratory, the effects of chronic increases in plasma levels of AVP on BP was investigated in intact rats, in rats with ABR denervation (SAD), and in rats with lesions of the area postrema *(59)*. The rationale for this study was to determine if maintained physiological levels of AVP would increase BP or alter the autonomic mechanisms maintaining BP. A second objective was to determine AVP effects on BP when mechanisms responsible for the apparent sympathoinhibitory response to AVP were eliminated. This was accomplished by evaluating the BP response to chronic infusion of AVP in SAD rats, or in rats with lesions of the area postrema. Previous studies indicated that, after SAD, the BP response to acute increases in AVP was enhanced *(16)*. Also, studies in dogs and rabbits indicate that lesioning of the area postrema prevents the sympathoinhibitory response to acute increases in AVP. In this study, chronic infusion of AVP (0.2 or 2.0 ng/ kg/min) for 10 d did not affect resting BP or the autonomic mechanisms contributing to resting blood. Also, in SAD or area postrema-lesioned rats, chronic infusion did not have a consistent effect on BP *(59)*. The authors concluded that chronic administration of AVP did not lead to an alteration of the neural humoral factors contributing to BP. These findings are surprising, as other studies show that AVP has acute actions on neural mechanisms, plays a role in maintenance of BP during chronic increases in osmolality, and increases BP through actions on renal V_1 receptors.

Increased daily salt intake can lead to a slow-developing HT in the absence of functional ABRs. Evidence suggests that AVP is involved in this HT *(60,61)*. In SAD rats, an 8% NaCl diet for 21 d increased MAP 30 mmHg *(60)*. In uninephrectomized SAD rabbits, iv infusions of 10% NaCl for 10 d resulted in a substantial increase in MAP, which was associated with an increase in sodium retention and plasma levels of AVP and norepinephrine (NE) *(61)*. Intravenous administration of AVP V_1 antagonists prevented

HT and the increase in plasma NE levels. The data suggests that the HT and increased NE observed in the SAD uninephrectomized rabbit, in response to an intake of 10% NaCl, involved an elevated AVP. Previous studies showed that the sympathoinhibitory response to AVP is dependent on a functional baroreflex. Consequently, in the absence of ABR, increases in circulating AVP will result in an augmented pressure response *(62)*. The increase in plasma NE may involve an interaction between sodium and AVP, which has been suggested in several studies, but has not been fully investigated *(63–65)*.

The observations in the above studies indicate an interaction between AVP and baroreflexes. Conditions that lead to augmented levels of AVP may result in an AVP-dependent HT. Using a 2-kidney, 1-clip hypertensive rabbit model, the potential roles of AVP, RAS, and SNS in the maintenance of BP were examined *(66)*. Blockade of the RAS with captopril had little effect on MAP or renal sympathetic nerve activity (RSNA) in the normotensive or hypertensive rabbit. However, in the hypertensive model, AVP increased substantially following captopril. Intravertebral infusion of the AVP V_1 antagonist also had little effect on MAP or RSNA, when administered alone. However, following AVP V_1 blockade, administration of captopril resulted in a fall in MAP of approx 10 mmHg, which was accompanied by an exaggerated increase in RSNA relative to the fall in MAP. This exaggerated response was not specific to the removal of the RAS, because reducing pressure by a similar amount with nicardipine resulted in a similar exaggerated response to RSNA. These observations suggest an interaction between AVP and the SNS when BP is reduced in this model of HT. Because the sum of the separate responses to the decrease in MAP with AVP V_1 antagonist and the decreases in MAP with captopril or nicardipine is less than the combined responses to captopril plus AVP V_1 or nicardipine plus AVP V_1, there appears to be a facilitory interaction between the ABR and AVP.

INTERACTION WITH ARTERIAL
AND CARDIOPULMONARY REFLEXES

There is considerable evidence in the dog and rabbit that circulating AVP interacts with central mechanisms involved in regulating the sensitivity of the arterial and cardio-pulmonary reflexes *(13,16,31)*. The resulting effect of the interaction is that AVP enhances the sympathoinhibitory response of the ABR to afferent input from baroreceptor afferent receptors. When AVP is elevated, the central response to increases in afferent activity is enhanced, resulting in a greater inhibition in renal *(16)* or lumbar sympathetic activity *(67)*. In the rabbit, infusion of AVP causes decreases in RSNA, which occur prior to detectable increases in MAP. Thus, although circulating levels of AVP may not be expressed in terms of basal BP, they may be affecting the sympathoexcitatory states. An example of this can be observed in renal hypertensive rabbits. For example, infusion of AVP V_1V_2 receptor antagonist into the vertebral or systemic circulation, in renal hypertensive rabbits, has little effect on basal BP. Blocking AVP resulted in an exaggerated increase in RSNA when BP was reduced, suggesting that AVP exerted a tonic inhibitory influence on the baroreflex control of RSNA *(66)*.

In addition to the effects of AVP on H_2O retention and vascular tone, increases in circulating AVP also alter the arterial and cardiopulmonary baroreflex regulation of the sympathetic and parasympathetic nervous system. As noted previously, even though AVP is a potent vasoconstrictor, large doses are required before significant pressor responses are observed *(13)*. It is now known that AVP acts in the hindbrain to enhance the sympathoinhibitory response of ABRs. Accordingly, this action of AVP in the central nervous system acts to buffer its vasoconstrictor actions *(16)*. In the absence of ABRs, the pressor response to a given dose of AVP is far greater than that observed with other agents *(13,16,18,68)*. Infusing AVP in conscious rabbits results in a much greater decrease in RSNA and HR than observed with other pressor agents for similar increases in MAP. Denervation of the ABRs prevents the sympathoinhibitory response to increasing doses of AVP, indicating that sympathoinhibition by AVP is mediated via the ABRs *(69)*. Additional studies have shown that area postrema is also critical to the central action of AVP. In area postrema-lesioned rabbits or dogs, increases in AVP produced dose/pressure-dependent decreases in sympathetic outflow similar to that observed with other pressor substances.

Studies examining the total ABR function, obtained by increasing and decreasing arterial pressure, showed that AVP produced a dose-dependent decrease in the maximum sympathetic nerve activity when BP was reduced, and shifted the operating point of the baroreflex function to a lower arterial pressure *(75)*. A similar observation was also reported for HR baroreflex function *(21,32,70)*. The importance of this resetting is that it provides a mechanism whereby the level of sympathetic outflow can be changed without a change in arterial pressure. With increases in AVP, the resetting results in a lower level of sympathetic outflow relative to MAP. This resetting not only appears to enhance the sympathoinhibitory influence of the ABR, but it also limits the level of sympathoexcitation. In dogs, the endogenous release of AVP in response to bilateral carotid occlusion acts to limit the activation of the SNS *(71)*. A similar finding is also observed during interruption of cardiopulmonary afferents. It should also be mentioned that osmotic-stimulated release of AVP can also modulate the arterial and cardiopulmonary reflexes *(23)*. Endogenous release of AVP to physiological stimuli may play a key role in modulating the arterial and cardiopulmonary reflex control of the autonomic nervous system. The importance of this action of AVP lies in the resetting of the reflexes toward lower pressures.

The principle site in the central nervous system, which is required for circulating AVP to modulate the arterial and cardiopulmonary reflexes, appears to be the area postrema. The area postrema is a circumventricular organ in the hindbrain. The neurons in this region project to areas of the brain involved in cardiovascular regulation, including the medial nucleus of the tractus solitarius (NTS). Because the area postrema has an incomplete blood–brain barrier, the neurons in this region are exposed to circulating factors, and thus can serve as afferent inputs to the areas to which they project. Neurons in the area postrema have receptors for AVP *(72)*. The functional significance of these AVP receptors is documented by studies showing that surgical lesions of the area postrema eliminate the effects of AVP in enhancing the ABR inhibition of sympathetic nerve activity (SNA), which, as noted previously, involves a resetting of the ABR toward lower pressures *(70)*. The effectiveness of the lesion of the area postrema is not simply limited to the destruction of fibers of passage, because destruction of the area postrema neurons with kainic acid also prevents the AVP modulation of the arterial and cardiopulmonary reflexes *(73)*.

Microinjections of AVP into the area postrema caused dose-dependent decreases in SNA, and also enhanced sympathoinhibitory responses to increases in arterial pressure *(74–76)*. Although these studies provide indirect evidence for an action of AVP on neurons in the area postrema, more direct evidence was shown by studies in which microinjections of the AVP V_1 receptor antagonist into the area postrema prevented circulating AVP from enhancing the sympathoinhibitory influence on the arterial and cardiopulmonary reflexes (75). Since microinjection of similar amounts of the AVP V_1 antagonist into the adjacent NTS did not prevent the effects of AVP on the arterial and cardiopulmonary reflexes, it was concluded that circulating AVP acts on V_1 receptors in the area postrema to reset the reflex control of the arterial and cardiopulmonary reflexes.

Electrophysiological studies provide additional support for the concept that circulating AVP acts on area postrema neurons, which project to neurons in the NTS, altering their response to afferent input. Studies in the dog reported that application of AVP excited 50% of area postrema neurons (77). Circulating AVP was shown to affect the activity of spontaneously active area postrema neurons via a V_1 receptor (78). Additional electrophysiological studies, using the in vitro rabbit brain-slice preparation, provide additional insight about the potential interaction between projections from the area postrema to NTS barosensitive neurons. The basic procedure involved the demonstration that simultaneous low-level stimulations of area postrema neurons and the solitary tract produced NTS action potentials more often than would be predicted by a simple summation. The facilitory interaction was prevented by perfusion of the slice with an α2-antagonist, yohimbine. This in vitro data was supported by in vivo studies showing that the effects of circulating AVP on the ABR could be prevented by infusion of an α2-antagonist (79). In vivo electrophysiological studies in anesthetized rabbits have also shown that stimulation of the area postrema facilitates the response of NTS neurons to baroreceptor afferents. More recent studies using the rabbit brain slice showed that microinjection of AVP on the area postrema increased the activity of spontaneously active NTS neurons, and enhanced the response to evoked responses to stimulation of the solitary tract. These studies provide compelling evidence for an action of AVP on area postrema neurons that project to NTS neurons. The resulting effect is to enhance the response of NTS to afferent input.

SUMMARY

AVP is a critical hormone in the regulation of body water. This action of AVP is mediated by V_2 receptors on renal tubules. AVP also has several other actions that make this hormone important in the regulation of the cardiovascular system. First, AVP is a potent vasoconstrictor. Increases in plasma levels of AVP can alter regional vascular resistance via V_1 vascular receptors. In addition, AVP causes relaxation of vascular smooth muscle via V_2 receptors. There appears to be an interaction between the V_1 and V_2 receptors, in which V_1 receptors may initially inhibit the response to V_2 receptor activation. There are also recent studies suggesting that one of the resulting actions of AVP on V_2 receptors enhances the agonist-stimulated increase in cAMP.

Recent studies indicate that AVP also acts on V_1 receptors in the renal medulla, restricting blood flow to this region. It is postulated that the resulting sustained HT is caused by a release of a vasoconstrictor substance or the inhibition of a vasodilator. Finally, the central action of circulating AVP on V_1 receptors in the area postrema is also important in the regulation of the cardiovascular system. The resulting modulation of cardiovascular reflexes provides an instantaneous mechanism for altering autonomic outflow to the heart and peripheral circulation.

REFERENCES

1. Starling EH, Verney EB. The secretion of urine as studied on the isolated kidney. Proc R Soc Lond (Biol) 1924;97:321–363.
2. Verney EB. The antidiuretic hormone and the factors which determine its release. Proc R Soc Lond (B) Biol Sci 1947;135:25–105.
3. Scher RW, Berl T, Anderson RJ. Osmotic and nonosmotic control of vasopressin release. Am J Physiol 1979;236:F321–F332.
4. Cowley AW Jr. Vasopressin and cardiovascular regulation. In: Guyton AC, Hall JE, eds. Cardiovascular Physiology IV: International Reviews of Physiology, vol. 26. University Park, Baltimore, MD, 1982, pp. 189–242.
5. Share L. Role of vasopressin in cardiovascular regulation. Physiol Rev 1988;68:1248-1284.
6. Share L, Levy MN. Carotid sinus pulse pressure, a determinant of plasma antidiuretic hormone concentration. Am J Physiol 1966;211:721–724.
7. Chien S, Peric B, Usami S. Reflex nature of release of antidiuretic hormone upon common carotid occlusion in vagotomized dogs. Proc Soc Exp Biol Med 1962;111:193–196.
8. Usami S, Peric B, Chien S. Release of antidiuretic hormone due to common carotid occlusion and its relation with vagus nerve. Proc Soc Exp Biol Med 1962;111:189–196.
9. Share L. Control of plasma ADH titer in hemorrhage: role of atrial and arterial receptors. Am J Physiol 1968;215:1384–1389
10. Schrier RW, Berl T, Anderson RJ. Osmotic and nonosmotic control of vasopressin release. Am J Physiol 1979;236:F321–F332.
11. Thrasher TN, Brown CJ, Keil LC, Ramsay DJ. Thirst and vasopressin release in the dog: an osmoreceptor or sodium receptor mechanism? Am J Physiol 1980;238:R333–R339.
12. Ericksson L, Fernandez O, Olsson K. Differences in the antidiuretic response to intracarotid infusions of various hypertonic solutions in the conscious goat. Acta Physiol Scand 1971;83:554–562.
13. Cowley AW, Monos E, Guyton AC. Interaction of vasopressin and the baroreceptor reflex system in the regulation of arterial blood pressure in the dog. Circ Res 1974;34:505–514.
14. Montani JP, Liard JF, Schoun JF, Möhring JM. Hemodynamic effects of exogenous and endogenous vasopressin at low plasma concentrations in conscious dogs. Circ Res 1980;47:346–355.
15. Cowley AW, Liard JF. Vasopressin and arterial pressure regulation. Hypertension Dallas 1988; 11(Suppl I):125–132.
16. Undesser KP, Hasser EM, Haywood JR, Johnson KA, Bishop VS. Interactions of vasopressin with the area postrema in arterial baroreflex function in conscious rabbits. Circ Res 1985;56:410–417.
17. Webb RL, Osborn JW Jr, Cowley AW Jr. Cardiovascular actions of vasopressin: baroreflex modulation in the conscious rat. Am J Physiol 1986;251:H1244–H1251.
18. Osborn JW, Liard JF, Cowley AW Jr. Effect of AVP on pressor responses to peripheral sympathetic stimulation in the rat. Am J Physiol 1987;252:H675–H680.
19. Hay M, Bishop VS. Interactions of the area postrema and the solitary tract in the nucleus tractus solitarius. Am J Physiol 1991;260:H1466–H1473.
20. Nishida Y, Bishop VS. Vasopressin-induced suppression of renal sympathetic outflow depends upon the number of baroafferent inputs in rabbits. Am J Physiol 1992;263:R1187–R1194.
21. Bishop VS, Hasser EM, Nair UC. Baroreflex control of renal nerve activity in conscious animals. Circ Res 1987;61:I-76–I-81.
22. Burnier M, Biollaz J, Brunner DB, Brunner HR. Blood pressure maintenance in awake dehydrated rats: renin, vasopressin, and sympathetic activity. Am J Physiol 1983;245:H203–H209.
23. Hasser EM, Bishop VS, Neurogenic and humoral factors maintaining arterial pressure in conscious dogs. Am J Physiol 1988;255:R693–R698.
24. Hasser EM, Haywood JR, and Bishop VS, Role of vasopressin and sympathetic nervous system during hypertonic NaCl infusion in conscious dogs. Am J Physiol 1985;248:H652–H657.
25. Trapani AJ, Undesser KP, Keeton TK, Bishop VS. Neurohumoral interactions in conscious dehydrated rabbit. Am J Physiol 1988;254:R338–R347.
26. Aisenbrey GA, Handelman WA, Arnold P, Manning M, Schrier RW. Vascular effects of arginine vasopressin during fluid deprivation in the rat. J Clin Invest 1981;67:961–968.
27. Andrews CE, Brenner BM. Relative contributions of arginine vasopressin and angiotensin II to maintenance of systemic arterial pressure in the anesthetized water-deprived rat. Circ Res 1981;48:254–258.

28. Liard JF. Atropine potentiates the pressor effect of arginine vasopressin in conscious dogs. J Cardiovasc Pharmacol 1984;6:867–871.

29. Caine AC, Lumbers ER, Reid IA. Effects and interactions of angiotensin and vasopressin on the heart of unanesthetized sheep. J Physiol 1985;367:l–11.

30. Brizzee BL, Walker BR. Vasopressinergic augmentation of the cardiac baroreceptor reflex in conscious rats. Am J Physiol 1990;258:R860–868.

31. Hasser EM, Bishop VS. Reflex effect of vasopressin after blockade of V1 receptors in the area postrema. Circ Res 1990;67:265–271.

32. Luk J, Ajaelo I, Wong V, Wong J, Chang D, Chou L, Reid IA. Role of V1 receptors in the action of vasopressin on the baroreflex control of heart rate. Am J Physiol 1993;265:R524–R529.

33. Scott JA, Konstam M, Kolodny GM. Absence of a direct chronotropic effect of vasopressin on the myocardial cell. Pharmacology 1982;24:57–60.

34. Walker BR, Childs M, Merrill E. Direct cardiac effects of vasopressin: role of V1 and V2 vasopressinergic receptors. Am J Physiol 1988;255:H261–H265.

35. Boyle WA, Segel LD. Direct cardiac effects of vasopressin and their reversal by a vascular antagonist. Am J Physiol 1986;251:734–741.

36. Matsuguchi H, Schmid PG. Acute interaction of vasopressin and neurogenic mechanisms in DOC-salt hypertension. Am J Physiol 1982;242:H37–H43.

37. Phillips MI. Functions of angiotensin in the central nervous system. Ann Rev Physiol 1987;49:413–435.

38. Smith MJ Jr, Cowley AW Jr, Guyton AC, Manning RD Jr. Acute and chronic effects of vasopressin on blood pressure, electrolytes, and fluid volumes. Am J Physiol 1979;237:F232–F240.

39. Cowley AW Jr, Merrill DC, Quillen EW Jr, Skelton MM. Long-term blood pressure and metabolic effects of vasopressin with servo-controlled fluid volume. Am J Physiol 1984;247:R537–R545.

40. Hall JE, Montani JP, Woods LL, Mizelle HL. Renal escape from vasopressin: role of pressure diuresis. Am J Physiol 1986;250:F907–F916.

41. Cowley AW Jr, Szczepanska-Sadowska E, Stepniakowski K, Mattson D. Chronic intravenous administration of V1 arginine vasopressin agonist results in sustained hypertension. Am J Physiol 1994;267: H751–H756.

42. Szczepanska-Sadowska E, Noszczyk B, Lon S, Stepniakowski K, Budzikowski A, Paczwa P. Central AVP and blood pressure regulation: relevance to interspecies differences and hypertension. Ann NY Acad Sci 1993;689:677–679.

43. Crofton JT, Share L, Shade RE, Allen C, Tarnowski D. Vasopressin in the rat with spontaneous hypertension. Am J Physiol 1978;235:H361–366.

44. Crofton JT, Share L, Wang BC, Shade RE. Pressor responsiveness to vasopressin in the rat with DOC-salt hypertension. Hypertension Dallas 1980;2:424–431.

45. Möhring J, Kintz J, Schoun J. Studies on the role of vasopressin in blood pressure control of spontaneously hypertensive rats with established hypertension (SHR, stroke-prone strain). J Cardiovasc Pharmacol 1979;1:593–608.

46. Sladek CD, Blair ML, Sterling C, Mangiapane ML. Attenuation of spontaneous hypertension in rats by a vasopressin antagonist. Hypertension Dallas 1988;12:506–512.

47. Filep J, Fejes-Toth G. Does vasopressin sustain blood pressure in conscious spontaneously hypertensive rats? Hypertension 1986;8:514–519.

48. Ganten U, Rascher W, Lang RE, Dietz R, Rettig R, Unger T, Taugner R, Ganten D. Development of a new strain of spontaneously hypertensive rats homozygous for hypothalamic diabetes insipidus. Hypertension 1983;5(Suppl l):I119–I128.

49. Crofton JT, Share L, Shade RE, Lee-Kwon WJ, Manning M, Sawyer WH. Importance of vasopressin in the development and maintenance of hypertension in the rat. Hypertension 1979;1:31–38.

50. Swords BH, Wyss JM, Berecek KH. Vasopressin and vasopressin receptors are enhanced in the central nervous system in deoxycorticosterone-NaCl hypertension. In: Jard S, Jamison R. eds. Vasopressin. John Libbey Eurotext, Paris, 1991, pp. 409–417.

51. Liard JF. Peripheral vasodilation induced by vasopressin analogue with selective V2 agonism in dogs. Am J Physiol 1989;256:H1621–H1626.

52. Liard JF. Interaction between V1 and V2 effects in hemodynamic response to vasopressin in dogs. Am J Physiol 1990;258:H482–H489.

53. Zhang J, Sato M, Duzic E, Kubalak SW, Lanier SM, Webb JG. Adenylyl cyclase isoforms and vasopressin enhancement of agonist-stimulated cAMP in vascular smooth muscle cells. Am J Physiol 1997; 273:H971–H980.

54. Vallotton MB, Gerber-Wicht C, Dolci W, Wuthrich RP. Interaction of vasopressin and angiotensin II in stimulation of prostacyclin synthesis in vascular smooth muscle cells. Am J Physiol 1989;257:E617–E624.
55. Wuthrich RP, Vallotton MB. Prostaglandin E2 and cyclic AMP response to vasopressin in renal medullary tubular cells. Am J Physiol 1986;251:F499–F505.
56. Liard JF. L-Name antagonizes vasopressin V2-induced vasodilation in dogs. Am J Physiol 1994; 266:H99–H106.
57. Szczepanska-Sadowska E, Stepniakowski K, Skelton MM, Cowley AW Jr. Prolonged stimulation of intrarenal V1 vasopressin receptors results in sustained hypertension. Am J Physiol 1994;267: R1217–R1225.
58. Mattson DL, Lu S, Nakanishi K, Papanek PE, Cowley AW Jr. Effect of chronic renal medullary nitric oxide inhibition on blood pressure. Am J Physiol 1994;266:H1918–H1926.
59. Pawloski CM, Eicker NM, Ball LM, Mangiapane ML, Fink GD. Effect of circulating vasopressin on arterial pressure regulation in rats. Am J Physiol 1989;257:H209–H218.
60. Osborn JW, Provo BJ. Salt-dependent hypertension in the sinoaortic-denervated rat. Hypertension 1992;19:658–662.
61. Ryuzaki M, Suzuki H, Kumagai K, Kumagai H, Ichikawa M, Matsumura Y, Saruta T. Role of vasopressin in salt-induced hypertension in baroreceptor-denervated uninephrectomized rabbits. Hypertension 1991;17:1085–1091.
62. Nishida Y, Bishop VS. Vasopressin-induced suppression of renal sympathetic outflow depends on the number of baroafferent inputs in rabbits. Am J Physiol 1992;263:R1187–R1194.
63. Matsuguchi H, Schmid PG, Van Orden D, Mark AL. Does vasopressin contribute to salt-induced hypertension in the Dahl strain? Hypertension 1981;3:174–181.
64. Berecek KH, Webb RL, Brody MJ. Evidence for a central role for vasopressin in cardiovascular regulation. Am J Physiol 1983;244:H852–H859.
65. Gavras H, Gavras I. Salt-induced hypertension: the interactive role of vasopressin and of the sympathetic nervous system. J Hypertens 1989;7:601–606.
66. Kumagai H, Suzuki H, Ichikawa M, Matsumura Y, Jimbo M, Ryuzaki M, Saruta T. Central and peripheral vasopressin interact differently with sympathetic nervous system and renin-angiotensin system in renal hypertensive rabbits. Circ Res 1993;72:1255–1265.
67. Scheuer DA, Bishop VS. Effect of vasopressin on baroreflex control of lumbar sympathetic nerve activity and hindquarter resistance. Am J Physiol 1996;270:H1963–H1971.
68. Montani JP, Liard JF, Schoun J, Möhring J. Hemodynamic effects of exogenous and endogenous vasopressin at low plasma concentrations in conscious dogs. Circ Res 1980;47:346–355.
69. Hay M, Hasser EM, Undesser KP, Bishop VS. Role of baroreceptor afferents on area postrema-induced inhibition of sympathetic activity. Am J Physiol 1991;260:H1353–H1358.
70. Nishida Y, Bishop VS. Vasopressin-induced suppression of renal sympathetic outflow depends upon the number of baroafferent inputs in rabbits. Am J Physiol 1992;263:R1187–R1194.
71. DiCarlo SE, Stahl LK, Hasser EM, Bishop VS. Role of vasopressin in the pressor response to bilateral carotid occlusion. J Autonom Nerv Syst 1989;27:1–10.
72. Phillips PA, Kelly JM, Abrahams JM, Gyzonka Z, Paxinos G, Mendelsohn FA, Johnston CI. Vasopressin receptors in rat brain and kidney: studies using a radio-iodinated V1 receptor antagonist. J Hypertension 1988;6(Suppl):S550–S553.
73. Cox B, Bishop VS. Neurons in area postrema mediate vasopressin-induced enhancement of the baroreflex. Am J Physiol 1990;258:H1943–H1946.
74. Suzuki S, Takeshita A, Imaizumi T, Hirook Y, Yoshida M, Ando S, Nakamura M. Central nervous system mechanisms involved in inhibition of renal sympathetic nerve activity induced by arginine vasopressin. Circ Res 1989;65:1390–1399.
75. Hasser EM, Bishop VS. Reflex effect of vasopressin after blockade of V1 receptors in the area postrema. Circ Res 1990;67:265–271.
76. Zhang X, Abdel-Rahman AR, Wooles WR. Vasopressin receptors in the area postrema differentially modulate baroreceptor responses in rats. Eur J Pharmacol 1992;222:81–91.
77. Carpenter DO, Briggs DBJ, Knox AP, Strominger N. Excitation of area postrema neurons by transmitters, peptides, and cyclic nucleotides. J Neurophysiol 1988;59:358–369.
78. Smith PM, Lowes VL, Ferguson AV. Circulating vasopressin influences area postrema neurons. Neuroscience 1993;59:185–195.
79. Hasser EM, Bishop VS. Role of alpha-adrenergic mechanisms on responses to area postrema stimulation and circulating vasopressin. Am J Physiol 1993;265:H530–H536.

8

Insulin and the Heart

*Roger W. Brownsey, Brian Rodrigues,
Subodh Verma, and John H. McNeill*

INTRODUCTION

This chapter outlines the aspects of heart function and metabolism that are modulated by insulin, and explores the biochemical mechanisms that account for the actions of the hormone. The actions of insulin on the heart must be viewed in the context of the constant and dynamic function of the organ, and also with respect to the complex set of endocrine, paracrine, and neural signals to which myocardial cells are exposed in vivo. The focus is on the metabolic responses, because these have been particularly well documented. The actions of insulin on heart metabolism have been established on the basis of studies in vitro with isolated cells or perfused tissue, as well as on clinical and experimental in vivo studies.

INSULIN AND MECHANICAL FUNCTION OF CARDIAC MUSCLE

Insulin contributes to acute and chronic regulation of the mechanical function of the heart. The importance of insulin (directly or indirectly) in the long-term maintenance of the mechanical function of the heart is revealed by the decline in heart function observed during chronic insulin deficiency, characterized by microangiopathy *(1)*, abnormalities in vascular sensitivity and reactivity to various ligands, altered cardiac autonomic function *(2)*, and an increased stiffness of the ventricular wall associated with perivascular

From: *Contemporary Endocrinology: Hormones and the Heart in Health and Disease*
Edited by: L. Share © Humana Press Inc., Totowa, NJ

thickening of basement membranes and interstitial accumulation of connective tissue and glycoproteins *(3,4)*. The systemic and vascular consequences of insulin deficiency are extremely important in this pathophysiology, but, in addition, there is compelling evidence for a specific diabetic cardiomyopathy that underlines long-term actions of insulin on the heart, which are crucial for maintenance of function, and which involve regulation of the expression of contractile and ion transport proteins *(3–6)*.

Rapid, positive inotropic effects of insulin on the heart were first observed using crude pancreatic extracts *(7)*, and have been confirmed in work using dog heart–lung preparations treated with partially purified insulin *(8)*, and, ultimately, in studies with homogeneous hormone in a variety of experimental models *(9,10)*. Positive inotropic effects also contribute to the cardioprotective effect of insulin during heart failure; effects that are enhanced in the presence of glucose and independent of changes in coronary flow *(11)*. The possibility that the positive inotropic effects of insulin might be mediated by hypoglycemia and subsequent sympathetic nerve function has been discounted *(12)*. It must be stressed that not all studies support the role of insulin as an inotropic agent in the heart. Thus, insulin has been shown to antagonize the positive inotropic effects of norepinephrine *(13)*, or to have no effects on cardiac output in rats or dogs during sustained infusion in euglycemic, hyperinsulinemic clamps *(14)*. On the other hand, several well-controlled clinical studies have revealed acute effects of insulin on cardiac output, notably caused by a rise in stroke volume at physiological insulin concentrations *(15)*.

Despite evidence indicating that insulin may exert a rapid and positive effect on cardiac contractility, it seems improbable that this effect will play a singular or dominant role in dictating the function of the heart physiologically, especially considering the slow time-course over which insulin concentrations change, and the rapid fluctuations in demands on the heart. It seems more reasonable to conclude that insulin modulates cardiac contractility by more permissive actions, being mediated by longer-term effects on expression of proteins involved in electrical and contractile activity, as well as rapid effects on ion transport, on the metabolic status of the heart, and perhaps on the blood flow through the myocardium.

INSULIN AND REGULATION OF MYOCARDIAL CONTRACTILE AND ION TRANSPORT PROTEINS

At the cellular level, chronic insulin deficiency results in changes in contractile proteins, and in subcellular organelles and proteins that control ion movements. The Ca^{2+}-ATPase activities of myosin and actomyosin are depressed following chronic hypoinsulinemia, and this depression is associated with a myosin isoenzyme shift (V1–V3). This is important, because the V3 isoenzyme exhibits lower specific ATPase activity, resulting in a decreased shortening velocity of cardiac muscle *(16–18)*. On a more general energetic level, mitochondrial oxidative capacity and Mg^{2+}-ATPase and Ca^{2+} uptake activities have all been demonstrated to be depressed in the diabetic myocardium *(19)*.

Several ion transport systems in the myocardium are also adversely impacted by chronic insulin deficiency. Sarcolemmal ion transport systems that develop defects during diabetes include Na^+-K^+-ATPase *(20)*, potassium currents *(21)*, and Ca^{2+} pump activity *(22)*. Calcium transport by the sarcoplasmic reticulum (SR) is another mechanism by which myocardial levels of Ca^{2+} are modulated. The SR participates in the relaxation of the heart by actively accumulating Ca^{2+} from the cytoplasmic space, and any alteration in the ability of this organelle to sequester Ca^{2+} ions efficiently would be expected to have an impact on relaxation. During diabetes, SR Ca^{2+} binding and Ca^{2+}-Mg^{2+}-ATPase activity are depressed, leading to a defect in SR Ca^{2+} transport, which then correlates with a slower relaxation *(23–25)*.

It should be noted that all of the above chronic changes were observed in isolated whole hearts obtained from animals that had been made moderately diabetic with low doses of streptozotocin (STZ, 55–60 mg/kg). More recently, it was demonstrated that more severe diabetes, induced with higher doses of STZ (100 mg/kg), led to rapid changes in shortening and relengthening of isolated myocytes, associated with impaired Ca^{2+} sequestration or extrusion, within 4–6 d after STZ treatment *(26)*. Comparable in vitro studies have revealed that culture of normal ventricular myocytes in the presence of high concentrations of glucose and low insulin, leads to abnormal ventricular relaxation similar to that observed following induction of diabetes in vivo. The effect of insulin deficiency, coupled with hyperglycemia in vitro, was inducible within 1 d, and was associated with impaired Ca^{2+} homeostasis *(27)*.

Insulin also exerts rapid effects on a number of additional ion transport mechanisms, which could play an important role in modulating cardiac contractility. These rapid effects of insulin must, of course, be considered within the context of complex external and intrinsic mechanisms involved in the regulation of cardiac electrical activity. On a global level, insulin influences membrane potential *(28)*, and induces a decline in plasma potassium *(29)* that is matched by corresponding uptake into tissues *(30)*. As a corollary, circulating potassium levels are elevated in diabetes *(31)*. The overall effects of insulin on ion balance reflect changes in the functions of several key membrane transport systems, although the truly primary actions are not always unambiguously defined. The ion transporters that are most notably responsive to insulin include the Na^+/H^+ antiporter *(32)*, the Na^+/K^+-ATPase *(33)*, a cation channel *(34)*, and a $Na^+/K^+/2Cl$-co-transporter *(35)*. A rapid and direct interaction between insulin receptor substrate (IRS) protein and Ca^{2+}-ATPase has also been observed *(36)*. The extent to which insulin leads to corresponding changes in the relevant transport systems in the heart merit concerted examination. Understanding the mechanisms by which insulin influences ion transport will also provide critical insights into insulin action generally, especially considering the power of patch-clamping techniques.

EFFECTS OF INSULIN ON MYOCARDIAL PERFUSION

Because of the reliance of the myocardium on oxidative metabolism, a significant restriction to myocardial blood flow has serious consequences for the function and, indeed, for the survival of cardiac myocytes. Acute and chronic effects of insulin may be significant in contributing to the adequacy of perfusion of the coronary circulation. There is increasing evidence that, in the short-term, insulin may stimulate blood flow through skeletal muscle beds *(15)* by enhancing the formation of nitric oxide in vascular endothelium *(37)*, and therefore inducing relaxation of the associated vascular smooth muscle. These local effects of insulin are compounded by central actions that lead to stimulation of sympathetic neural activity *(38)*. It will be important to establish whether similar local effects are induced directly in myocardial vascular smooth muscle. Appropriate response systems are certainly present, and there appear to be complex functions for nitric oxide within the myocardium *(39)*. More generally, insulin may contribute to tonic control of vascular smooth muscle and peripheral blood pressure (and therefore the load against which the heart must pump). Certainly, insulin resistance is frequently associated with hypertension *(40)*, and agents directed at correcting insulin resistance may correct defects in blood pressure *(41)*.

In addition to rapid effects on vascular wall function, defects in insulin secretion or action may contribute significantly to development of impaired tissue perfusion, as a result of the pathogenesis of macrovascular (atherosclerosis) and microvascular disease *(40)*. The decline in vascular function progresses over many years, ranging from modest changes in responsiveness and permeability to loss of elasticity and outright occlusion. The consequences of this process include compromised perfusion and function of the heart, and finally necrosis of tissue significantly deprived of blood flow. A detailed discussion is beyond the scope of this chapter, but there is compelling evidence to suggest that loss of insulin sensitivity may play a key role in the development of abnormalities that are major risk factors for atherosclerosis, notably hyperinsulinemia, hypertriglyceridemia, elevated very low density lipoprotein, reduced high-density lipoprotein (and associated cholesterol levels), impaired glucose tolerance or frank hyperglycemia, and hypertension *(40,41)*. The association between insulin resistance and atherosclerosis has also been noted in major prospective clinical studies *(42)*.

ROLES OF INSULIN IN DELIVERY OF METABOLIC FUELS TO THE HEART

The perpetual functional demand on the heart is reflected by dense vascularization of the myocardium and a reliance on oxidative metabolism, indicated by abundance of mitochondria, which occupy close to 30% of myocardial cell volume *(43)*. The oxidative capacity of the heart provides the ability to utilize long-chain fatty acids as a predominant metabolic fuel, and also to oxidize glucose and lactate under most conditions, as well as ketones when available *(44)*.

Insulin plays a major role in regulating the balance of metabolic fuels received by the myocardium, principally through its actions on adipose tissue, skeletal muscle, and liver, in counterpoint to the catabolic effects of glucagon, catecholamines, and other hormones (Fig. 1). The effects of insulin on protein metabolism may be especially significant in regulating substrate availability to the heart. The ability of insulin to suppress protein degradation, notably in skeletal muscle, profoundly affects overall carbohydrate and nitrogen economy *(45,46)*. In insulin deficiency, therefore, the increase in supply of amino acids from net protein catabolism provides precursors for hepatic gluconeogenesis and ketogenesis, and contributes to the balance of substrates delivered to the myocardium.

Another critical action of insulin is inhibition of adipose tissue triglyceride hydrolysis (regulating the actions of lipolytic hormones), because this action dictates levels of long-chain fatty acids released to enter a complex with circulating serum albumin. The loss of regulation of adipose tissue lipolysis is most exaggerated in poorly controlled insulin-dependent diabetes or cachexia, but is also evident in postabsorptive metabolism in the normal 24-h cycle *(45–47)*. The increased availability of fatty acids leads to enhanced β-oxidation at the expense of pyruvate oxidation in cardiac myocytes and other cells with sufficient oxidative capacity. The glucose–fatty acid cycle *(48)*, therefore, provides a critical mechanism to conserve glucose for cells with less metabolic flexibility (neurons and blood cells, for example).

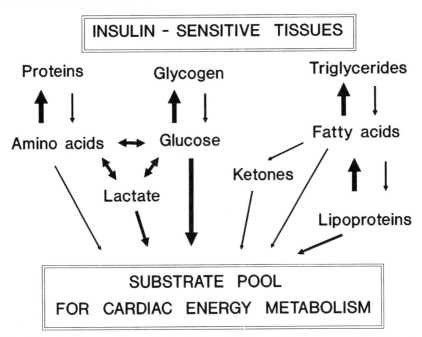

Fig. 1. Insulin and delivery of metabolic fuels to the heart. This summary illustrates the major actions of insulin on a range of insulin-sensitive tissues, which establish the balance of metabolic fuels carried in the blood as the substrate pool for cardiac energy metabolilsm. Quantitatively, the most important noncardiac targets for insulin action are skeletal muscle, white fat, and liver. Under most conditions, the heart is exposed to a constant concentration of glucose. Long-chain fatty acids represent the dominant metabolic fuel consumed in the myocardium; long-chain acyl-CoA esters are derived from circulating fatty acid–albumin complexes, circulating lipoproteins, or intramyocardial triacylglycerols. Prominent rapid effects of insulin on the noncardiac tissues include suppression (thin arrows) of fatty acid release from white fat, of glycogenolysis (in liver and skeletal muscle), of gluconeogenesis (in liver), and of proteolysis (most significantly in skeletal muscle). Furthermore, the anticatabolic effects of insulin are complemented by positive stimulation (bold arrows) of fuel storage in fat, liver, and skeletal muscle. Significant sources of lactate include exercising skeletal muscle, gut, and adipose tissue. Circulating ketones are likely to accumulate only during extended starvation or catabolic states, such as uncontrolled Type I diabetes. Lipoprotein supply to the heart is restriacted by effects of insulin on hepatic VLDL synthesis and secretion, and by effects on adipose tissue LPL and hormone-sensitive lipase.

Increases in circulating free fatty acids in insulin deficiency have important effects on the liver that also contribute to changes in substrate delivery to the heart. Particularly important is the stimulation of synthesis and export of complex lipoproteins by elevated delivery of free fatty acids to the liver *(49,50)*. During starvation, the circulating lipoprotein-triglycerides are predominantly accessed by skeletal and cardiac muscles, because lipoprotein lipase activity is maintained in these tissues, but declines in adipose tissue *(51)*. In diabetes, however, functional lipoprotein lipase declines in skeletal muscle and heart, as well as in adipose tissue, thus contributing significantly to diabetic hyperlipoproteinemia *(52)*.

DIRECT ACTIONS OF INSULIN ON CARDIAC METABOLISM

The actions of insulin on the metabolism of cardiac myocytes involves effects on the expression of proteins and on the acute control of enzyme and transport protein activity. In general, increases in insulin concentrations lead to enhanced uptake and oxidation of

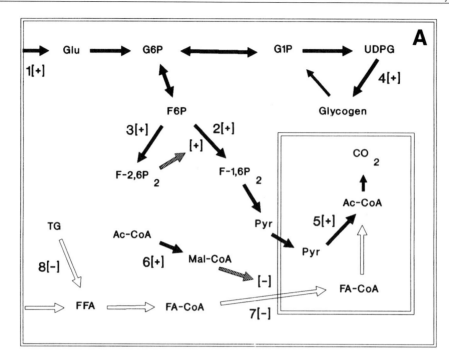

Fig. 2. Rapid effects of insulin on myocardial energy metabolism. Primary effects of insulin include the activation (+) of glucose transport, glycolysis, glycogen synthesis, and pyruvate oxidation. Insulin also leads to increased production of malonyl-CoA (Mal-CoA), therefore leading to inhibition of transport of fatty acyl-CoA esters (FA-CoA) across the mitochondrial membrane, via carnitine palmitoyltransferase-I. The supply of FA-CoA is also restricted by inhibition of myocardial hormone-sensitive lipase. (**A**) An overview of some of the principal steps in myocardial energy metabolism; (**B**) the numbering of the insulin-sensitive proteins discussed.

B

Protein	Proposed mechanism of response to insulin	References
1. Glucose transporters (GLUTs)	Principally GLUT-4, but also GLUT-1, are activated by translocation to sarcolemma/T-tubules.	[62-78]
2. 6-Phosphofructo-1-kinase (PFK-1)	Activated by increase in fructose 2,6-bisphosphate (via PFK-2). Increases in [5'-AMP] & decreases in [citrate] may also contribute.	[83-85]
3. 6-Phosphofructo-2-kinase (PFK-2)	Increased substrate supply via GLUTs and hexokinase, plus direct phosphorylation and activation by PKB etc	[85-89]
4. Glycogen synthase	Enhanced substrate supply and allosteric activation via G6P, plus dephosphorylation of multiple sites.	[111-121]
5. Pyruvate dehydrogenase complex (PDC)	PDC activation via decreased [acetyl-CoA]/[CoA] and [NADH/NAD]. Insulin effects apparently do not persist in isolated mitochondria.	[93-106]
6. Acetyl-CoA carboxylase (ACC)	Distinct cardiac isoform not fully characterized. Activation may involve specific site phosphorylation/dephosphorylation and allosteric control.	[155-161]
7. Carnitine palmitoyltransferase (CPT-I)	Inhibited by increase in [malonyl-CoA], the product of ACC. Sensitivity to malonyl-CoA may be increased.	[150-154]
8. Hormone-sensitive lipase	Presumed to be via dephosphorylation of one or more PKA sites. Activation of PDE-III may contribute to counter effects of PKA. Control of re-esterification may also dictate net flux.	[140-147]

Insulin

Synthesis, secretion, vascular transit, clearance

⬇

Insulin Receptor

Insulin-induced conformational activation,
autophosphorylation, kinase activation

⬇

Insulin Receptor Substrate Proteins

Tyrosyl phosphorylation of multiple receptor substrates

⬇

Recruitment and Activation of Enzyme Complexes

Receptor substrates provide nucleus for protein-protein complexes,
involving lipid and protein kinases and phosphatases, adaptors etc

⬇

Signalling Pathways to Functional Responses

Multiple pathways mediated by :
(i) activation of PI 3-kinases and generation of phosphoinositides,
(ii) activation of Ras-GTPases and their targets, (iii) others ?

⬇

Regulation and Crosstalk Controls

Multiple steps of regulation involve :
(i) Covalent controls via PTPases, Ser/Thr kinases, etc
(ii) Steric controls via small mediators and proteins
(iii) intracellular re-localization/traffic

Fig. 3. Overview of insulin signaling.

carbohydrates at the expense of fatty acid oxidation. In concert, insulin suppresses protein catabolism, while stimulating net synthesis of specific proteins, and of glycogen and lipid reserves (Fig. 2). Proteins important in energy metabolism, which are rapidly activated in response to insulin, include glucose transporters, phosphofructokinases, and glycogen synthase. Flux through pyruvate dehydrogenase and acetyl-CoA carboxylase also increase in response to insulin, and contributes importantly to enhanced pyruvate oxidation with restriction of fatty acid β-oxidation (notably at the level of the carnitine palmitoyltransferase-1) (Fig. 2). Mechanisms by which signals from the insulin receptor are transmitted to intracellular targets have been extensively reviewed, but are still not completely understood (Fig. 3). Specific details of insulin signaling in the heart are even more fragmentary. Here, the authors focus on a specific set of insulin target proteins in the heart that play critical roles in acute metabolic control. A detailed consideration of the multiple and complex effects of insulin action on gene expression and protein synthesis are beyond the scope of this chapter, but have been reviewed recently (46,53–55).

Glucose Transport

Early studies in the laboratories of Neely and Morgan (44) established that insulin stimulated the uptake of glucose by perfused rat hearts. Furthermore, perfused hearts from diabetic animals display markedly depressed rates of basal glucose utilization *(44,56)*. In many earlier studies, hearts were perfused by the non-working Langendorff method, with glucose as the sole substrate. Intracellular concentrations of glucose were low in the absence of insulin (less than 1 mM), rising markedly following insulin stimulation (as high as 12 mM), and therefore exceeding the K_m of hexokinase. This suggested that glucose metabolism was limited by glucose transport in the absence of insulin, and that hexokinase (or further downstream metabolic enzymes) made important contributions to flux control following insulin stimulation. This concept has been reinforced by others, and was recently confirmed in studies of individual myocardial cells *(57)*, and in studies with isolated, working, perfused hearts *(58)*.

An important caveat to the interpretation of the studies with glucose as sole exogenous substrate became evident with the recognition that fatty acids suppress glucose utilization by heart and skeletal muscle *(59–61)*. Quantitative aspects of insulin action on glucose transport are therefore most reliably reflected in studies in vivo, or in which physiologically relevant concentrations of fatty acids are also supplied in vitro. Even so, basal rates of glucose transport into heart cells are markedly higher, and effects of insulin appreciably smaller, than in skeletal muscle or adipose tissue *(62)*.

Compared to other insulin-responsive tissues, heart muscle expresses among the highest levels so far detected of the insulin-sensitive glucose transporter (GLUT)-4 isoform *(62–64)*. The level of expression of GLUT-4 in heart muscle is equivalent to that seen in brown adipose tissue, 2–5-fold higher than in several subtypes of red skeletal muscle, and substantially higher than in white skeletal muscle and adipose tissue. The ratio of GLUT-1:GLUT-4 in heart muscle (approx 1:3) means that the expression of the GLUT-1 isoform is also substantial in the heart. GLUT-1 probably accounts for the high rates of glucose transport in the absence of insulin, and to the fact that the proportional increase on insulin stimulation (not more than three- or fourfold) is substantially smaller than the stimulation observed in skeletal muscle or adipose tissue (10–40-fold).

Another important characteristic of muscle cells is exercise-induced stimulation of glucose transport, which is insulin-independent *(65)*. Similarly, increases in cardiac work are associated with increased glucose consumption *(44)*, and contraction-induced stimulation appears to preclude further activation by insulin *(66)*. The significance of insulin stimulation of myocardial glucose transport must therefore be considered in the context of the effects dictated by mechanical demands of the heart, especially because catecholamines and Ca^{2+} ions may also activate glucose transport independently of insulin *(67)*.

The stimulation of glucose transport in fat cells by insulin is mostly accounted for by the translocation of GLUT-4 from intracellular membranes to the plasma membrane *(68,69)*. Similarly, translocation of GLUT-1 and GLUT-4 has been demonstrated in perfused hearts *(70)* and in isolated cardiac myocytes *(71)*. In muscle cells, the intracellular reserve of GLUTs appears in tubulovesicular structures associated with the trans Golgi *(71,72)*. Further, the T-tubule system of muscle cells may contribute significantly as a destination for insulin-stimulated relocation of GLUTs *(73)*.

GLUT traffic probably proceeds by membrane-trafficking mechanisms similar to those established for secretion and neurotransmission *(74)*. Proteins important in membrane fusion, which may be involved in GLUT traffic in the heart, include NEM-sensitive factor and soluble NSF attachment protein 25, the plasma membrane SNAP receptors syntaxin-1A and -1B, the GLUT-4 vesicle-associated membrane protein (VAMP)2, cellubrevin/VAMP3, synaptobrevin-2, and the vp165/aminopeptidase *(74–77)*.

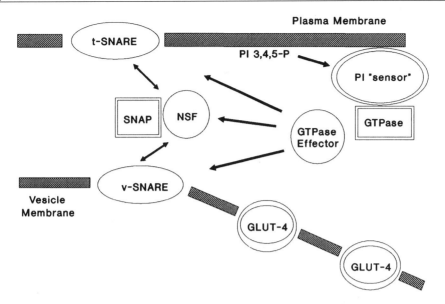

Fig. 4. Possible scenario for insulin signaling to glucose transport. Plasma membrane and GLUT-containing vesicle membranes must be brought into contact to allow GLUT protein translocation. In this scenario, membrane contacts require target (t) and vesicle (v) membrane SNAREs, bridged by NSF/SNAP complexes. Candidate t-SNAREs include syntaxins-1A, -1B; v-SNAREs might include VAMPs-2,-3, synaptobrevin-2 and Vp165. The building and/or stabilization of this membrane–membrane contact, and subsequent steps required for fusion and GLUT relocation, are sensitive to switch controls exerted by GTPases (perhaps including Rabs, ARFs, or dynamin). The insulin signals might intercede at the level of these GTPase via proteins such as Grp1 or centaurin-α, which are receptors for the polyphosphoinositide products of insulin-activated PI 3-kinases (PI "Sensor" in figure). Grps may then regulate trafficking GTPases, which, in turn, influence the SNAP/SNARE assembly. The dominant effect of insulin is to stimulate recruitment of GLUTs into the plasma membrane. However, control of endocytosis and recycling through complex intracellular membrane pools (here omitted) must also be defined.

Insulin signaling to GLUT traffic systems is not yet completely understood, though rapid progress is being made (Fig. 4). GLUT-4 activation is mediated by signaling via IRS proteins to p85/p110 isoform of phosphatidylinositol-3'-OH-kinase (PI 3-kinase) *(78)*. Beyond the production of 3-phospho-inositides, the picture of signaling to GLUT-4 is less clear. A link from PI 3-kinase to the traffic machinery might be provided by polyphosphoinositide-binding proteins that are able to interact with GTPases. Candidates identified so far include general receptor for phosphoinositides (Grp)1, which can potentially act as a guanine nucleotide exchange factor for GTPases such as Rab and ARF protein *(74)*. These GTPases must then interface with the budding and fusion apparatus to effect GLUT flux between membrane sites (Fig. 4).

Besides inducing rapid GLUT translocation, insulin also contributes to the longer-term expression of GLUTs. The expression of GLUT-1 and basal glucose transport rates declined in the heart with 48-h starvation, but GLUT-4 levels and maximal stimulation by insulin were not appreciably affected *(62,64)*. Chronic diabetes following STZ treatment leads to reduced myocardial GLUT-4 expression *(79,80)*, although no changes in expression were detected up to several days after STZ treatment *(64)*. Clinically, in Type I (insulin-dependent) or Type II diabetics, glucose uptake into skeletal muscle displays insulin resistance during euglycemic, hyperinsulinemic clamps, but uptake into heart muscle is normal *(81,82)*.

Glycolysis and Pyruvate Oxidation

In addition to its effects on glucose transport, insulin also induces activation of phosphofructokinases, hexokinase, and the pyruvate dehydrogenase complex (PDC), all of which contribute notably to control of glucose metabolism. Changes in flux through glycolysis are broadly coordinated with rates of pyruvate oxidation; both are increased as the workload of glucose-perfused hearts is increased, and also stimulated, in response to insulin *(44)*. Uncoupling of glycolysis and pyruvate oxidation is possible: This is most apparent in hypoxia or anoxia, when glycolysis is markedly activated, but terminal oxidation of pyruvate and fatty acids is precluded. In fact, even under normoxic conditions, flux through glycolysis is not perfectly coordinated with that through glucose oxidation and conditions such as cardiac hypertrophy and ischemia/reperfusion may further disrupt the balance between glycolysis and glucose oxidation, *(61,83)*.

The regulation of 6-phosphofructo-1-kinase (PFK-1) is critical in the control of glycolysis. In the presence of normal tissue levels of ATP and citrate, the enzyme is substantially inhibited *(84)*. Activation of PFK-1 is achieved by the generation of activators (deinhibitors), rather than by removal of citrate or ATP. One activator, 5'-AMP is likely to be sufficiently abundant only when oxidative metabolism cannot match energy demand. Fructose 2,6-*bis*-phosphate, the product of the dual-function 6-phoshofructo-2-kinase (PFK-2): fructose 2,6-*bis*-phosphatase, is a critical modulator of cardiac PFK-1, because it is able to overcome the inhibitory effects of ATP *(85)*. Intramyocardial concentrations of fructose 2,6-bisphosphate are increased in response to insulin and epinephrine, and also during increases in cardiac workload, thereby contributing to the corresponding increases in rates of glycolysis *(86–88)*. The cardiac form of PFK-2 therefore plays a significant role in the activation of glycolysis in response to insulin. Because both PFK isoforms are inhibited by citrate, the accumulation of this one tricarboxylic acid cycle intermediate during fatty acid and before oxidation serves the dual role of directly inhibiting PFK-1, and also suppressing the formation of the PFK-1 activator, fructose-2,6-*bis*-phosphate *(85)*.

In vitro, the cardiac PFK-2 isoform is activated by phosphorylation, mediated in vitro by several protein kinases, including PKA, PKB, p70 S6 kinase, and MAP kinase-activated protein kinase (MAPKAP-K1) *(89)*. Because the effects of insulin on cardiac PFK-2 are blocked by wortmannin, but not by rapamycin (therefore excluding a role for p70 S6 kinase), or by blocking the activation of MAPKAP-K1 (with PD98059), it is likely that PKB is the relevant PFK-2 kinase *(85*; Fig. 5*)*.

Insulin treatment leads, indirectly, to activation of hexokinase; notably through activation of GLUT-4, and by reduction in the concentration of glucose-6-phosphate (through activation of PFK-1 and glycogen synthase). Hexokinase may also be controlled by translocation to the outer surface of the mitochondrial membrane *(90)*. Insulin also influences expression of hexokinase (principally the hexokinase-II isoform), which is decreased in hearts from alloxan- or STZ-diabetic rats *(91)*, probably accounting for the parallel decline in activity of the hexose monophosphate pathway in experimental diabetes *(92)*.

The pyruvate dehydrogenase complex, another major target for insulin action, is subject to a complex set of control mechanisms involving covalent phosphorylation and noncovalent mechanisms *(93–95)*. The rise in intramitochondrial acetyl-CoA (and fall

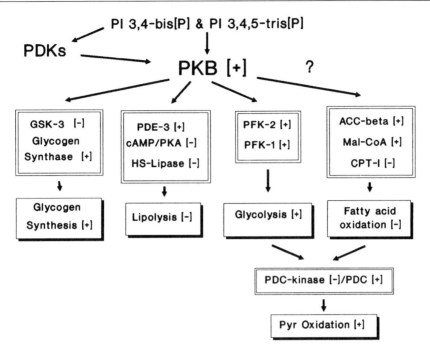

Fig. 5. Phosphoinositides and PKB in insulin metabolic signaling. Phosphatidylinositol (PI) 3,4-biphosphate and PI 3,4,5-trisphosphate are generated rapidly following activation of PI 3-kinase(s) in response to insulin. The 3-phosphoinositides exert dual effects – directly activating protein kinase B (PKB) and also its upstream (activating) kinases PDKs (phosphoinositide-dependent kinases). PKB appears to serve several key roles in mediating insulin signaling to the indicated metabolic responses (shadowed boxes). Other abbreviations: GSK, glycogen synthase kinase, PDE, phosphodiesterase, PFK, phosphofructokinase; ACC, acetyl-CoA carboxylase; CPT, carnitine palmitoyl transferase; Mal, malonyl; HS, hormone-sensitive; PDC, pyruvate dehydrogenase complex.

in free CoA), occasioned by enhanced rates of oxidation of fatty acids or ketones, causes product inhibition of PDC *(94,95)*. In addition, the associated PDC kinase becomes activated by a high ratio of acetyl-CoA:CoA. PDC kinase phosphorylates three sites on the α-subunit-acetyl of the pyruvate dehydrogenase (E1) components of the complex, converting the complex into a phosphorylated form with very low specific activity *(93,96,97)*. A major mechanism for regulation of PDC by insulin, therefore, relies on the complex intertissue factors that lead to diminished availability of fatty acyl-CoA esters within the myocardium.

Insulin-mediated activation of PDC persists in mitochondria isolated from hormone-treated adipocytes; however, the mechanism for the effect of insulin is still not fully understood, and persistent activation has not been observed with heart mitochondria *(98)*. The activation of PDC in adipose tissue is probably explained by increases in PDC-phosphate phosphatase *(99)*, which is dependent on Mg^{2+} for activity, and is further stimulated by Ca^{2+} *(100)*. Similarly, PDC can be activated by increases in cytoplasmic, and hence mitochondrial, Ca^{2+} in the heart *(101)*. The rapid cycling of Ca^{2+} in the heart, even at basal levels of heart rate, therefore provides an important mechanism for sustained activation of mitochondrial TCA cycle activity, which is insulin-independent, and which may be enhanced following activation of contractility by catecholamines *(98,101,102)*.

The dramatic suppression of PDC function in diabetes is explained, in part, by exaggerated rates of fatty acid metabolism, but there are also important controls mediated by altered gene and protein expression. The expression of PDC itself does not change appreciably in starvation, and has generally been found to decrease only marginally in diabetes *(103–105)*. A major factor in the suppression of PDC is the dramatic increase in expression and activity of PDC kinase in starvation and experimental diabetes, suggesting that insulin plays a critical and tonic-inhibitory role in the expression of this intramitochondrial protein kinase *(103–105)*, notably the PDK-4 isoform *(106)*.

Glycogen Metabolism

The regulation of glycogen metabolism in the heart differs in important respects from that of hepatic and skeletal muscle reserves, indicating distinct roles for myocardial glycogen *(83)*. It has long been recognized that the concentration of glycogen in the heart is increased in insulin-deficient diabetes, but the corresponding reserves in liver and skeletal muscle become markedly depleted *(107)*. Despite the maintenance of steady-state levels of glycogen in the diabetic heart, when β-oxidation accounts for a major proportion of the energy demand of the whole heart, the myocardial glycogen pool still turns over rapidly *(108–110)*. Rates of glycogen accumulation in the heart can be increased even without increases in glucose uptake, provided an alternate fuel is available to allow redirection of glucose from glycolysis to glycogen synthase *(111)*. This may be an important mechanism to allow glycogen conservation and repletion in the heart during and following exercise, when lactate release from skeletal muscles is increased, and also when the supply of fatty acids and ketones is increased in starvation or insulin-dependent diabetes *(112)*.

Another important feature of myocardial glycogen metabolism is that the glucose-6-phosphate derived from glycogenolysis is preferentially oxidized, compared with exogenous glucose *(108–110)*. The role of insulin in regulating glycogen turnover and the mechanism for preferential oxidation of glycogen–glucose are still not fully understood. It is clear, however, that preferential oxidation of glycogen-glucose offers an immediate energetic advantage (sparing the ATP required for initial substrate phosphorylation), and this may confer a selective advantage when energy demand is altered abruptly *(83,110)*. Cardiac glycogen metabolism is further complicated by a marked transmural gradient of glycogen concentration and glucose metabolism: Glycogen concentrations and rates of glucose uptake are highest in the innermost layers of muscle *(113)*. The differential distribution of glycogen may suggest a critical function in domains of muscle that may be forced to rely less on β-oxidation, and indicates that the actions of insulin and other hormones may be expressed differentially through the myocardium.

The impact of insulin on glycogen metabolism is mediated by several complementary mechanisms. Stimulation of GLUT-4 leads to increased intracellular concentration of glucose-6-phosphate, which not only provides the carbon source for glycogen chain extension, but also acts as an activator of glycogen synthase by a direct allosteric binding, and by promoting the net dephosphorylation of glycogen synthase *(114)*. Insulin treatment does not appear to alter the proportion of glycogen phosphorylase in the active form in perfused hearts *(115,116)*, and this probably contributes to the high rates of glycogen turnover, even when net glucose oxidation is suppressed.

Insulin also stimulates the dephosphorylation and activation of glycogen synthase independent of glucose metabolism. The activation of glycogen synthase by insulin is inhibited by wortmannin, but is little affected by rapamycin or PD98059 *(117,118)*, suggesting that a signaling pathway involving PI 3-kinase plays a major role. In fact, it appears that PKB, one of the downstream targets of 3-phosphoinositides, is able to directly phosphorylate and inactivate GSK-3, thus providing a mechanism to promote net dephosphorylation of glycogen synthase (119; Fig. 5).

In diabetes, the ability of insulin to induce glycogen synthase activation is severely blunted (115,120,121), and this defect is associated with decreases in the levels and insulin-mediated activation of glycogen synthase phosphatase (116). This observation further underlines the importance of the activation of protein serine/threonine phosphatases in insulin action.

Fatty Acid Metabolism

Under normal aerobic conditions, the heart derives from 50% to greater than 95% of its metabolic energy from the oxidation of long-chain fatty acids. Physiologically, the combination of elevated plasma insulin and glucose restricts myocardial fatty acid oxidation to the lower end of its range. This chapter has discussed the roles of insulin in regulating the supply of exogenous fatty acids to the myocardium, notably at the level of adipose tissue and liver, to control circulating levels of free fatty acids, and the level and tissue targeting of lipoprotein triglycerides. Insulin also regulates fatty acid metabolism within the heart itself. The impact of insulin on glucose transport and subsequent metabolism generates competition for fuel selection at the level of PDC, which is strikingly revealed by the actions of pyruvate and dichloroacetate (122). Additional factors that contribute to the regulation of fuel selection in the myocardium include the metabolism of triglycerides by triglyceride lipases and the formation of long chain acylcarnitines catalyzed by carnitine palmitoyl transferase (CPT-I).

Fatty acids may be generated in the myocardium by release from triglycerides in the plasma lipoproteins, as well as from endogenous-tissue triglyceride stores. The hydrolysis of plasma triglycerides is effected at the luminal surface of vascular endothelial cells by lipoprotein lipase (LPL), which is synthesized in cardiac myocytes (123,124). Insulin does not induce rapid mobilization of LPL (125), but does have important actions on LPL in the longer term. The expression of cardiac LPL is sustained during moderate starvation (when the adipose tissue enzyme is repressed), and this contributes to the channeling of lipid fuels from adipose tissue to muscle (51,123). Studies of the expression of LPL in the heart in experimental diabetes have yielded differing results. A number of studies have demonstrated a decline in LPL enzyme activity, immunoreactive protein and/or mRNA levels in STZ diabetes (52,126–128). Heparin-releasable LPL at the vascular endothelium has also been shown to be reduced in perfused hearts from diabetic rats (51). The decline in LPL levels, coupled with altered properties of the circulating lipoproteins, combines to markedly reduce the utilization of circulating triglycerides by the diabetic heart (129). The LPL activity recovered from cardiomyocytes is also reduced by STZ diabetes (130), which is explained partly by a decline in general protein synthesis and partly by a defect in processing of the enzyme to the fully active form. No changes in LPL mRNA abundance or turnover were detected during 4–5 d of STZ diabetes (131). In contrast to the studies just described, several reports have concluded that STZ diabetes leads to no decrease in cardiac LPL, or even an increase (132–134). Experimental protocols are probably critical, for example, acute diabetes, or the induction of moderate diabetes, by injection of low doses of STZ (55 mg/kg), led to enhanced pools of heparin-releasable LPL (135,136).

Control of LPL gene transcription and mRNA translation, and of protein maturation and trafficking, are all likely to be important features of the action of insulin on this critical enzyme *(123,130,131,136)*. The effects of insulin may be evident only in the presence of additional factors, such as steroid hormones *(137)*.

The role of endogenous myocardial triglycerides as an energy fuel was directly demonstrated from mass measurements *(138)*, and from release of $^{14}CO_2$ from triglycerides prelabeled with (^{14}C)palmitate *(139)*. The size and turnover of the cardiac triglyceride reserve are both increased in hearts from diabetic rats *(138,140,141)*, and in cardiomyocytes from diabetic rats *(142)*, reflecting enhanced hydrolysis and re-esterification. Myocardial triglyceride lipolysis is limited by the activity of hormone-sensitive lipase, which is similar to the adipose tissue enzyme in that it is activated by catecholamines and inhibited by insulin and nicotinic acid *(143–145)*.

The rapid effects of insulin on lipolysis are mediated by a wortmannin-sensitive pathway that leads to activation of a relevant lipase-phosphatase and/or to PKB-dependent activation of PDE-3 *(146;* Fig. 5). In addition to regulation via lipase phosphorylation and dephosphorylation, feedback inhibition of hormone-sensitive lipase by fatty acids might account for the conservation of myocardial triglycerides when exogenous fatty acids are abundant *(141,147,148)*. Furthermore, increases in esterification rates, normally limited by availability of fatty acyl-CoA esters, would also offer an attractive explanation of the maintenance of triglyceride reserves with high turnover *(138,149)*.

Fatty acid oxidation is also regulated in the heart, especially by control of CPT-I. A critical mechanism for regulating CPT-I, through allosteric inhibition by malonyl-CoA, was elucidated as a result of studies of hepatic fatty acid oxidation and ketogenesis *(150)*. The distinct M (muscle) isoform of CPT-I represents 98% of the total activity in adult heart *(151)*; it exhibits a higher K_m for carnitine and lower IC50 for malonyl-CoA than the liver (L) isoform *(152)*. The sensitivity of CPT-I to malonyl-CoA is diminished in the liver in starvation and in STZ diabetes *(153)*, but opinions are divided about the importance of this mechanism in the heart *(152–154)*.

The rapid effects of insulin on CPT-I activity are mediated by changes in the concentration of malonyl-CoA in cells. The only source of malonyl-CoA in mammalian cells is the reaction catalyzed by acetyl-CoA carboxylase, an enzyme that is activated by insulin in adipose tissue and liver *(155)*. The heart expresses a distinct 280-kDa isoform of acetyl-CoA carboxylase *(156,157)*, which appears to play a significant role in regulating fatty acid oxidation in the heart, judging by the inverse relationship between rates of fatty acid oxidation and tissue concentrations of malonyl-CoA *(61,158)*. The 280-kDa isoform of acetyl-CoA carboxylase is the product of a distinct gene and displays distinct properties, compared with the 265-kDa isoform found predominantly in adipose tissue and liver *(156,157,159–161)*. The mechanism by which acetyl-CoA carboxylase might be regulated by insulin in the heart is not resolved.

Because the heart expresses no fatty acid synthase *(162)*, a mechanism for malonyl-CoA removal must be available and may be regulated. Malonyl-CoA decarboxylase has been described in mitochondria from various rat tissues *(163)*, but removal of cytoplasmic malonyl-CoA is not understood.

CONCLUDING COMMENTS

The actions of insulin on the heart must be viewed within the context of dynamic mechanical function and complex interactions with multiple extracellular signals. The basal activity of the heart is itself formidable, and further increases in workload and mechanical stretch have dramatic effects on energy demand, metabolism, and signal transduction pathways. Defining the significance of the roles of insulin within these contexts remains an important challenge. The potentially devastating impact of the withdrawal of insulin or loss of cellular insulin sensitivity on heart structure, metabolism, and function indicates that this challenge is worth meeting.

Much of this discussion has dealt with cardiac myocytes, but the role of endothelial and other cells should not be underestimated, as indicated by the crucial need to regulate blood flow and pressure. Examples of the complex interplay between myocyte and endothelium are revealed by the way in which insulin must transit the endothelium to reach the myocytes, and by features of the control of LPL: It is synthesized in myocytes, processed and translocated to endothelial lining, and plays a vital and dynamically controlled gatekeeper function in dictating lipoprotein metabolism in the heart.

The interactions of insulin with other extracellular and intrinsic control systems may involve either antagonistic, overlapping, or complementary mechanisms. Moreover, these interactions may be evident within specific developmental, nutritional, or pathological contexts. Overall, understanding of insulin action on the heart may have come a long way, but, clearly, it is faced with many intriguing and important problems.

ACKNOWLEDGMENTS

Work in these laboratories has been supported by grants from the Medical Research Council of Canada, the Heart and Stroke Foundation of British Columbia and Yukon, and the Canadian Diabetes Association (with an award in the memory of Dorothea Riddell Minnis). B.R. is a scholar of the Canadian Diabetes Association. S.V. is a Fellow of the Medical Research Council of Canada. The authors are also grateful to co-workers and colleagues for many helpful comments and discussions.

REFERENCES

1. Shapiro LM. Diabetes-induced heart-muscle disease and left ventricular dysfunction. Pract Cardiol 1985;11:79–91.
2. Friedman JJ. Vascular sensitivity and reactivity to norepinephrine in diabetes mellitus. Am J Physiol 1989;256:1134–1138.
3. Hulper B, Wilms B. Investigations of autonomic diabetic neuropathy of the cardiovascular system. In: Gries FA, Freund F, Rabe F, and Berger H, eds. Aspects of Autonomic Neuropathy in Diabetes. Georg Thieme Verlag, Stuttgart, 1980, pp. 77–80.
4. Regan TJ, Lyons MM, Ahmed SS. Evidence for cardiomyopathy in familial diabetes mellitus. J Clin Invest 1977;60:885–889.
5. Regan TJ, Ettinger PO, Khan MI, Jesran MU, Lyons MM, Oldewurtel HA, Weber M. Altered myocardial function and metabolism in chronic diabetes mellitus without ischemia in dogs. Circ Res 1974; 35:222–237.
6. Dhalla NS, Pierce GN, Innes IR, Beamish RE. Pathogenesis of cardiac dysfunction in diabetes mellitus. Can J Cardiol 1985;1:263–281.
7. Clark AH. Interrelation of the surviving heart and pancreas of the dog in sugar metabolism. J Exp Med 1916;24:621–650.
8. Visscher MB, Muller EA. Influence of insulin upon the mammalian heart. J Physiol 1927;62:341–348.
9. Lucchesi BR, Medina M. Positive inotropic action of insulin in the canine heart. Eur J Pharmacol 1972; 18:107–115.
10. Christensen NJ. Acute effects of insulin on cardiovascular function and noradrenaline uptake and release. Diabetologia 1983;25:377–381.

11. Sheldon MB. Braimbridge MV, Clement AJ. Effects of glucose and insulin on failing myocardium in an isolated heart preparation. Br Heart J 1969;31:393–398.

12. Downing SE, Lee JC. Myocardial and coronary vascular responses to insulin in the diabetic lamb. Am J Physiol 1979;237:H514–H519.

13. Lee JC, Downing SE. Effects of insulin on cardiac muscle contraction and responsiveness to norepinephrine. Am J Physiol 1976;230:1360–1365.

14. Brands MW, Lee WF, Keen HL, Alonso-Galicia M, Zappe DH, Hall JE. Cardiac output and renal function during insulin hypertension in Sprague-Dawley rats. Am J Physiol 1996;271:R276–R281.

15. Baron AD. Hemodynamic actions of insulin. Am J Physiol 1994;267:E187–E202.

16. Dillmann WH. Diabetes mellitus induces changes in cardiac myosin of the rat. Diabetes 1980;29:579–582.

17. Malhotra A, Penpargkul S, Fein FS, Sonnenblick EH, Scheuer J. Effect of streptozotocin-induced diabetes in rats on cardiac contractile proteins. Circ Res 1981;49:1243–1250.

18. Akella AB, Ding XL, Cheng R, Gulati J. Diminished Ca^{2+} sensitivity of skinned cardiac muscle contractility coincident with troponin T-band shifts in the diabetic rats. Circ Res 1995;76:600–606.

19. Pierce GN, Dhalla NS. Mitochondrial abnormalities in diabetic cardiomyopathy. Can J Cardiol 1985;1:48–54.

20. Pierce GN, Dhalla NS. Sarcolemmal Na^+-K^+ ATPase activity in diabetic rat heart. Am J Physiol 1983;245:241–247.

21. Shimoni Y, Ewart HS, Severson D. Type I and II models of diabetes produce different modifications of K^+ currents in rat heart: role of insulin. J Physiol 1998;507:485–496.

22. Heyliger CE, Prakash A, McNeill JH. Alterations in cardiac sarcolemmal Ca^{2+} pump activity during diabetes mellitus. Am J Physiol 1987;252:540–544.

23. Lopaschuk GD, Tahiliani A, Vadlamudi RVSV, Katz S, McNeill JH. Cardiac sarcoplasmic reticulum function in insulin or carnitine-treated diabetic rats. Am J Physiol 1983;245:969–976.

24. Ganguly PK, Pierce GN, Dhalla KS, Dhalla NS. Defective sarcoplasmic reticular calcium transport in diabetic cardiomyopathy. Am J Physiol 1983;244:528–535.

25. Bouchard RA, Bose D. Influence of experimental diabetes on sarcoplasmic reticulum function in rat ventricular muscle. Am J Physiol 1991;260:341–354.

26. Ren J, Davidoff AJ. Diabetes rapidly induces contractile dysfunctions in isolated ventricular myocytes. Am J Physiol 1997;272:148–158

27. Davidoff AJ, Ren J. Low insulin and high glucose induce abnormal relaxation in cultured adult rat ventricular myocytes. Am J Physiol 1997;272:159–167.

28. Zierler KL. Electrical events in transduction of insulin action and insulin action on electrical events. Prog Endocr Res Ther 1988;4:91–103.

29. Briggs AP, Koechig I, Doisy EA, Weber CJ. Some changes in the composition of blood due to injection of insulin. J Biol Chem 1924;58:721–730.

30. Agius L, Peak M, Beresford G, Al-Habori M, Thomas TH. Role of ion content and cell volume in insulin action. Biochem Soc Trans 1994;22:516–522.

31. Bedford JJ, Leader JP. Response of tissues of the rat to anisosmolality in vivo. Am J Physiol 1993;264:R1164–R1179.

32. Moore RD. Stimulation of Na^+:H^+ exchange by insulin. Biophys J 1981;33:203–210.

33. Clausen T, Kohn PG. Effect of insulin on the transport of sodium and potassium in rat soleus muscle. J Physiol 1977;265:19–42.

34. McGeoch JEM, Guidotti G. Insulin-stimulated cation channel in skeletal muscle—inhibition by calcium causes oscillation. J Biol Chem 1992;267:832–841.

35. Weil-Maslansky E, Gutman Y, Sasson S. Insulin activates furosemide-sensitive K^+ and Cl^- uptake system in BC3H1 cells. Am J Physiol 1994;267:C932–C939.

36. Bennett AM, Tonks NK. Regulation of distinct stages of skeletal muscle differentiation by mitogen-activated protein kinases. Science 1997;278:1288–1291.

37. Steinberg HO, Brechtel G, Johnson A, Fineberg N, Baron AD. Insulin-mediated skeletal muscle vasodilation is nitric oxide dependent. A novel action of insulin to increase nitric oxide release. J Clin Invest 1994;94:1171–1179.

38. Scherrer U, Sartori C. Insulin as a vascular and sympathoexcitatory hormone: implications for blood pressure regulation, insulin sensitivity and cardiovascular morbidity. Circulation 1997;96:4104–4113.

39. Kelly RA, Balligand J-L, Smith TW. Nitric oxide and cardiac function. Circ Res 1996;79:363–380.

40. Reaven GM. Pathophysiology of insulin resistance in human disease. Physiol Rev 1995;75:473–486.

41. Buchanan TA, Meehan WP, Jeng YY, Yang D, Chan TM, Nadler JL, et al. Blood pressure lowering by pioglitazone. Evidence for a direct vascular effect. J Clin Invest 1995;96:354–360.

42. Howard G, O'Leary DH, Zaccaro D, Haffner S, Rewers M, Hamman R, et al. Insulin sensitivity and atherosclerosis. Circulation 1996;93:1809–1817.

43. Williams A. Mitochondria. In: Noble AJ, ed. Cardiac Metabolism. John Wiley, New York 1983, p. 151.

44. Neely JR, Morgan HE. Relationship between carbohydrate and lipid metabolism and the energy balance of heart muscle. Annu Rev Physiol 1974;36:413–459.

45. Cahill GF. Physiology of insulin in man. Diabetes 1971;20:785–799.

46. Kimball SR, Vary TC, Jefferson LS. Regulation of protein synthesis by insulin. Annu Rev Physiol 1994;56:321–348.

47. Beutler B, Cerami A. Cachectin: more than a tumor necrosis factor. N Engl J Med 1987;316:379–385.

48. Randle PJ, Hales CN, Garland PB, Newsholme EA. Glucose fatty acid cycle. Its role in insulin sensitivity and the metabolic disturbances of diabetes mellitus. Lancet 1963;I:785–789.

49. Dashti N, Wofbauer G. Secretion of lipids, apolipoproteins and lipoproteins by human hepatoma cell line, HepG2: effects of oleic acid and insulin. J Lipid Res 1987;28:423–426.

50. Lewis GF, Uffelman KD, Szeto LW, Weller B, Steiner G. Interaction between free fatty acids and insulin in the acute control of very low density lipoprotein production in humans. J Clin Invest 1995; 95:158–166.

51. Bjorensztajn J, Otway S, Robinson DS. Effect of fasting on the clearing factor lipase (lipoprotein lipase) activity of defatted preparations of rat heart muscle. J Lipid Res 1970;11:102–110.

52. Deshaies Y, Geloen A, Paulin A, Bukowieki LJ. Restoration of lipoprotein lipase activity in insulin-deficient rats by insulin infusion is tissue-specific. Can J Physiol Pharmacol 1991;69:746–751.

53. O'Brien RM, Granner DK. Regulation of gene expression by insulin. Physiol Rev 1996;76:1109–1161.

54. Pain VM. Initiation of protein synthesis in eukaryotic cells. Eur J Biochem 1996;236:747–771.

55. Proud CG, Denton RM. Molecular mechanisms for the control of translation by insulin. Biochem J 1997;328:329–341.

56. Knowlton FP, Starling EH. Experiments on the consumption of sugar in the normal and the diabetic heart. J Physiol 1912;45:146–163.

57. Manchester J, Kong X, Nerbonne J, Lowry OH, Lawrence JC. Glucose transport and phosphorylation in single cardiac myocytes: rate-limiting steps in glucose metabolism. Am J Physiol 1994;266: E326–E333.

58. Kashiwaya Y, Sato K, Tsuchiya N, Thomas S, Fell DA, Veech RL, Passonneau JV. Control of glucose utilization in working perfused rat heart. J Biol Chem 1994;269:25,502–25,514.

59. Shipp JC, Opie LH, Challoner DR. Fatty acid and glucose metabolism in the perfused heart. Nature 1961;189:1018–1019.

60. Newsholme EA, Randle PJ, Manchester KL. Inhibition of the phosphofructokinase reaction in perfused rat heart by respiration of ketone bodies, fatty acids and pyruvate. Nature 1962;193:270–271.

61. Lopaschuk GD, Belke DD, Gamble J, Itoi T, Schonekess BO. Regulation of fatty acid oxidation in the mammalian heart in health and disease. Biochim Biophys Acta 1994;1213:263–276.

62. Kraegen EW, Sowden JA, Halstead MB, Clark PW, Rodnick KJ, Chisholm DJ, James DE. Glucose transporters and in vivo glucose uptake in skeletal and cardiac muscle: fasting, insulin stimulation and immunoisolation studies of GLUT1 and GLUT4. Biochem J 1993;295:287–293.

63. James DE, Strube M, Mueckler M. Molecular cloning and characterization of an insulin-regulatable glucose transporter. Nature 1989;338:83–87.

64. Camps M, Castello A, Munoz P, Monfar M, Testar X, Palacin M, Zorzano A. Effect of diabetes and fasting on GLUT-4 (muscle/fat) glucose-transporter expression in insulin-sensitive tissues. Biochem J 1992;282:765–772.

65. Hayashi T, Wojtaszewski JF, Goodyear LJ. Exercise regulation of glucose transport in skeletal muscle. Am J Physiol 1997;273:E1039–E1051.

66. Kolter T, Uphues I, Wichelhaus A, Reinauer H, Eckel J. Contraction-induced translocation of the glucose transporter GLUT4 in isolated ventricular cardiomyocytes. Biochem Biophys Res Commun 1992;189:1207–1214.

67. Rattigan S, Appleby GJ, Clark MG. Insulin-like action of catecholamines and Ca^{2+} to stimulate glucose transport and GLUT4 translocation in perfused rat heart. Biochim Biophys Acta 1991;1094:217–223.

68. Cushman SW, Wardzala LJ. Potential mechanism of insulin action on glucose transport in isolated rat adipose cells: apparent translocation of intracellular transport systems to the plasma membrane. J Biol Chem 1980;255:4758–4762.

69. Suzuki K, Kono T. Evidence that insulin causes the translocation of glucose transport activity to the plasma membrane from an intracellular storage site. Proc Natl Acad Sci USA 1980;77:2542–2545.

70. Watanabe T, Smith MM, Robinson FW, Kono T. Insulin action on glucose transport in cardiac muscle. J Biol Chem 1984;259:13,117–13,122.

71. Slot JW, Geuze HJ, Gigengack S, James DE, Lienhard GE. Translocation of the glucose transporter GLUT-4 in cardiac myocytes of the rat. Proc Natl Acad Sci USA 1991;88:7815–7819.

72. Rodnick KJ, Slot JW, Studelska DR, Hanpeter DE, Robinson LJ, Geuze HJ, James DE. Immunocyto-chemical and biochemical studies of GLUT4 in rat skeletal muscle. J Biol Chem 1992;267:6278–6285.

73. Burdett E, Beeler T, Klip A. Distribution of glucose transporters and insulin receptors in the plasma membrane and transverse tubules of skeletal muscle. Arch Biochem Biophys 1987;253:279–286.

74. Holman GD, Kasuga M. From receptor to transporter: insulin signaling to glucose transport. Diabeto-logia 1997;40:991–1003.

75. Timmers K.I, Clark AE, Omatsu-Kanabe M, Whiteheart SW, Bennett MK, Holman GD, Cushman SW. Identification of SNAP receptors in rat adipose cell membrane fractions and in SNARE complexes co-immunoprecipitated with epitope-tagged NSF. Biochem J 1996;320:429–436.

76. Martin LB, Shewan A, Millar CA, Gould GW, James DE. Vesicle-associated membrane protein 2 plays a specific role in the insulin-dependent trafficking of the facilitative glucose transporter GLUT4 in 3T3-L1 adipocytes. J Biol Chem 1998;273:1444–1452.

77. Cain CC, Trimble WS, Lienhard GE. Members of the VAMP family of synaptic vesicle proteins are components of glucose transporter-containing vesicles from rat adipocytes. J Biol Chem 1992;267:11,681–11,684.

78. Hara K, Yonezawa K, Sakaue H, Ando A, Kotani K, Kitamura T, et al. Phosphatidylinositol 3-kinase activity is required for insulin-stimulated glucose transport but not Ras activation in CHO cells. Proc Natl Acad Sci USA 1994;91:7415–7419.

79. Garvey TW, Huecksteadt TP, Birnbaum MJ. Pretranslational suppression of an insulin-responsive glucose transporter in rats with diabetes mellitus. Science 1989;245:60–63.

80. Berger JC, Diswas C, Vicario P, Strout HV, Saperstein R, Pilch PF. Decreased expression of the insulin-responsive glucose transporter in diabetes and fasting. Nature 1989;340:70–72.

81. Nuutila P, Knuuti J, Ruotsalainen U, Koivisto VA, Eronen E, Teras M, et al. Insulin resistance is localized to skeletal but not heart muscle in type 1 diabetes. Am J Physiol 1993;264:E756–E762.

82. Maki M, Nuutila P, Laine H, Voipio-Pulkki L-M, Haaparanta M, Solin O, Knuuti JM. Myocardial glucose uptake in patients with NIDDM and stable coronary artery disease. Diabetes 1997;46:1491–1496.

83. Taegtmeyer H. Energy metabolism in the heart: from basic concepts to clinical applications. Curr Probl Cardiol 1994;19:57–116.

84. Pogson CI, Randle PJ. Control of rat heart phosphofructokinase by citrate and other regulators. Biochem J 1966;100:683–693.

85. Hue L, Depre C, Lefebvre V, Rider MH, Veitch K. Regulation of glucose metabolism in cardiac muscle. Biochem Soc Trans 1995;23:311–314.

86. Hue L, Blackmore PF, Shikama H, Robinson-Steiner A, Exton JH. Regulation of fructose-2,6-bisphosphate content in rat hepatocytes, perfused hearts and perfused hind limbs. J Biol Chem 1982;257:4308–4314.

87. Rider MH, Hue L. Activation of rat heart phosphofructokinase-2 by insulin in vivo. FEBS Lett 1984;176:484–488.

88. Lawson JWR, Uyeda K. Effects of insulin and work on fructose 2,6-bisphosphate content and phos-phofructokinase activity in perfused rat hearts. J Biol Chem 1987;262:3165–3173.

89. Deprez J, Vertommen D, Alessi DR, Hue L, Rider MH. Phosphorylation and activation of heart 6-phosphofructo-2-kinase by protein kinase B and other protein kinases of the insulin signaling cascades. J Biol Chem 1997;272:17,269–17,275.

90. Vogt C, Yki-Jarvinen H, Iozzo P, Pipek R, Pendergrass M, Koval J, et al. Effects of insulin on subcellular localization of hexokinase II in human skeletal muscle in vivo. J Clin Endocrinol Metab 1998;83:230–234.

91. Printz RL, Koch S, Potter LR, O'Doherty RM, Tiesinga JJ, Moritz S, Evanauer DK. Hexokinase II mRNA and gene structure, regulation by insulin and evolution. J Biol Chem 1993;268:5209–5219.

92. Sochor M, Gonzalez A-M, McLean P. Regulation of alternative pathways of glucose metabolism in rat heart by alloxan diabetes: changes in pentose phosphate pathway. Biochem Biophys Res Commun 1984;118:110–116.

93. Linn TC, Pettit FH, Reed LJ. Regulation of the activity of the pyruvate dehydrogenase complex from beef kidney mitochondria by phosphorylation and dephosphorylation. Proc Natl Acad Sci USA 1969; 62:234–241.

94. Garland PB, Randle PJ. Control of pyruvate dehydrogenase in perfused rat heart by intracellular concentrations of acetyl CoA. Biochem J 1964;91:6C–7C.

95. Kerbey AL, Randle PJ, Cooper RH, Whitehouse S, Pask HT, Denton RM. Regulation of pyruvate dehydrogenase in rat heart. Mechanism of regulation of proportions of dephosphorylated and phosphorylated enzyme by oxidation of fatty acids and ketone bodies and effects of diabetes: role of coenzyme A, acetyl-coenzyme A and reduced and oxidised nicotinamide adenine dinucleotide. Biochem J 1976; 154:327–348.

96. Cooper RH, Randle PJ, Denton RM. Regulation of heart muscle pyruvate dehydrogenase kinase. Biochem J 1974;143:625–641.

97. Hughes WA, Brownsey RW, Denton RM. Studies on the incorporation of ^{32}P phosphate into pyruvate dehydrogenase in intact rat fat cells. Biochem J 1980;192:469–481.

98. McCormack JG, Denton RM. Role of intramitochondrial Ca^{2+} in the regulation of oxidative phosphorylation in mammalian tissues. Biochem Soc Trans 1993;21:793–799.

99. Hughes WA, Denton RM. Incorporation of ^{32}Pi into pyruvate dehydrogenase phosphate in mitochondria from control and insulin-treated adipose tissue. Nature 1976;264:471–473.

100. Severson DL, Denton RM, Pask HT, Randle PJ. Calcium and magnesium ions as effectors of adipose tissue pyruvate dehydrogenase phosphate phosphatase. Biochem J 1974;140:225–237.

101. McCormack GJ, England PJ. Ruthenium red inhibits the activation of pyruvate dehydrogenase caused by positive inotropic agents in the perfused heart. Biochem J 1983;214:581–585.

102. McCormack GJ, Halestrap AP, Denton RM. Role of calcium ions in regulation of mammalian intramitochondrial metabolism. Physiol Rev 1990;70:391–425.

103. Kerbey AL, Richardson LJ, Randle PJ. Roles of intrinsic kinase and of kinase/activator protein in the enhanced phosphorylation of pyruvate dehydrogenase complex in starvation. FEBS Lett 1984;176: 115–119.

104. Priestman DA, Mistry SC, Halsall A, Randle PJ. Role of protein synthesis and of fatty acid metabolism in the longer-term regulation of pyruvate dehydrogenase kinase. Biochem J 1994; 300:659–664.

105. Jones BS, Yeaman SJ. Long-term regulation of pyruvate dehydrogenase complex. Evidence that kinase activator protein (KAP) is free pyruvate dehydrogenase kinase. Biochem J 1991;275:780–783.

106. Wu P, Sato J, Zhao Y, Jaskiewicz J, Popov KM, Harris RA. Starvation and diabetes increase the amount of pyruvate dehydrogenase kinase isoenzyme 4 in rat heart. Biochem J 1998;329:197–201.

107. Cruickshank EWH, Kosterlitz HW. Utilization of fat by the aglycaemic mammalian heart. J Physiol 1941;99:208–223.

108. Henning SL, Wambolt RB, Schonekess BO, Lopaschuk GD, Allard MF. Contribution of glycogen to aerobic myocardial glucose metabolism. Circulation 1996;93:1549–1555.

109. Goodwin GW, Arteaga JR, Taegtmeyer H. Glycogen turnover in the isolated working rat heart. J Biol Chem 1995;270:9234–9240.

110. Goodwin G, Ahmad F, Taegtmeyer H. Preferential oxidation of glycogen in isolated working rat heart. J Clin Invest 1996;97:1409–1416.

111. Laughlin MR, Taylor JF, Chesnick AS, Balaban RS. Non-glucose substrates increase glycogen synthesis in vivo in dog heart. Am J Physiol 1994;267:H217–H223.

112. Russell RR, Cline GW, Guthrie PH, Goodwin GW, Shulman GI, Taegtmeyer H. Regulation of exogenous and endogenous glucose metabolism by insulin and acetoacetate in the isolated working rat heart. J Clin Invest 1997;100:2892–2899.

113. De Tata V, Bergamini C, Gori Z, Locci-Cubeddu T, Bergamini E. Transmural gradient of glycogen metabolism in the normal rat left ventricle. Pflugers Arch ges Physiol 1983;396:60–65.

114. Villar-Palasi C, Guinovart JJ. Role of glucose 6-phosphate in the control of glycogen synthase. FASEB J 1997;11:544–558.

115. Miller TB. Dual role for insulin in the regulation of cardiac glycogen synthase. J Biol Chem 1978; 253:5389–5394.

116. Nuttall FQ, Gannon MC, Corbett VA, Wheeler MP. Insulin stimulation of glycogen synthase D phosphatase (protein phosphatase). J Biol Chem 1976;251:6724–6729.

117. Cross DAE, Alessi DR, Vandenheede JR, McDowell HE, Hundal HS, Cohen P. Inhibition of glycogen synthase kinase-3 by insulin or insulin-like growth factor I in the reat skeletal muscle cell line L6

is blocked by wortmannin but not by rapamycin. Evidence that wortmannin blocks activation of the mitogen-activated protein kinase pathway in L6 cells between Ras and Raf. Biochem J 1994;303: 21–26.

118. Robinson LJ, Razzack Z. F, Lawrence JC. Jr James DE. Mitogen-activated protein kinase activation is not sufficient for stimulation of glucose transport or glycogen synthase in 3T3-L1 adipocytes. J Biol Chem 1993;268:26,422–26,427.

119. Cross DAE, Alessi DR, Cohen P, Andjelkovich M, Hemmings BA. Inhibition of glycogen synthase kinase-3 by insulin mediated by protein kinase B. Nature 1995;378:785–789.

120. Laughlin MR, Petit WA, Shulman RG, Barrett EJ. Measurement of myocardial glycogen synthesis in diabetic and fasted rats. Am J Physiol 1990;258:E184–E190.

121. Thorburn AW, Gumbiner B, Bulacan F, Brechtel G, Henry RR. Multiple defects in muscle glycogen synthase activity contribute to reduced glycogen synthesis in non-insulin dependent diabetes mellitus. J Clin Invest 1991;87:489–495.

122. Whitehouse S, Cooper RH, Randle PJ. Mechanism of activation of pyruvate dehydrogenase by dichloroacetate and other halogenated carboxylic acids. Biochem J 1974;141:761–774.

123. Olivecrona T, Hultin M, Bergo M, Olivecrona G. Lipoprotein lipase: regulation and role in lipoprotein metabolism. Proc Nutr Soc 1997;56:723–729.

124. O'Brien KD, Ferguson M, Gordon D, Deeb SS, Chait A. Lipoprotein lipase is produced by cardiac myocytes rather than interstitial cells in human myocardium. Arterioscler Thromb 1994;14:1445–1451.

125. Braun JEA, Severson DL. Lipoprotein lipase release from cardiac myocytes is increased by decavanadate but not insulin. Am J Physiol 1992;262:663–670.

126. Tavangar K, Murata Y, Pedersen ME, Goers JF, Hoffman AR, Kraemer FB. Regulation of lipoprotein lipase in the diabetic rat. J Clin Invest 1992;90:1672–1678.

127. Liu L, Severson DL. Myocardial lipoprotein lipase activity: regulation by diabetes and fructose-induced hypertriglyceridemia. Can J Physiol Pharmacol 1995;73:369–377.

128. Taskinen M-R. Lipoprotein lipase in diabetes. Diabetes Metab Rev 1987;3:551–570.

129. O'Looney P, Irwin D, Briscoe P, Vahouny GV. Lipoprotein composition as a component in the lipoprotein clearance defect in experimental diabetes. J Biol Chem 1985;260:428–432.

130. Braun JEA, Severson DL. Diabetes reduces the heparin- and phospholipase C-releasable lipoprotein lipase from cardiomyocytes. Am J Physiol 1991;260:E477–E485.

131. Carroll R, Liu L, Severson DL. Post-transcriptional mechanisms are responsible for the reduction in lipoprotein lipase activity in cardiomyocytes from diabetic rat hearts. Biochem J 1995;310:67–72.

132. Inadera H, Tashiro J, Okubo Y, Ishikawa K, Shirai K, Saito Y, Yoshida S. Response of lipoprotein lipase to calorie intake in streptozotocin-induced diabetic rats. Scand J Clin Invest 1992;52:797–802.

133. Stam H, Schoonderwoerd K, Breeman W, Hulsman W. Effects of hormones, fasting and diabetes on triglyceride lipase activity in rat heart and liver. Horm Metab Res 1984;16:293–297.

134. Nomura T, Hagino H, Gotoh M, Iguchi A, Sakamoto N. Effects of streptozotocin diabetes on tissue specific lipase activities in the rat. Lipids 1984;19:594–599.

135. Rodrigues B, Severson DL. Acute diabetes does not reduce heparin-releasable lipoprotein lipase activity in perfused hearts from Wistar-Kyoto rats. Can J Physiol Pharmacol 1993;71:657–661.

136. Rodrigues B, Cam MC, Jian K, Lim F, Sambandam N, Shepherd G. Differential effects of streptozotocin-induced diabetes on cardiac lipoprotein lipase activity. Diabetes 1997;46:1346–1353.

137. Ewart HS, Carroll R, Severson DL. Lipoprotein lipase activity in rat cardiomyocytes is stimulated by insulin and dexamethasone. Biochem J 1997;327:439–442.

138. Denton RM, Randle PJ. Hormonal control of lipid concentration in rat heart and gastrocnemius. Nature 1965;208:488.

139. Olson RE, Hoeschen RJ. Utilization of endogenous lipid by the isolated perfused rat heart. Biochem J 1967;108:796–801.

140. Murthy VK, Bauman MD, Shipp JC. Regulation of triacylglycerol lipolysis in the perfused hearts of normal and diabetic rats. Diabetes 1983;32:718–722.

141. Saddik M, Lopaschuk GD. Triacylglycerol turnover in isolated working hearts of acutely diabetic rats. Can J Physiol Pharmacol 1994;72:1110–1119.

142. Kenno KA, Severson DL. Lipolysis in isolated myocardial cells from diabetic rat hearts. Am J Physiol 1985;249:1024–1030.

143. Kreisberg RA. Effect of epinephrine on myocardial triglyceride and free fatty acid utilization. Am J Physiol 1966;210:385–389.

144. Brownsey RW, Brunt RV. Effect of adrenaline-induced endogenous lipolysis upon the mechanical and metabolic performance of ischaemically-perfused rat hearts. Clin Sci Mol Med 1977;53:513–521.
145. Crass MF, Shipp JC, Pieper GM. Effects of catecholamines on myocardial endogenous substrates and contractility. Am J Physiol 1975;228:618–627.
146. Wijkander J, Landstrom TR, Manganiello V, Belfrage P, Degerman E. Insulin-induced phosphorylation and activation of phosphodiesterase 3B in rat adipocytes: possible role for protein kinase B but not mitogen-activated protein kinase or p70 S6 kinase. Endocrinology 1998;139:219–227.
147. Severson DL. Regulation of lipid metabolism in adipose tissue and heart. Can J Physiol Pharmacol 1979;57:923–937.
148. Crass MF. Exogenous substrate effects on endogenous lipid metabolism in the working rat heart. Biochim Biophys Acta 1972;280:71–81.
149. Denton RM, Randle PJ. Concentrations of glycerides and phospholipids in rat heart and gastrocnemius muscles. Effects of alloxan-diabetes and perfusion. Biochem J 1967;104:416–422.
150. McGarry JD, Mannaerts GP, Foster DW. A possible role for malonyl-CoA in the regulation of hepatic fatty acid oxidation and ketogenesis. J Clin Invest 1977;60:265–270.
151. Weis BC, Cowan AT, Brown N, Foster DW, McGarry JD. Use of a selective inhibitor of liver carnitine palmitoyltransferase I (CPT I) allows quantification of its contribution to total CPT I activity in rat heart. J Biol Chem 1994;269:26,443–26,448.
152. McGarry JD, Mills SE, Long CS, Foster DW. Observations on the affinity of carnitine, and malonyl-CoA sensitivity of carnitine palmitoyltransferase I in animal aand human tissues. Demonstration of the presence of malonyl-CoA in nonhepatic tissues of the rat. Biochem J 1983;214:21–28.
153. Cook GA, Gamble MS. Regulation of carnitine palmitoyltransferase by insulin results in decreased activity and decreased apparent Ki values for malonyl-CoA. J Biol Chem 1987;262:2050–2055.
154. Hudson EK, Liu M-H, Buja LM, McMillin JB. Insulin-associated changes in carnitine palmitoyltransferase in cultured neonatal rat cardiac myocytes. J Mol Cell Cardiol 1995;27:599–613.
155. Brownsey RW, Denton RM. Acetyl CoA carboxylase. In: Boyer P, Krebs EG, eds. The Enzymes: Control by Phosphorylation, Part B, vol. 18. Academic, New York, 1987, pp. 123–146.
156. Thampy KG. Formation of malonyl-CoA in rat heart. J Biol Chem 1989;264:17,631–17,634.
157. Bianchi A, Evans JL, Iverson AJ, Nordlund AC, Watts TD, Witters LA. Identification of an isozymic form of acetyl-CoA carboxylase. J Biol Chem 1990;265:1502–1509.
158. Saddik M, Gamble J, Witters LA, Lopaschuk GD. Acetyl-CoA carboxylase regulation of fatty acid oxidation in the heart. J Biol Chem 1993;268:25,836–25,845.
159. Winz R, Hess D, Aebersold R, Brownsey RW. Unique structural features and differential phosphorylation of the 280-kDa component (isozyme) of rat liver acetyl-CoA carboxylase. J Biol Chem 1994;269:14,438–14,445.
160. Ha J, Lee J-K, Kim K-S, Witters LA, Kim K-H. Cloning of human acetyl-CoA carboxylase-β and its unique features. Proc Natl Acad Sci USA 1996;93:11,466–11,470.
161. Abu-Elheiga L, Almarza-Ortega DB, Baldini A, Wakil SJ. Human acetyl-CoA carboxylase 2–molecular cloning, characterization, chromosomal mapping and evidence for two isoforms. J Biol Chem 1997;272:10,669–10,677.
162. Shipp JC, Matos OE, Knizely H, Crevasse LE. CO_2 formed from endogenous and exogenous substrates in perfused rat heart. Am J Physiol 1964;207:1231–1236.
163. Kim YS, Kolattukudy PE. Purification and properties of malonyl-CoA decarboxylase from rat liver mitochondria and its immunological comparison with the enzymes from rat brain, heart and mammary gland. Arch Biochem Biophys 1978;190:234–246.

9 Kinins in the Heart

Oscar A. Carretero

CONTENTS

OVERVIEW
KININ-GENERATING SYSTEM
ROLE OF KININS IN PATHOGENESIS OF HYPERTENSION
    AND IN THE ANTIHYPERTENSIVE EFFECT OF ACE INHIBITORS
CARDIOPROTECTIVE EFFECTS OF KININS
CARDIAC ISCHEMIA
REFERENCES

OVERVIEW

Kinins are polypeptides that contain the sequence of the nonapeptide, bradykinin, in their structure. In mammals, the main kinins are bradykinin and lysine-bradykinin. They are generated by a group of enzymes known as kininogenases, which include plasma and tissue kallikrein. Kininogenases release kinins from low- (LMWK) and high-molecular-weight kininogen (HMWK), which are present in high concentrations in plasma. Kinins are rapidly hydrolyzed in various tissues and plasma by a group of enzymes known as kininases; the best known are angiotensin-converting enzyme (ACE) and neutral endopeptidase 24.11 (NEP). Kinins release various endothelial autacoids, particularly nitric oxide (NO), endothelium-derived hyperpolarizing factor (EDHF), eicosanoids, and tissue plasminogen activator (tPA). These substances exert a cardioprotective effect by causing hemodynamic changes and/or by a direct effect on the heart. The heart and vascular tissue contain the components of the kallikrein-kinin system, and kinins are also present in the venous effluent of isolated hearts perfused with saline buffers. Myocardial ischemia increases local release of kinins, which is enhanced further by ACE inhibitors. Kinins are also found in vascular and cardiac tissue in higher concentrations than in plasma. In isolated cardiac arteries and microvessels, angiotensin stimulates the formation of cyclic guanosine 3',5'-monophosphate (cGMP), and this effect is mediated by the release of kinins and NO. The beneficial cardiovascular effects of ACE inhibitors, which are well documented, have generally been attributed to blockade of the renin-angiotensin system (RAS); however, there is a significant amount of evidence suggesting that kinins also participate in the cardioprotective effects of ACE inhibitors, especially in myocardial infarction (MI) induced by ischemia and reperfusion, left ventricular remodeling

From: *Contemporary Endocrinology: Hormones and the Heart in Health and Disease*
Edited by: L. Share © Humana Press Inc., Totowa, NJ

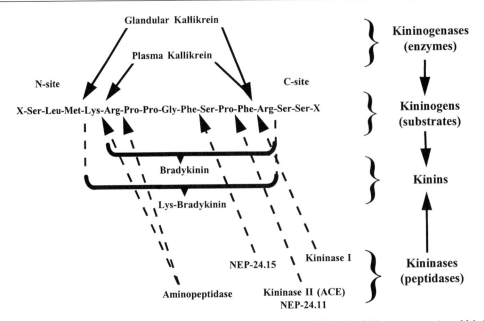

Fig. 1. Sites of kininogen cleavage by glandular and plasma kallikrein (full arrows, top) and kinin hydrolysis by kininase I or carboxypeptidase, kininase II or ACE, NEP 24.11, NEP 24.15, and aminopeptidases (broken arrows, bottom). Adapted with permission from ref. *126*.

after MI, and heart failure (HF). Recent evidence suggests that some of the effects of angiotensin (ANG) type 1 receptor (AT_1) antagonists are caused by activation of type 2 receptors, which may act via release of kinins and NO. This chapter will address the role of kinins within the heart, with emphasis on their role in the reduction of MI by ischemic preconditioning and the cardioprotective effect of ACE inhibitors in hypertension, as well as during MI induced by ischemia-reperfusion, left ventricular remodeling after MI, and HF post-MI.

KININ-GENERATING SYSTEM

Kinins are polypeptides that contain the sequence of the nonapeptide bradykinin in their structure. In mammals, the chief kinins are bradykinin and lysine (Lys)-bradykinin, which are generated by a group of enzymes known as kininogenases, including plasma and tissue (glandular) kallikreins. Tissue kallikrein releases Lys-bradykinin from low-(LMWK) and high-molecular-weight kininogen (HMWK) (kallikrein substrate); plasma kallikrein only hydrolyzes HMWK, releasing bradykinin. Plasma contains high concentrations of kininogens. Components of the kallikrein-kinin system, including a kallikrein-like enzyme, tissue kallikrein, and kininogen and their mRNAs, have been found in the heart and vascular tissue *(1–6)*. Kinins probably act as local hormones (paracrine systems) via the release of various autacoids; they are found in vascular and cardiac tissue in much higher concentrations than in plasma *(7)*, consistent with kinin production in tissue and their function as paracrine hormones. Kinins are rapidly hydrolyzed by a group of kininases, such as kininase II or angiotensin-converting enzyme (ACE), neutral endo-peptidase 24.11 (NEP), and aminopeptidase P *(8–10*; Fig. 1).

The effects of kinins are mediated by stimulation of at least two known subtypes of kinin receptors, B_1 and B_2, which have been classified based on their responses to various

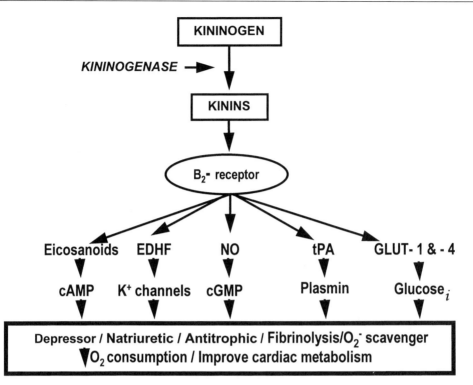

Fig. 2. Mechanism of kinin generation, and the multiple and complex effects of kinins via various intermediaries and their second messengers. Adapted with permission from ref. *19.*

agonists, and more recently have been cloned *(11–13)*. The B_1 receptor is the principal receptor for des-Arg[9] bradykinin; the B_2 receptor is more sensitive to bradykinin and Lys-bradykinin. Investigations using kinin analogs with agonistic and antagonistic actions in various tissues suggest that other subtypes of receptors also exist *(11,14)*; however, the vasodilator and cardiovascular protective effects of kinins appear to be mediated by the B_2 receptor. Acting through this receptor, kinins stimulate the release of endothelium-derived relaxing factors such as nitric oxide (NO), endothelium-derived hyperpolarizing factor (EDHF, the identity of which remains unclear), prostacyclin, and tissue plasminogen activator (tPA) *(15–18)*. These autacoids probably cause vasodilatation and cardiovascular protection by different mechanisms: NO, by stimulating soluble guanylate cyclase and production of cyclic guanosine 3',5'-monophosphate (cGMP); prostacyclin (the principal endothelial prostaglandin), by stimulating adenyl guanyl cyclase and the formation of cyclic adenosine monophosphate (cAMP); EDHF, by stimulating the opening of K^+-channels; and tPA, by activating plasminogen *(19)*. In addition, kinins interacting with insulin facilitate the translocation of glucose transporters (GLUT-1 and GLUT-4) to surface membranes, and consequently glucose uptake *(20–23)*. Thus, kinins acting via these autacoids have multiple and complex effects (Fig. 2). Because of these complex effects of kinins, because ACE inhibitors block not only the hydrolysis of kinins but also other peptides, and because ACE inhibitors also block the conversion of angiotensin I to II (ANG I or II), the effects of these inhibitors are likewise complex (Fig. 3). In the absence of endothelial autacoids, kinins cause vasoconstriction and stimulate cell growth and proliferation. In the past few years, the availability of potent and stable kinin

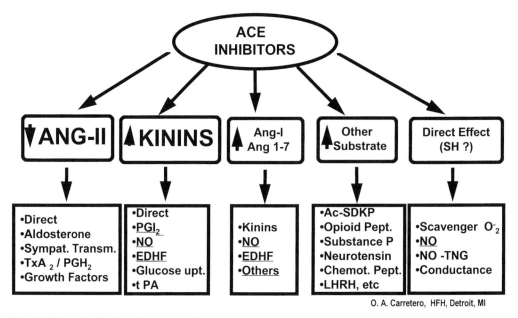

Fig. 3. Hypothetical mechanisms of action of ACE inhibitors. ACE has multiple substrates, and inhibition of their hydrolysis may explain the cardioprotective effect of ACE inhibitors.

receptor antagonists has allowed delineation of the role of kinins as endogenous cardioprotective substances more clearly, and also determination of their contribution to the therapeutic effects of ACE and NEP inhibitors.

ROLE OF KININS IN THE PATHOGENESIS OF HYPERTENSION AND IN THE ANTIHYPERTENSIVE EFFECT OF ACE INHIBITORS

Kinins in the Pathogenesis of Hypertension

In the kidney, kallikrein and kininogen are synthesized in the distal nephron, where receptors are located and kinins are released. The author and others have provided evidence that the renal kallikrein-kinin system may act as an endogenous diuretic and natriuretic system (24,25). Decreased activity of the renal kallikrein-kinin system may play a role in salt-sensitive hypertension (HT). Frequently, urinary kallikrein has been measured as an indicator of renal activity; however, the amount of kininogen and kininases, pH, and expression of kinin receptors in the distal nephron may all affect the activity of this system (26). Urinary kallikrein excretion is decreased in patients with essential HT, and in various animal models of genetic HT (27–29). Low urinary kallikrein excretion in children is a genetic marker associated with a family history of essential HT, and children with high urinary kallikrein excretion are less likely to have a genetic background of HT (30–32).

In rat models of genetic HT, urinary kallikrein excretion is also decreased, and a restriction-fragment-length polymorphism for the kallikrein gene family in spontaneously hypertensive rats (SHR) is linked to high BP (33). However, in renovascular HT urinary and arterial tissue, kallikrein are also decreased (3,28). Thus, the decrease in urinary kallikrein excretion can be both an alteration of kallikrein gene expression and/or secondary to increased BP. With mineralocorticoid HT or treatment, urinary kallikrein excretion and plasma kinins are increased *(27,34)*; however, it is not known whether these increases partially attenuate the rise in BP caused by volume expansion. Using the first generation of kinin antagonists, it was found that at very high doses they acutely increase BP in normal rats *(35)*. However, the significance of these studies is hampered by the very high dose of the antagonist, which in itself may have produced some non-specific effect.

In kininogen-deficient Brown Norway rats, and in rats receiving either a kallikrein inhibitor (aprotinin) or a kinin receptor antagonist (icatibant or Hoe 140), hypertensinogenic stimuli, such as high salt intake, a mineralocorticoid and salt, or ANG II, reportedly cause BP to increase faster and higher than in rats with a normal kallikrein-kinin system *(36,37)*. However, N.-E. Rhaleb et al. in this laboratory (unpublished results), have not been able to confirm these studies. Mice in which the bradykinin B_2 receptor is deleted (B_2 −/−) by homologous recombination (gene knock-out) have normal BP, compared to 129/SvEv Tac controls *(38)*; however, it has also recently been reported that they have higher BP than 129/SvJ *(39)*. The reason for this disparity may be related to the use of different controls; according to a recent publication investigating the relationships between various 129 substrains *(40)*, there should be fewer allelic polymorphisms between the original B_2−/− and 129/SvEvTac than between B_2−/− and 129/SvJ. Independent of this difference, both studies reported that B_2−/− develop HT when fed a high-sodium diet. Dahl salt-sensitive rats also have low urinary kallikrein excretion, even prior to the development of HT *(41)*. Rats inbred for low urinary kallikrein excretion developed HT when placed on high sodium *(42)*. The role of kinins in the regulation of normal BP and the pathogenesis of essential HT remains controversial; however, they may contribute to the development of salt-sensitive HT. This is important because in blacks urinary kallikrein excretion is low and the prevalence of salt-sensitive HT is high *(43)*.

Role of Kinins in the Antihypertensive Effect of ACE Inhibitors

Increased tissue kinin concentrations and potentiation of their effect may be involved in the therapeutic effect of ACE inhibitors. This hypothesis is supported by the following: ACE is one of the chief peptidases that hydrolyzes kinins, and has a higher affinity for kinins than for angiotensin; although plasma kinins are unchanged or moderately increased after treatment with ACE inhibitors, tissue and urinary kinins increase, possibly promoting vasodilatation and increased sodium and water excretion; inhibition of the kallikrein-kinin system with kinin antibodies, aprotinin, or kinin antagonists partially blocks the acute hypotensive effects of ACE inhibitors; and in kininogen- and kinin-deficient Brown Norway rats with experimental renovascular HT, the acute antihypertensive effect of ACE inhibitors is significantly reduced in both magnitude and duration *(44–48)*.

The role of kinins in the chronic antihypertensive effect of ACE inhibitors is unclear. The author has not been able to block the effect of ACE inhibitors on BP with the kinin antagonist, icatibant, in either HT or heart failure (HF; *49,50*). Linz and Schölkens *(51)*, using the same model of HT (aortic coarctation) and the same ACE inhibitor and kinin antagonist at the same doses, found complete reversal of the effect of the ACE inhibitor on both BP and left ventricular hypertrophy (LVH). The reason for these disparate results is not clear; however, it is surprising that the effect of ACE inhibitors can be completely reversed in this model, because HT is highly dependent on the renin-angiotensin system (RAS) *(52)*. In two-kidney, one-clip renovascular hypertensive rats (2K1C), Bao et al. *(53)* showed that approx 25% of the chronic antihypertensive effect of an ACE inhibitor was hindered by chronic kinin B_2 receptor blockade. The same investigators found that in 2K1C Brown Norway Katholiek rats, which are deficient in kininogen and kinins, none of the effect of the ACE inhibitor was altered by the kinin antagonist, suggesting that part of the chronic effect of the ACE inhibitor was mediated by kinins. In SHR, they found that none of the chronic antihypertensive effect of the ACE inhibitor was caused by kinins. Numerous reports suggest that a modest part of the acute antihypertensive effect of ACE inhibitors is mediated by kinins. The role of kinins in the chronic antihypertensive effect of ACE inhibitors depends on the model of HT studied; in HT induced by aortic coarctation between the renal arteries, its role is controversial; in 2K1C renovascular HT, approx 25% of the effect of the ACE inhibitor could be caused by kinins, and in SHR none of the effect was mediated by kinins.

CARDIOPROTECTIVE EFFECTS OF KININS

Left Ventricular Hypertrophy

ACE inhibitors administered in antihypertensive doses appear to be more effective than other antihypertensive drugs in reducing LVH (54). ACE inhibitors may diminish hypertrophy by decreasing afterload and preload (hemodynamic changes); inhibiting the conversion of ANG I to II, thereby blocking the direct cardiotrophic effect of ANG II; and/or increasing cardiac kinins, which may have an antitrophic effect via NO and prostaglandins. Using rats with ascending aortic stenosis, Weinberg et al. (55) reported that ACE inhibitors improved survival, decreased the extent of LVH, and improved cardiac function, despite persistent elevation of LV systolic pressure. They concluded that the favorable effect of ACE inhibitors may be related in part to inhibition of the effects of cardiac ACE on myocyte hypertrophy. The same group (56) reported that they could not obtain similar effects using an AT_1-antagonist (ant), suggesting that the effect of ACE inhibitors may be related not to inhibition of ANG II formation, but rather suppression of kinin hydrolysis.

Linz et al. (57) reported that nonantihypertensive doses of ramipril were effective in reducing hypertrophy caused by aortic banding in rats; antihypertensive doses of an ANG II blocker were less effective. Using the same model, they later demonstrated that the antihypertensive and antihypertrophic effects of high doses of this ACE inhibitor, as well as the antihypertrophic effects of low, nonantihypertensive doses, were reversed by a specific kinin B_2 receptor antagonist (51), suggesting that bradykinin participates in the beneficial effects of ACE inhibitors and that this effect is not hemodynamic, because doses that did not decrease BP had a similar effect. However, the inhibitor was given in the drinking water, and rats are nocturnal animals that eat and drink during the night, but BP was measured during the day; thus, a low dose of the ACE inhibitor may decrease BP during the night, and this will not be detected when BP is measured during the day. Furthermore, the use of nondepressor doses of ACE inhibitors does not exclude changes in other hemodynamic parameters, such as pulse pressure, preload, and/or cardiac output, all of which may contribute to decreased LVH.

In contrast, using the same aortic coarctation model as Linz and Schölkens (51), the same ACE inhibitor and B_2 kinin receptor antagonist, and the same doses, the author was unable to reproduce their results (49). It was found that left ventricular (LV) weight correlated significantly with BP (Fig. 4), only antihypertensive doses of the ACE inhibitor produced an antihypertrophic effect, and the kinin antagonist did not block either the

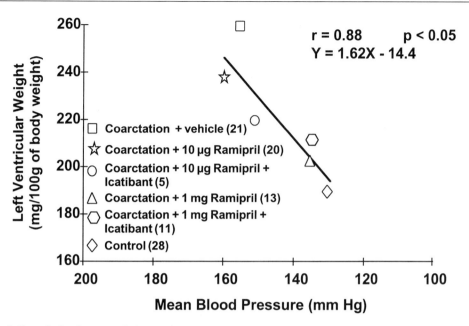

Fig. 4. Correlation between left ventricular weight and mean BP in hypertensive rats (aortic coarctation between renal arteries) treated with: (1) vehicle (square), (2) ramipril (10 μg) at nonantihypertensive doses (star), (3) ramipril (10 mg) plus the kinin antagonist icatibant (circle), (4) ramipril (1 μg) at antihypertensive doses (triangle), (5) ramipril (1 mg) plus icatibant (hexagon), and (6) control (sham aortic coarctation) (diamond). Note that ramipril at nonantihypertensive doses did not affect LV weight; furthermore, icatibant did not reverse either the antihypertensive or antihypertrophic effects of ramipril. Adapted with permission from ref. *49.*

antihypertensive or antihypertrophic effects of the inhibitor. Similarly, using an experimental model of genetic HT, the stroke-prone spontaneously hypertensive rat (SPSHR), Gohlke et al. *(58)* determined that chronic treatment with low, nonantihypertensive doses of ramipril did not alter LVH. In this study, antihypertensive doses of the ACE inhibitor decreased BP and hypertrophy, but chronic blockade of the B_2 kinin receptor did not abolish the antihypertensive or antihypertrophic effects of the ACE inhibitor. They found that hearts from untreated SPSHR had evidence of ischemia, including low coronary flow and abnormal metabolic parameters, compared with normotensive controls. Low doses of the ACE inhibitor resulted in increased LV contractility and improved flow and metabolism. Thus, the improvements in cardiac function were independent of reductions in afterload or hypertrophy. Using SHR, Harrap and O'Sullivan *(59)* studied the role of kinins in the effect of ACE inhibitors on the weight of transplanted (not pumping blood) and native hearts. They found that at antihypertensive doses the ACE inhibitor decreased heart weight in both native and transplanted hearts; however, in the transplanted hearts this effect was reversed by a kinin B_2 receptor antagonist, but in the native hearts it was not. The mechanisms by which kinins improve cardiac metabolism are not known; however, kinins increase glucose uptake by myocytes *(60)* and mediate the improvement in insulin sensitivity during treatment with ACE inhibitors *(61,62).* Acting via kinins, ACE inhibitors increase myocardial capillary length and density, which, together with local vasodilatation, may improve cardiac tissue perfusion *(58).* Thus, ACE inhibitors acting via an increase in tissue kinins, NO, and glucose uptake, together with increased perfusion and decreased cardiac workload, may improve cardiac metabolism and function (63,64).

The above data suggest that in HT, increasing kinin concentrations in the heart are an unlikely cause of ACE inhibitor-induced reductions in LVH. Reductions in heart size are likely to be determined primarily by the decrease in BP and preload afforded by the ACE inhibitor. On the other hand, a kinin-dependent mechanism appears to participate in the antitrophic effects of ACE inhibitors in transplanted nonpumping hearts, thus separating hemodynamic from nonhemodynamic effects. Furthermore, Gohlke's study (58) suggests that in SPSHR, cardiac kinins are responsible for improving the metabolic and functional status of the ischemic and hypertrophic heart, thereby contributing to the cardioprotective effects of ACE inhibitors but not the antihypertrophic effect.

CARDIAC ISCHEMIA

According to several experimental models, cardiac ischemia increases the release of local bradykinin, which is further enhanced by administration of an ACE inhibitor (65–67). Such a response appears to favorably influence cardiodynamic and metabolic events during ischemic episodes, and to protect against postischemic reperfusion arrhythmia and injury. During the past few years, a series of experiments suggested that kinins have a protective effect in the ischemic heart. In isolated working hearts with acute myocardial ischemia and subsequent reperfusion, administration of bradykinin or an ACE inhibitor resulted in a similar pattern of improved myocardial function and metabolism, as well as a significant reduction in the incidence and duration of ventricular fibrillation (68–70). In dogs with occlusion/reperfusion injury, intracoronary infusion of bradykinin in doses too low to improve hemodynamics reduced reperfusion injury and normalized myocardial metabolism (69).

Increasing cardiac kinins by infusing bradykinin or ACE inhibitors reduces myocardial infarct (MI) size caused by ischemia or ischemia/reperfusion in animals (71–73). In humans, Hashimoto et al. (74) found that kinin levels in the peripheral circulation were increased soon after MI, perhaps limiting infarct size. The author studied the role of kinins in the cardioprotective effects of ACE inhibitors using ischemia/reperfusion injury in rats, and found that an ACE inhibitor reduced infarct size and arrhythmia; this effect was reversed by a kinin B_2 receptor antagonist, a NO synthesis inhibitor, or a cyclooxygenase inhibitor (73; Figs. 5 and 6). A NEP 24.11 inhibitor also reduced ischemia/reperfusion infarct size, and this cardioprotective effect was blocked completely by a kinin B_2 receptor antagonist and partially by an atrial natriuretic factor receptor antagonist (75). During ischemia/reperfusion, kinins acting via prostaglandins and NO are involved in the reduction of MI size and the effect of ACE inhibitors.

Myocardial Ischemic Preconditioning

Repeated brief coronary occlusion renders the myocardium more resistant to injury from subsequent prolonged ischemia, a process called ischemic preconditioning. As indicated previously, ischemia results in the release of kinins. Furthermore, a kinin B_2 receptor antagonist diminished the cardioprotective effect of preconditioning (76,77), suggesting that kinins are important in reducing MI size after preconditioning. The author tested the hypothesis that kinins mediate the effect of preconditioning by studying MI size induced by ischemia/reperfusion, using mice lacking the gene encoding for

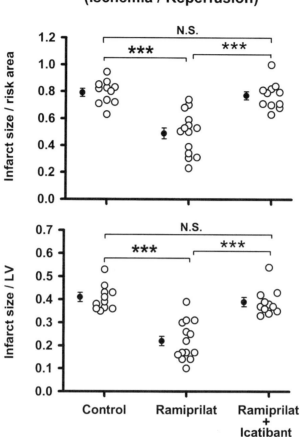

Fig. 5. Infarct size (caused by ischemia/reperfusion) as a percentage of the area at risk (top) and left ventricle (bottom), and effect of treatment with: (1) vehicle (control), (2) an ACE inhibitor (ramiprilat), and (3) ACE inhibitor plus kinin receptor antagonist (icatibant). Open circles represent individual animals; filled circles represent the mean for the group. *** $p < 0.001$ vs ramiprilat. Reproduced with permission from ref. *127*.

the B_2 kinin receptor as well as rats deficient in the kinin precursor kininogen (Brown Norway Katholiek rats) *(78)*. In both models, the reduction in MI size as an effect of preconditioning was completely absent. Figure 7 shows the effect of preconditioning on MI size in mice with intact B_2 receptors (+/+), and in mice with the B_2 receptor knocked out (-/-). There is also evidence that NO is involved in the cardioprotective effect of preconditioning *(79)*. Kinins, perhaps acting via release of NO, participate in the cardioprotective effect of preconditioning; the mechanism behind this protection is not known, but may include hyperpolarization caused by activation of K^+ channels *(80,81)*. Kinins acting via release of NO may be scavengers of free radicals during ischemia/reperfusion and/or reduce O_2 consumption *(63,82)*.

Left Ventricular Remodeling Following Myocardial Damage

ACE inhibitors improve cardiac function and remodeling and prolong survival in patients with HF *(83–88)*. This cardioprotective effect may result from blockade of the

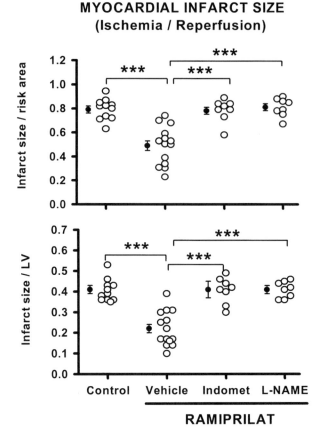

Fig. 6. Effects of the cyclooxygenase inhibitor indomethacin (Bayer Pharmaceuticals, Lever Keusen, Germany) or the NO synthase inhibitor L-NAME on reduction of MI size by treatment with an ACE inhibitor (ramiprilat). MI size is shown as a percentage of the area at risk (top) and the LV (bottom). **** $p < 0.001$ vs ramiprilat. Reproduced with permission from ref. *127.*

RAS and/or inhibition of kinin destruction. McDonald et al. *(89)* studied the role of kinins in the remodeling effect of ACE inhibitors in dogs after discrete transmural myocardial necrosis caused by direct current shock. They found that treatment for 4 wk with an ACE inhibitor, starting immediately after induction of myocardial necrosis, prevented the early increase in LV mass, and that this effect was abolished by the B_2 antagonist, icatibant; however, the hypotensive effect of the ACE inhibitor was not blunted. They did not observe any significant change in ventricular volume or hemodynamics. Also, using this model, these investigators have shown that an AT_1-ant was ineffective in attenuating remodeling *(90)*, further supporting the hypothesis that the effects of ACE inhibitors during cardiac remodeling caused by myocardial damage are mediated by kinins, and not necessarily caused by a decrease in ANG II.

Stauss et al. *(91)* reported that, in rats administration of ACE inhibitors before coronary ligation resulted in reduced infarct size, heart weight, and end-diastolic pressure. All of these effects were blocked by concomitant administration of icatibant. Losartan, an AT_1-ant, did not affect any of these parameters. In this study, the cardioprotective effect of the ACE inhibitor was again the result of reduced degradation of kinins, rather than reduced synthesis of ANG II; however, from this study it is not possible to determine

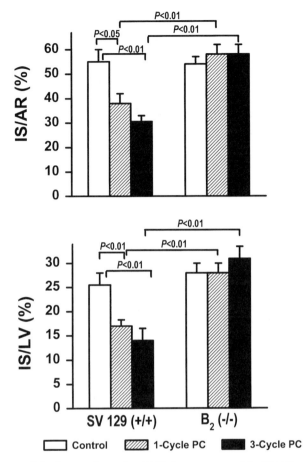

Fig. 7. Effect of preconditioning on the ratio of MI size to area at risk (IS/AR, upper panel) and left ventricle (IS/LV, lower panel) in 129SvEvTac mice (SV 129) and B_2 kinin receptor knock-out mice ($B_2-/-$). Control indicates without preconditioning; PC, preconditioning. Reproduced with permission from ref. *78*.

whether ACE inhibitors acting via kinins prevented remodeling and HF after MI, because the ACE inhibitor was administered prior to induction of infarction, so that the infarcted area was 61% smaller than in untreated rats. Ventricular remodeling is influenced by three interdependent factors: infarct size, infarct healing, and ventricular wall stress *(92)*. Collectively, these studies suggest that kinins mediate part of the effect of ACE inhibitors during cardiac remodeling, and consequently prevent the development of HF.

Heart Failure

In patients and experimental models of HF, ACE inhibitors reduce morbidity and mortality and improve cardiac function *(84–87,93–97)*. There is also evidence that AT_1-ants improve cardiac function in HF *(98–100)*. Thus, because both ACE inhibitors and AT_1-ants block the RAS at different levels, and both have a cardioprotective effect, various investigators interpreted these data as implying that the cardioprotective effect of ACE inhibitors is a result of blockade of the conversion of ANG I to II, not inhibition of kinin hydrolysis. However, as mentioned before there is evidence that some of the effects of ACE inhibitors are mediated by an increase in kinin tissue concentrations, which may

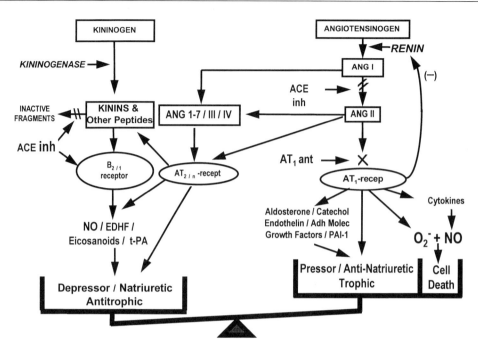

Fig. 8. Hypothetical mechanism of action of ACEi and AT_1-ant in HF. ACEi act by blocking both conversion of ANG I to ANG II and hydrolysis of kinins. Acting via the B_2 receptor, kinins stimulate the release of various autacoids, such as NO, endothelium-derived hyperpolarizing factor (EDHF), eicosanoids, and t-PA; AT_1-ant blocks the corresponding receptor, causing increased renin release, which results in the formation of angiotensins. These angiotensins act on the AT_2 receptor, which induces the release of autacoids similar to those stimulated by kinins. Adapted with permission from ref. *50*.

act through the release of NO and eicosanoids *(50,89)*. To explain this apparent incongruity, the author postulated that the effects of the AT_1-ant are not entirely caused by blockade of the AT_1 receptor. Angiotensin receptors comprise two major subtypes, AT_1 and AT_2 *(101)*. When the AT_1 receptor is blocked, plasma renin and angiotensins increase; angiotensin may act on AT_2 receptors, which could have an antitrophic effect *(102)* either directly or by the release of autacoids such as kinins and NO *(103,104)*, and consequently may contribute to the therapeutic effect of AT_1-ant by a mechanism similar to kinins. The author tested the hypothesis that in HF the chronic therapeutic effect of ACE inhibitors is not only caused by inhibition of formation of ANG II but is mediated in part by kinins, whereas that of AT_1-ants is caused not only by blockade of the AT_1 receptor, but also by activation of the AT_2 receptor. Activation of the AT_2 receptor may exert protection via kinins and other autacoids (Fig. 8). This hypothesis was tested using a model of HF induced by MI in Lewis inbred rats *(50)*. In this strain, ligation of the left anterior descending coronary artery produces uniformly large infarcts with low mortality *(105)*. In addition, 2 mo after MI both ventricular volume and end-diastolic pressure are significantly increased, but the ejection fraction (EF) is decreased. To assess LV dilatation and performance, the author used a direct angiographic method *(106)*. This model of HF was used to investigate whether the kinin antagonist icatibant blocks the beneficial effect of an ACE inhibitor, and whether the beneficial effects of an AT_1-ant (L158809) are blocked by either an AT_2-ant (PD123319) or icatibant. The author found that the rats with MI had a significant increase in LV end-diastolic (LVEDV), and end-systolic volume (LVESV)

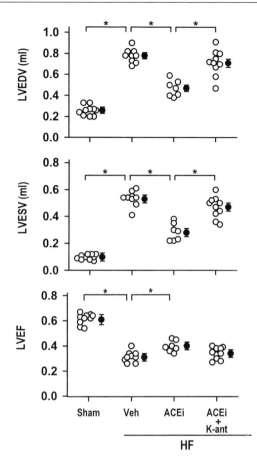

Fig. 9. Effect of the angiotensin-converting enzyme inhibitor ramipril (ACEi) and ACEi plus the kinin antagonist icatibant (K-ant) on LVEDV (top), LVESV (middle), and left ventricular ejection fraction (bottom) in sham-operated rats (Sham) and rats with chronic HF. $p < 0.05$; Veh, vehicle. Reproduced with permission from ref. *50.*

as well as interstitial collagen deposition and cardiomyocyte size, but EF was decreased. As expected, chronic treatment with an ACE inhibitor improved LV function and attenuated remodeling. Some of the changes caused by the ACE inhibitor were small, as for example the increase in LVEF; however, this increase occurred simultaneously with decreases in LV end-diastolic pressure (LVEDP), suggesting that the pumping ability of the LV was significantly improved. Cardiomyocyte cross-sectional area (an indicator of myocyte volume), as well as interstitial collagen fraction and oxygen diffusion distance, were all decreased by the ACE inhibitor; capillary density was increased, indicating that LV remodeling at the cellular level may have been attenuated as well. It was observed that part of the cardioprotective effect of the ACE inhibitor was blocked by the kinin B_2-ant icatibant (Fig. 9), supporting the hypothesis that inhibition of kinin hydrolysis contributes to the therapeutic effect of ACE inhibitors in chronic HF. Treatment with the B_2-ant by itself did not have any effect on function and remodeling, suggesting either that, in the absence of the ACE inhibitor, kinins are present at concentrations that do not affect the progression of HF, or else that blockade of the RAS is necessary in order for kinins to have a cardioprotective effect, or both.

The mechanism by which activation of the kinin B_2 receptor may produce cardio-protection is not well established. Farhy et al. *(107)*, in this laboratory, have shown that ACE inhibitors reduce neointima formation after carotid injury, and that this effect is mediated by kinins, eicosanoids, and NO. Their study suggests that ACE inhibitors, acting via kinins-eicosanoids-NO, have an antitrophic effect. The author's study further supports the hypothesis that ACE inhibitors, acting via kinins, have an antitrophic effect in chronic HF, because ventricular volume, myocyte size, and interstitial fibrosis were decreased by the ACE inhibitor, and these effects were partially blocked by the B_2-ant *(50)*. Although blockade of the effect of the ACE inhibitor on myocyte size, capillary density, and oxygen diffusion distance by the B_2-ant did not reach statistical significance, it tended to change in the anticipated direction. The effects of ACE inhibitors on these parameters could be caused mainly by a decrease in ANG II concentrations, and increased tissue kinins may play primarily a modulatory role.

Two major ANG II receptor subtypes have been identified, AT_1 and AT_2 *(101)*. Of the total number of ANG II receptors found in the normal rat ventricle, roughly 31% are AT_2; during LVH, AT_2 increases to approx 60% *(108)*. In the author's study, the AT_1-ant exhibited a cardioprotective effect similar to ACE inhibitors *(50)*. To study the role of AT_2 receptors in the effects of AT_1-ant, the author used an AT_2-ant, which blocked many of the beneficial effects of the AT_1-ant (Fig. 10). The mechanism by which activation of the AT_2 receptor may produce cardioprotection is not known. Most known effects of ANG II, such as increasing BP, stimulating myocyte hypertrophy, and increasing colla-gen synthesis, are attributed to the AT_1 receptor; AT_2 receptors, which are primarily embryonic, may be activated during development of cardiac hypertrophy and HF *(108–111)*. There is evidence that the AT_2 receptor antagonizes both the pressor and growth effects of the AT_1 receptor; however, neither the mediator nor the second messenger of this receptor is well established *(102)*. It could be that the AT_2 receptor exerts its bene-ficial effects on HF by stimulating local release of NO either directly or via kinins *(50,103,104,112)*, which, together with blockade of the AT_1 receptor, may have an anti-trophic effect; consequently, LV remodeling regresses and LV function improves. In endothelial cells in culture, ANG II increased the release of cGMP; this effect was blocked by a kinin antagonist and a NO synthesis inhibitor, and was markedly inhibited by an AT_2-ant but only marginally inhibited by an AT_1-ant *(113)*, suggesting that ANG II-stimulated release of NO is predominantly caused by stimulation of the AT_2 receptor, and may lead to an increase in the effect of kinins, stimulation of NO, and increased cGMP formation. Also, in isolated microvessels of the dog heart, it has been shown that angiotensin stimulates cGMP via either the AT_2 and/or a non-AT_1 or AT_2 receptor (AT_n), kinins, and NO *(104)*. Brosnihan et al. *(114)* recently reported that ANG 1–7 dilates canine coronary arteries through kinins and NO via AT_n. Also, Siragy and Carey *(103)* recently reported that during low sodium intake, angiotensin stimulates increased renal interstitial cGMP via the AT_2 receptor. Thus, it is possible that during blockade of the AT_1 receptor, activation of the AT_2 or AT_n receptor may mediate some of the cardiovascular effects of AT_1-ants, either directly or via kinins and/or NO and cGMP. The author also tested whether the effects of the AT_1-ant are mediated by kinins, and found that the kinin B_2-ant partially blocked the effects of the AT_1-ant on LVEDV and LVESV (Fig. 11), but not its other effects. These data suggest that during blockade of the AT_1 receptor, kinin levels normally present in tissue exert an effect that leads to reduction of ventricular

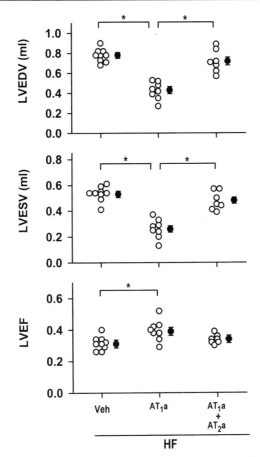

Fig. 10. Effect of the AT_1 antagonist L158809 (AT_{1a}) and AT_{1a} + the AT_2 antagonist PD123319 (AT_{2a}) on LVEDV (top), LVESV (middle), and LVEF (bottom) in rats with chronic HF. $* p < 0.05$; Veh, vehicle. Reproduced with permission from ref. *50*.

volume. Another explanation could be that during AT_1 blockade, activation of AT_2 receptors may lead to an increase in the effect of kinins *(114)*.

ACE inhibitors and AT_1-ants may exert a cardioprotective effect by causing hemodynamic changes, and/or by a direct effect on the heart. In the author's study, both ACE inhibitors and AT_1-ant decreased BP, and this hypotensive effect was not blocked by either B_2-ant or AT_2-ant; however, the cardioprotective effect was partially blocked. These data were interpreted as indicating that a decrease in afterload was not the chief cause of the cardioprotective effect. However, an effect on preload cannot be excluded, especially because both ACE inhibitors and AT_1-ants may result in natriuresis and diuresis (acting via blockade of the RAS, an increase in tissue kinins, and/or activation of the AT_2 receptor) *(25,115)*. In addition, by increasing NO they may cause venous dilatation. All of these actions may lead to a decrease in preload and LV chamber radius, and consequently decrease end-diastolic stress *(116–118)*. Because LVEDP was decreased by both ACE inhibitors and AT_1-ant, it could be that decreased preload is important for the therapeutic effects that were observed *(116)*. Also, the B_2-ant blocked the effect of the AT_1-ant on LV volume, but not its effect on cardiocyte hypertrophy or collagen deposition,

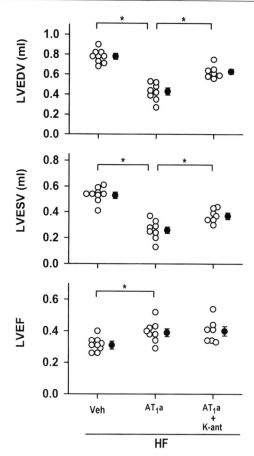

Fig. 11. Effect of the AT_1 antagonist L158809 (AT_{1a}) and AT_{1a} + the kinin antagonist icatibant (K-ant) on LVEDV (top), LVESV (middle), and LVEF (bottom) in rats with chronic HF. $*p < 0.05$; Veh, vehicle. Reproduced with permission from ref. *50*.

suggesting that some of the observed effects may be caused by a decrease in preload secondary to diuresis and/or venous dilatation caused by kinins. It has been shown that diuretics decrease LV mass principally by reducing chamber diameter; however, they failed to decrease LV wall thickness and prevent remodeling *(116,118)*. This could be because diuretics stimulate the RAS; the potent vasoconstrictor and myocardial growth-promoting action of ANG II may offset the cardiac benefit of diuretics.

On the other hand, the components of both renin-angiotensin *(119–121)* and kalli-krein-kinin systems *(5,6,122,123)* are present in the heart, so that some of the effects of ACE inhibitors and AT_1-ants may be local. Furthermore, decreasing afterload does not necessarily result in cardiac remodeling in HF. Cohn *(124)* showed that in patients with chronic HF, the vasodilator prazosin failed to exert an antiremodeling effect. Similar results were obtained by McDonald et al. *(90)* in a canine model of remodeling, in which the α-blocker terazosin failed to inhibit remodeling, but ACE inhibitors and nitrates did. Additionally, in the Cooperative North Scandinavian Enalapril Survival Study *(84)*, the decreased mortality that occurred during treatment with ACE inhibitors was also observed in patients treated with vasodilators (nitrates and hydralazine), suggesting that the bene-fit of ACE inhibitors goes beyond hemodynamic effects. Taken together, these data may suggest that the beneficial cardiac effects of ACE inhibitors and AT_1-ant are not only dependent on their hemodynamic action, but also probably interfere with autocrine/paracrine actions involving the cardiac renin-angiotensin and kallikrein-kinin systems. Nevertheless, at present it is not well established whether the effects of ACE inhibitors and AT_1-ants on cardiac function and remodeling are caused by changes in autacoids acting either directly on the heart or secondary to hemodynamic effects, or (more probably) both.

The effect of kinins may be mediated by the release of prostaglandins and/or NO. In patients with coronary artery disease and HF, treatment with salicylate (a cyclooxygenase inhibitor) reduced some of the beneficial effects of the ACE inhibitor *(125)*. The authors interpreted these data as showing that part of the effect of ACE was caused by kinins (which stimulate prostaglandins), and that this effect was blocked by salicylate. However, only a small number of patients was studied, making any conclusions premature.

In summary in chronic HF caused by MI, both ACE inhibitors and AT_1-ant have a cardioprotective effect, manifested by attenuation of LV chamber remodeling. The effects of ACE inhibitors are mediated in part by kinins; those of AT_1-ants are triggered by activation of the AT_2 receptor. The decrease in ventricular volume caused by the AT_1-ant is also mediated in part by kinins. The author speculates that in HF, blockade of AT_1 receptors increases both renin and angiotensin; these stimulate the AT_2 receptor, which in turn may play an important role in the therapeutic effect of AT_1-ants via kinins and other autacoids. Thus, the mechanisms by which ACE inhibitors and AT_1-ant work in HF are similar, in that both block the RAS, and both may induce the release of similar autacoids.

ACKNOWLEDGMENTS

This work was supported by National Institutes of Health grant HL28982 and a grant from the Fujimoto Corporation, Osaka, Japan. The author is grateful to Pharmacia Upjohn (Kalamazoo, MI) for donating ramipril and Hoechst (Somerville, NJ) for donating icatibant.

REFERENCES

1. Nolly H, Scicli AG, Scicli G, Carretero OA. Characterization of a kininogenase from rat vascular tissue resembling tissue kallikrein. Circ Res 1985;56:816–821.
2. Nolly H, Scicli AG, Scicli G, Lama MC, Guercio AM, Carretero OA. Kininogenase from rat vascular tissue. Adv Exp Med Biol 1986;198A:11–17.
3. Nolly H, Carretero OA, Scicli G, Madeddu P, Scicli AG. A kallikrein-like enzyme in blood vessels of one-kidney, one-clip hypertensive rats. Hypertension 1990;16:436–440.
4. Nolly HL, Saed G, Scicli G, Carretero OA, Scicli AG. The kallikrein-kinin system in cardiac tissue. Agents Actions Suppl 1992;38/III:62–72.
5. Nolly H, Carretero OA, Scicli AG. Kallikrein release by vascular tissue. Am J Physiol 1993;265: H1209–H1214.
6. Nolly H, Carbini LA, Scicli G, Carretero OA, Scicli AG. A local kallikrein-kinin system is present in rat hearts. Hypertension 1994;23:919–923.
7. Campbell DJ, Kladis A, Duncan A-M. Bradykinin peptides in kidney, blood, and other tissues of the rat. Hypertension 1993;21:155–165.
8. Erdös EG. Angiotensin I converting enzyme and the changes in our concepts through the years. Lewis K. Dahl memorial lecture. Hypertension 1990;16:363–370.
9. Ura N, Carretero OA, Erdös EG. Role of renal endopeptidase 24.11 in kinin metabolism in vitro and in vivo. Kidney Int 1987;32:507–513.
10. Kitamura S, Carbini LA, Carretero OA, Simmons WH, Scicli AG. Potentiation by aminopeptidase P of blood pressure response to bradykinin. Br J Pharmacol 1995;114:6–7.

11. Regoli D. Pharmacology of bradykinin and related kinins. Adv Exp Med Biol 1983;156:569–584.
12. Menke JG, Borkowski JA, Bierilo KK, MacNeil T, Derrick AW, Schneck KA, et al. Expression cloning of a human B_1 bradykinin receptor. J Biol Chem 1994;269:21,583–21,586.
13. Borkowski JA, Ransom RW, Seabrook GR, Trumbauer M, Chen H, Hill RG, Strader CD, Hess JF. Targeted disruption of a B_2 bradykinin receptor gene in mice eliminates bradykinin action in smooth muscle and neurons. J Biol Chem 1995;270:13,706–13,710.
14. Regoli D, Rhaleb N-E, Dion S, Drapeau G. New selective bradykinin receptor antagonists and bradykinin B_2 receptor characterization. Trends Pharmacol Sci 1990;11:156–161.
15. Moncada S, Palmer RMJ, Higgs EA. Nitric oxide: physiology, pathophysiology, and pharmacology. Pharmacol Rev 1991;43:109–142.
16. Vane JR, Änggård EE, Botting RM. Regulatory functions of the vascular endothelium. N Engl J Med 1990;323:27–36.
17. Mombouli J-V, Illiano S, Nagao T, Scott-Burden T, Vanhoutte PM. Potentiation of endothelium-dependent relaxations to bradykinin by angiotensin I converting enzyme inhibitors in canine coronary artery involves both endothelium-derived relaxing and hyperpolarizing factors. Circ Res 1992;71:137–144.
18. Smith D, Gilbert M, Owen WG. Tissue plasminogen activator release in vivo in response to vasoactive agents. Blood 1985;66:835–839.
19. Carretero OA, Scicli AG. The kallikrein-kinin system as a regulator of cardiovascular and renal function. In: Laragh JH, Brenner BM, eds. Hypertension: Physiology, Diagnosis, and Management. Raven, New York, 1995, pp. 983–999.
20. Miyata T, Taguchi T, Uehara M, Isami S, Kishikawa H, Kaneko K, Araki E, Shichiri M. Bradykinin potentiates insulin-stimulated glucose uptake and enhances insulin signal through the bradykinin B_2 receptor in dog skeletal muscle and rat L6 myoblasts. Eur J Endocrinol 1998;138:344–352.
21. Rett K, Maerker E, Renn W, van Gilst W, Haering HU. Perfusion-independent effect of bradykinin and fosinoprilate on glucose transport in Langendorff rat hearts. Am J Cardiol 1997;80:143A–147A.
22. Rett K, Wicklmayr M, Dietze GJ, Häring HU. Insulin-induced glucose transporter (GLUT1 and GLUT4) translocation in cardiac muscle tissue is mimicked by bradykinin. Diabetes 1996;45(Suppl 1): S66–S69.
23. Thomas J, Linssen M, van der Vusse GJ, Hirsch B, Rosen P, Kammermeier H, Fischer Y. Acute stimulation of glucose transport by histamine in cardiac microvascular endothelial cells. Biochim Biophys Acta 1995;1268:88–96.
24. Marin-Grez M, Cottone P, Carretero OA. Evidence for an involvement of kinins in regulation of sodium excretion. Am J Physiol 1972;223:794–796.
25. Saitoh S, Scicli AG, Peterson E, Carretero OA. Effect of inhibiting renal kallikrein on prostaglandin E_2, water, and sodium excretion. Hypertension 1995;25:1008–1013.
26. Brukman J, Murray RD, Churchill PC, Scicli AG, Carretero OA. Effect of urinary alkalinization on the intrarenal formation of kinins. Am J Physiol 1985;249:F827–F831.
27. Margolius HS, Horwitz D, Geller RG, Alexander RW, Gill JR Jr, Pisano JJ, Keiser HR. Urinary kallikrein excretion in normal man. Relationships to sodium intake and sodium-retaining steroids. Circ Res 1974;35:812–818.
28. Keiser HR, Geller RG, Margolius HS, Pisano JJ. Urinary kallikrein in hypertensive animal models. Fed Proc 1976;35:199–202.
29. Carretero OA, Polomski C, Hampton A, Scicli AG. Urinary kallikrein, plasma renin and aldosterone in New Zealand genetically hypertensive (GH) rats. Clin. Exp. Pharmacol. Physiol. 1976;3(Suppl): 55–59.
30. Williams RR, Hunt SC, Hasstedt SJ, Berry TD, Wu LL, Barlow GK, Stults BM, Kuida H. Definition of genetic factors in hypertension: a search for major genes, polygenes, and homogeneous subtypes. J Cardiovasc Pharmacol 1988;12:S7–S20.
31. Berry TD, Hasstedt SJ, Hunt SC, Wu LL, Smith JB, Ash KO, Kuida H, Williams RR. A gene for high urinary kallikrein may protect against hypertension in Utah kindreds. Hypertension 1989;13:3–8.
32. Zinner SH, Margolius HS, Rosner B, Kass EH. Stability of blood pressure rank and urinary kallikrein concentration in childhood: an eight-year follow-up. Circulation 1978;58:908–915.
33. Pravenec M, Křen V, Kuneš J, Scicli AG, Carretero OA, Simonet L, Kurtz TW. Cosegregation of blood pressure with kallikrein gene family polymorphism. Hypertension 1991;17:242–246.
34. Nakagawa M, Nasjletti A. Plasma kinin concentration in deoxycorticosterone-salt hypertension. Hypertension 1988;11:411–415.

35. Carbonell LF, Carretero OA, Madeddu P, Scicli AG. Effects of a kinin antagonist on mean blood pressure. Hypertension 1988;11(Suppl I):I-84–I-88.
36. Majima M, Mizogami S, Kuribayashi Y, Katori M, Oh-Ishi S. Hypertension induced by a nonpressor dose of angiotensin II in kininogen-deficient rats. Hypertension 1994;24:111–119.
37. Madeddu P, Parpaglia PP, Demontis MP, Varoni MV, Fattaccio MC, Tonolo G, Troffa C, Glorioso N. Bradykinin B_2-receptor blockade facilitates deoxycorticosterone-salt hypertension. Hypertension 1993;21:980–984.
38. Alfie ME, Sigmon DH, Pomposiello SI, Carretero OA. Effect of high salt intake in mutant mice lacking bradykinin-B_2 receptors. Hypertension 1997;29:483–487.
39. Emanueli C, Angioni GR, Anania V, Spissu A, Madeddu P. Blood pressure responses to acute or chronic captopril in mice with disruption of bradykinin B_2-receptor gene. J Hypertens 1997;15:1701–1706.
40. Simpson EM, Linder CC, Sargent EE, Davisson MT, Mobraaten LE, Sharp JJ. Genetic variation among 129 substrains and its importance for targeted mutagenesis in mice. Nat Genet 1997;16:19–27.
41. Carretero OA, Amin VM, Ocholik T, Scicli AG, Koch J. Urinary kallikrein in rats bred for their susceptibility and resistance to the hypertensive effect of salt. A new radioimmunoassay for its direct determination. Circ Res 1978;42:727–731.
42. Madeddu P, Varoni MV, Demontis MP, Chao J, Simson JA, Glorioso N, Anania V. Kallikrein-kinin system and blood pressure sensitivity to salt. Hypertension 1997;29:471–477.
43. Kailasam MT, O'Connor DT, Parmer RJ. Hereditary intermediate phenotypes in African American hypertension. Ethn Health 1996;1:117–128.
44. Carretero OA, Miyazaki S, Scicli AG. Role of kinins in the acute antihypertensive effect of the converting enzyme inhibitor, captopril. Hypertension 1981;3:18–22.
45. Carretero OA, Scicli AG, Maitra SR. Role of kinins in the pharmacological effects of converting enzyme inhibitors. In: Horovitz ZP, ed. Angiotensin Converting Enzyme Inhibitors. Mechanisms of Action and Clinical Implications. Urban & Schwarzenberg, Baltimore, 1981, pp. 105–121.
46. Ørstavik TB, Carretero OA, Johansen L, Scicli AG. Role of kallikrein in the hypotensive effect of captopril after sympathetic stimulation of the rat submandibular gland. Circ Res 1982;51:385–390.
47. Carbonell LF, Carretero OA, Stewart JM, Scicli AG. Effect of a kinin antagonist on the acute antihypertensive activity of enalaprilat in severe hypertension. Hypertension 1988;11:239–243.
48. Danckwardt L, Shimizu I, Bönner G, Rettig R, Unger T. Converting enzyme inhibition in kinin-deficient Brown Norway rats. Hypertension 1990;16:429–435.
49. Rhaleb N-E, Yang X-P, Scicli AG, Carretero OA. Role of kinins and nitric oxide in the antihypertrophic effect of ramipril. Hypertension 1994;23:865–868.
50. Liu Y-H, Yang X-P, Sharov VG, Nass O, Sabbah HN, Peterson E, Carretero OA. Effects of angiotensin-converting enzyme inhibitors and angiotensin II type 1 receptor antagonists in rats with heart failure: role of kinins and angiotensin II type 2 receptors. J Clin Invest 1997;99:1926–1935.
51. Linz W, Schölkens BA. A specific B_2-bradykinin receptor antagonist HOE 140 abolishes the antihypertrophic effect of ramipril. Br J Pharmacol 1992;105:771–772.
52. Carretero OA, Kuk P, Piwonska S, Houle JA, Marin-Grez M. Role of the renin-angiotensin system in the pathogenesis of severe hypertension in rats. Circ Res 1971;29:654–663.
53. Bao G, Gohlke P, Unger T. Role of bradykinin in chronic antihypertensive actions of ramipril in different hypertension models. J Cardiovasc Pharmacol 1992;20(Suppl 9):S96–S99.
54. Dahlöf B, Pennert K, Hansson L. Reversal of left ventricular hypertrophy in hypertensive patients. A metaanalysis of 109 treatment studies. Am J Hypertens 1992;5:95–110.
55. Weinberg EO, Schoen FJ, George D, Kagaya Y, Douglas PS, Litwin SE, et al. Angiotensin-converting enzyme inhibition prolongs survival and modifies the transition to heart failure in rats with pressure overload hypertrophy due to ascending aortic stenosis. Circulation 1994;90:1410–1422.
56. Weinberg EO, Lee MA, Weigner M, Lindpaintner K, Bishop SP, Benedict CR, et al. Angiotensin AT_1 receptor inhibition. Effects on hypertrophic remodeling and ACE expression in rats with pressure-overload hypertrophy due to ascending aortic stenosis. Circulation 1997;95:1592–1600.
57. Linz W, Henning R, Schölkens BA. Role of angiotensin II receptor antagonism and converting enzyme inhibition in the progression and regression of cardiac hypertrophy in rats. J Hypertens 1991;9(Suppl 6):S400–S401.
58. Gohlke P, Linz W, Schölkens BA, Kuwer I, Bartenbach S, Schnell A, Unger T. Angiotensin-converting enzyme inhibition improves cardiac function. Role of bradykinin. Hypertension 1994;23:411–418.
59. Harrap SB, O'Sullivan JB. Cardiac transplantation, perindopril, and left ventricular hypertrophy in spontaneously hypertensive rats. Hypertension 1996;28:622–626.

60. Dietze G, Maerker E, Lodri C, Schifman R, Wicklmayr M, Geiger R, et al. Possible involvement of kinins in muscle energy metabolism. Adv Exp Med Biol 1984;167:63–71.

61. Tomiyama H, Kushiro T, Abeta H, Ishi T, Takahashi A, Furukawa L, et al. Kinins contribute to the improvement of insulin sensitivity during treatment with angiotensin converting enzyme inhibitor. Hypertension 1994;23:450–455.

62. Kohlmann O Jr, Neves F de A, Ginoza M, Tavares A, Cezaretti ML, Zanella MT, et al. Role of bradykinin in insulin sensitivity and blood pressure regulation during hyperinsulinemia. Hypertension 1995;25:1003–1007.

63. Zhang X, Xie Y-W, Nasjletti A, Xu X, Wolin MS, Hintze TH. ACE inhibitors promote nitric oxide accumulation to modulate oxygen consumption. Circulation 1997;95:176–182.

64. Xie YW, Shen W, Zhao G, Xu X, Wolin MS, Hintze TH. Role of endothelium-derived nitric oxide in the modulation of canine myocardial mitochondrial respiration in vitro. Implications for the development of heart failure. Circ Res 1996;79:381–387.

65. Hashimoto K, Hirose M, Furukawa H, Kimura E. Changes in hemodynamics and bradykinin concentration in coronary sinus blood in experimental coronary occlusion. Jpn Heart J 1977;18:679–689.

66. Matsuki T, Shoji T, Yoshida S, Kudoh Y, Motoe M, Inoue M, et al. Sympathetically induced myocardial ischaemia causes the heart to release plasma kinin. Cardiovasc Res 1987;21:428–432.

67. Baumgarten CR, Linz W, Kunkel G, Schölkens BA, Wiemer G. Ramiprilat increases bradykinin outflow from isolated hearts of rat. Br J Pharmacol 1993;108:293–295.

68. Linz W, Wiemer G, Schölkens BA. ACE inhibition induces NO-formation in cultured bovine endothelial cells and protects isolated ischemic rat hearts. J Mol Cell Cardiol 1992;24:909–919.

69. Linz W, Martorana PA, Schölkens BA. Local inhibition of bradykinin degradation in ischemic hearts. J Cardiovasc Pharmacol 1990;15(Suppl 6):S99–S109.

70. Linz W, Schölkens BA, Kaiser J, Just M, Qi BY, Albus U, Petry P. Cardiac arrhythmias are ameliorated by local inhibition of angiotensin formation and bradykinin degradation with the converting-enzyme inhibitor ramipril. Cardiovasc Drugs Ther 1989;3:873–882.

71. Martorana PA, Kettenbach B, Breipohl G, Linz W, Schölkens BA. Reduction of infarct size by local angiotensin-converting enzyme inhibition is abolished by a bradykinin antagonist. Eur J Pharmacol 1990;182:395–396.

72. Hartman JC, Wall TM, Hullinger TG, Shebuski RJ. Reduction of myocardial infarct size in rabbits by ramiprilat: reversal by the bradykinin antagonist HOE 140. J Cardiovasc Pharmacol 1993;21:996–1003.

73. Liu Y-H, Yang X-P, Sharov VG, Sabbah HN, Scicli AG, Carretero OA. Role of kinins, nitric oxide and prostaglandins in the protective effect of ACE inhibitors on ischemia/reperfusion myocardial infarction in rats. Hypertension 1994;24:380 (abstract).

74. Hashimoto K, Hamamoto H, Honda Y, Hirose M, Furukawa S, Kimura E. Changes in components of kinin system and hemodynamics in acute myocardial infarction. Am Heart J 1978;95:619–626.

75. Yang X-P, Liu Y-H, Peterson E, Carretero OA. Effect of neutral endopeptidase 24.11 inhibition on myocardial ischemia/reperfusion injury: the role of kinins. J Cardiovasc Pharmacol 1997;29:250–256.

76. Wall TM, Sheehy R, Hartman JC. Role of bradykinin in myocardial preconditioning. J Pharmacol Exp Ther 1994;270:681–689.

77. Parratt JR, Vegh A, Papp JG. Bradykinin as an endogenous myocardial protective substance with particular reference to ischemic preconditioning—a brief review of the evidence. Can J Physiol Pharmacol 1995;73:837–842.

78. Yang X-P, Liu Y-H, Scicli GM, Webb CR, Carretero OA. Role of kinins in the cardioprotective effect of preconditioning. Study of myocardial ischemia/reperfusion injury in B$_2$ kinin receptor knockout mice and kininogen-deficient rats. Hypertension 1997;30:735–740.

79. Vegh A, Papp JG, Szekeres L, Parratt JR. Evidence that bradykinin contributes to the pronounced antiarrhythmic effects of ischaemic preconditioning. Br J Pharmacol 1994;111:193P (abstract).

80. Grover GJ, D'Alonzo AJ, Parham CS, Darbenzio RB. Cardioprotection with the KATP opener cromakalim is not correlated with ischemic myocardial action potential duration. J Cardiovasc Pharmacol 1995;26:145–152.

81. Wall TM, Farrell AL, Hartman JC. Temporal relationship between bradykinin and KATP channels in the mechanism of cardioprotective ischemic preconditioning. Circulation 1995;92(Suppl I):I–252 (abstract).

82. Katori M, Majima M. Preventive role of renal kallikrein-kinin system in the early phase of hypertension and development of new antihypertensive drugs. Adv Pharmacol 1998;44:147–224.

83. Gavras H, Faxon DP, Berkoben J, Brunner HR, Ryan TJ. Angiotensin converting enzyme inhibition in patients with congestive heart failure. Circulation 1978;58:770–776.

84. CONSENSUS Trial Study Group. Effects of enalapril on mortality in severe congestive heart failure. The results of the Cooperative North Scandinavian Enalapril Survival Study (CONSENSUS). N Engl J Med 1987;316:1429–1435.

85. Pfeffer MA, Braunwald E, Moyé LA, Basta L, Brown EJ Jr, Cuddy TE, et al. on behalf of the SAVE Investigators. Effect of captopril on mortality and morbidity in patients with left ventricular dysfunction after myocardial infarction. Results of the survival and ventricular enlargement trial. N Engl J Med 1992;327:669–677.

86. The SOLVD Investigators. Effect of enalapril on mortality and the development of heart failure in asymptomatic patients with reduced left ventricular ejection fractions. N Engl J Med 1992;327:685–691.

87. Ball SG, Acute Infarction Ramipril Efficacy (AIRE) study investigators. Effect of ramipril on mortality and morbidity of survivors of acute myocardial infarction with clinical evidence of heart failure. Lancet 1993;342:821–828.

88. Gavras H, Gavras I. Cardioprotective potential of angiotensin converting enzyme inhibitors. J Hypertens 1991;9:385–392.

89. McDonald KM, Mock J, D'Aloia A, Parrish T, Hauer K, Francis G, Stillman A, Cohn JN. Bradykinin antagonism inhibits the antigrowth effect of converting enzyme inhibition in the dog myocardium after discrete transmural myocardial necrosis. Circulation 1995;91:2043–2048.

90. McDonald KM, Garr M, Carlyle PF, Francis GS, Hauer K, Hunter DW, et al. Relative effects of α_1-adrenoceptor blockade, converting enzyme inhibitor therapy, and angiotensin II subtype 1 receptor blockade on ventricular remodeling in the dog. Circulation 1994;90:3034–3046.

91. Stauss HM, Zhu Y-C, Redlich T, Adamiak D, Mott A, Kregel KC, Unger T. Angiotensin-converting enzyme inhibition in infarct-induced heart failure in rats: bradykinin versus angiotensin II. J Cardiovasc Risk 1994;1:255–262.

92. Pfeffer MA, Braunwald E. Ventricular remodeling after myocardial infarction. Experimental observations and clinical implications. Circulation 1990;81:1161–1172.

93. GISSI-3 Study Group. Effects of lisinopril and transdermal glyceryl trinitrate singly and together on 6-week mortality and ventricular function after acute myocardial infarction. Lancet 1994;343:1115–1122.

94. Garg R, Yusuf S, for the Collaborative Group on ACE Inhibitor Trials. Overview of randomized trials of angiotensin-converting enzyme inhibitors on mortality and morbidity in patients with heart failure. JAMA 1995;273:1450–1456 (review).

95. Pfeffer JM, Fischer TA, Pfeffer MA. Angiotensin-converting enzyme inhibition and ventricular remodeling after myocardial infarction. Annu Rev Physiol 1995;57:805–826.

96. Pfeffer JM, Pfeffer MA, Braunwald E. Influence of chronic captopril therapy on the infarcted left ventricle of the rat. Circ Res 1985;57:84–95.

97. McDonald KM, Rector T, Carlyle PF, Francis GS, Cohn JN. Angiotensin-converting enzyme inhibition and beta-adrenoceptor blockade regress established ventricular remodeling in a canine model of discrete myocardial damage. J Am Coll Cardiol 1994;24:1762–1768.

98. Dickstein K, Chang P, Willenheimer R, Haunso S, Remes J, Hall C, Kjekshus J. Comparison of the effects of losartan and enalapril on clinical status and exercise performance in patients with moderate or severe chronic heart failure. J Am Coll Cardiol 1995;26:438–445.

99. Dickstein K, Gottlieb S, Fleck E, Kostis J, Levine B, DeKock M, LeJemtel T. Hemodynamic and neurohumoral effects of the angiotensin II antagonist losartan in patients with heart failure. J Hypertens 1994;12(Suppl):S31–S35.

100. Pitt B, Segal R, Martinez FA, Meurers G, Cowley AJ, Thomas I, et al, on behalf of ELITE Study Investigators. Randomised trial of losartan versus captopril in patients over 65 with heart failure (Evaluation of Losartan in the Elderly Study, ELITE). Lancet 1997;349:747–752.

101. Whitebread S, Mele M, Kamber B, de Gasparo M. Preliminary biochemical characterization of two angiotensin II receptor subtypes. Biochem Biophys Res Commun 1989;163:284–291.

102. Nakajima M, Hutchinson HG, Fujinaga M, Hayashida W, Morishita R, Zhang L, et al. The angiotensin II type 2 (AT_2) receptor antagonizes the growth effects of the AT_1 receptor: gain-of-function study using gene transfer. Proc Natl Acad Sci USA 1995;92:10,663–10,667.

103. Siragy HM, Carey RM. The subtype-2 (AT_2) angiotensin receptor regulates renal cyclic guanosine 3',5'-monophosphate and AT_1 receptor-mediated prostaglandin E_2 production in conscious rats. J Clin Invest 1996;97:1978–1982.

104. Seyedi N, Xu X, Nasjletti A, Hintze TH. Coronary kinin generation mediates nitric oxide release after angiotensin receptor stimulation. Hypertension 1995;26:164–170.

105. Liu Y-H, Yang X-P, Nass O, Sabbah HN, Peterson E, Carretero OA. Chronic heart failure induced by coronary artery ligation in Lewis inbred rats. Am J Physiol 1997;272:H722–H727.

106. Yang X-P, Sabbah HN, Liu Y-H, Sharov VG, Mascha EJ, Alwan I, Carretero OA. Ventriculographic evaluation in three rat models of cardiac dysfunction. Am J Physiol 1993;266:H1946–H1952.

107. Farhy RD, Carretero OA, Ho K-L, Scicli AG. Role of kinins and nitric oxide in the effects of angiotensin converting enzyme inhibitors on neointima formation. Circ Res 1993;72:1202–1210.

108. Lopez JJ, Lorell BH, Ingelfinger JR, Weinberg EO, Schunkert H, Diamant D, Tang S-S. Distribution and function of cardiac angiotensin AT_1- and AT_2-receptor subtypes in hypertrophied rat hearts. Am J Physiol 1994;267:H844–H852.

109. Nio Y, Matsubara H, Murasawa S, Kanasaki M, Inada M. Regulation of gene transcription of angiotensin II receptor subtypes in myocardial infarction. J Clin Invest 1995;95:46–54.

110. Suzuki J, Matsubara H, Urakami M, Inada M. Rat angiotensin II (type 1A) receptor mRNA regulation and subtype expression in myocardial growth and hypertrophy. Circ Res 1993;73:439–447.

111. Everett AD, Tufro-McReddie A, Fisher A, Gomez RA. Angiotensin receptor regulates cardiac hypertrophy and transforming growth factor-β_1 expression. Hypertension 1994;23:587–592.

112. Hecker M, Porsti I, Busse R. Mechanisms involved in the angiotensin II-independent hypotensive action of ACE inhibitors. Braz J Med Biol Res 1994;27:1917–1921.

113. Korth P, Fink E, Linz W, Schölkens BA, Wohlfart P, Wiemer G. Angiotensin II receptor subtype-stimulated formation of endothelial cyclic GMP and prostacyclin is accompanied by an enhanced release of endogenous kinins. Pharm Pharmacol Lett 1995;3:124–127.

114. Brosnihan KB, Li P, Ferrario CM. Angiotensin-(1–7) dilates canine coronary arteries through kinins and nitric oxide. Hypertension 1996;27:523–528.

115. Lo M, Liu K-L, Lantelme P, Sassard J. Subtype 2 of angiotensin II receptors controls pressure-natriuresis in rats. J Clin Invest 1995;95:1394–1397.

116. Dahlöf B. Regression of left ventricular hypertrophy—are there differences between antihypertensive agents? Cardiology 1992;81:307–315.

117. Liebson PR, Grandits GA, Dianzumba S, Prineas RJ, Grimm RH Jr, Neaton JD, Stamler J, for the Treatment of Hypertension Study Research Group. Comparison of five antihypertensive monotherapies and placebo for change in left ventricular mass in patients receiving nutritional-hygienic therapy in the Treatment of Mild Hypertension Study (TOMHS). Circulation 1995;91:698–706.

118. Sharpe N, Murphy J, Smith H, Hannan S. Preventive treatment of asymptomatic left ventricular dysfunction following myocardial infarction. Eur Heart J 1990;11(Suppl B):147–156.

119. Lindpaintner K, Ganten D. The cardiac renin-angiotensin system. An appraisal of present experimental and clinical evidence. Circ Res 1991;68:905–921.

120. Dzau VJ, Re RN. Evidence for the existence of renin in the heart. Circulation 1987;75(Suppl I):I-134–I-136.

121. Sadoshima J, Xu Y, Slayter HS, Izumo S. Autocrine release of angiotensin II mediates stretch-induced hypertrophy of cardiac myocytes in vitro. Cell 1993;75:977–984.

122. Linz W, Schölkens BA. Role of bradykinin in the cardiac effects of angiotensin-converting enzyme inhibitors. J Cardiovasc Pharmacol 1992;20(Suppl 9):S83–S90.

123. Minshall RD, Nakamura F, Becker RP, Rabito SF. Characterization of bradykinin B_2 receptors in adult myocardium and neonatal rat cardiomyocytes. Circ Res 1995;76:773–780.

124. Cohn JN. Structural basis for heart failure. Ventricular remodeling and its pharmacological inhibition. Circulation 1995;91:2504–2507 (editorial).

125. Baur LH, Schipperheyn JJ, van der Laarse A, Souverijn JH, Frolich M, de Groot A, et al. Combining salicylate and enalapril in patients with coronary artery disease and heart failure. Br Heart J 1995;73:227–236.

126. Carretero OA, Scicli AG. Kinins paracrine hormone. Kidney Int 1988;34(Suppl 26):S-52–S-59.

127. Liu Y-H, Yang X-P, Sharov VG, Sigmon DH, Sabbah HN, Carretero OA. Paracrine systems in the cardioprotective effect of angiotensin-converting enzyme inhibitors on myocardial ischemia/reperfusion injury in rats. Hypertension 1996;27:7–13.

10

Endothelin and the Heart

David P. Brooks and Eliot H. Ohlstein

The death of Cleopatra some 2000 years prior to the discovery of endothelin *(1)* provides an historical insight into the potential importance of the cardiac effects of endothelin and its isopeptides. It is thought that the snake used by Cleopatra to kill herself was the Israeli burrowing asp, *Atractaspis engaddensis*, and that coronary vasospasm is the primary cause of death from the venom of this snake (*vida infra*). One of the components of this venom is sarafotoxin 6c, whose human homolog is endothelin (ET). The death of Cleopatra seems to have foreshadowed the discovery of ET and its possible role in cardiac function and dysfunction.

INTRODUCTION: ENDOTHELIN AND ITS RECEPTORS

Endothelin-1, originally termed porcine endothelin by Yanagisawa et al. *(1)*, is a 21-amino-acid peptide with 2 intrachain disulfide bonds and a mol wt of 2492 Daltons. The isopeptides, ET-1, ET-2, and ET-3, are separate gene products with a high degree of homology (Fig. 1; *2*). There is some evidence that ET isopeptides can be differentially expressed in a tissue-specific manner. The four cardiotoxic sarafotoxins, 6a, b, c, and d, show a significant degree of sequence homology with the ETs, and interact with ET receptors *(3,4)*. The production of human ET involves expression of the 212-amino-acid precursor, preproendothelin (preproET), which is cleaved proteolytically to a 38-amino-acid residue precursor peptide, "big endothelin" *(1)*. Cleavage of the Trp 21-Val-22 big ET by ET-converting enzyme (ECE) results in the biologically active ET peptide (Fig. 2). Shortly after the discovery of ET, a human ET cDNA, which indicated that ET-1 is derived from a 212-amino-acid peptide human preproET-1, was reported *(5)*. Subsequently, ECE was purified *(6)*, sequenced, cloned, and characterized *(7)*.

From: *Contemporary Endocrinology: Hormones and the Heart in Health and Disease*
Edited by: L. Share © Humana Press Inc., Totowa, NJ

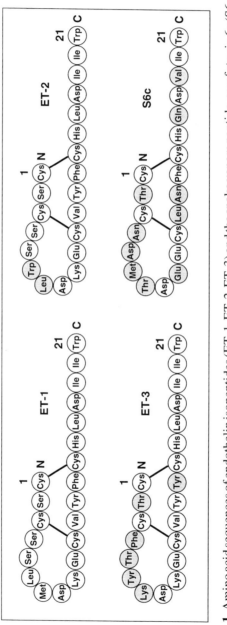

Fig. 1. Amino acid sequences of endothelin isopeptides (ET-1, ET-2, ET-3) and the snake venom peptide, sarafotoxin 6c (S6c).

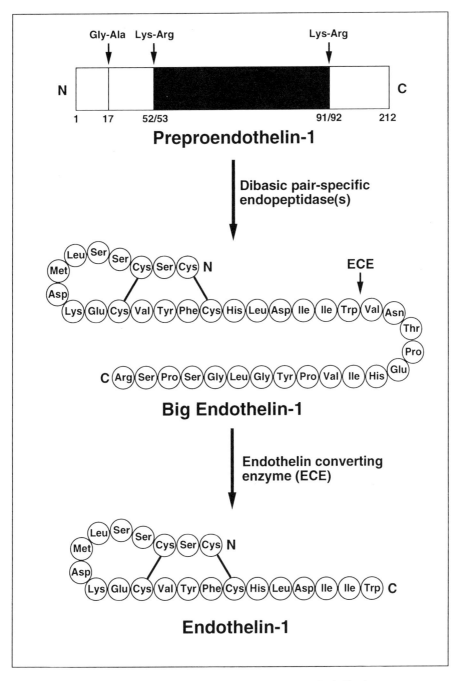

Fig. 2. Biosynthetic processing of human endothelin-1.

To date, only two ET receptor subtypes have been cloned and sequenced: the ET_A and ET_B receptors *(8,9)*. Both receptors are G-protein-coupled, 7-transmembrane-spanning receptors, which can be distinguished by their relative affinities for the ET and sarafotoxin isopeptides. The ET_A receptor has greater selectivity for ET-1 and ET-2, compared to ET-3 and sarafotoxin 6c; the ET_B receptor has an equal affinity for all the isopeptides (Fig. 3). A third receptor, ET_C, which has higher affinity for ET-3 and sarafotoxin 6c

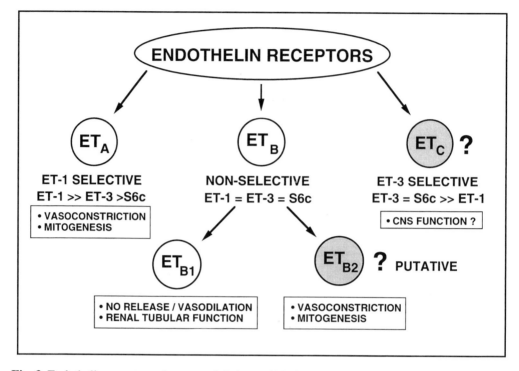

Fig. 3. Endothelin receptor subtypes and their possible function. Endothelin ET_A and ET_B (ET_{B1}) receptors have been cloned. Existence of ET_C and ET_{B2} receptors is postulated, based on binding and functional data.

compared to ET-1, has been postulated, but not identified to date. In addition, evidence is growing that there are two subtypes of ET_B receptors: one that mediates nitric oxide-induced vasodilation (ET_{B1}), and one that causes vasoconstriction (ET_{B2}).

CARDIAC ENDOTHELIN

In addition to being under the influence of circulating ET, cardiac cells can synthesize the peptide. Thus, ET-1 is released by both cardiac myocytes *(10)* and endothelial cells (ECs) *(11)*. Furthermore, epicardial mesothelial cells in culture have been shown to release ET *(12)*. PreproET mRNA has been demonstrated in cardiac ECs *(11)* and myocytes *(13,14)*, as well as in transplanted human hearts *(15)*.

A number of different stimuli can increase ET release or preproET mRNA expression in cardiac ECs and myocytes; these include hypoxia *(10)*, pressure overload *(14)*, and angiotensin II *(13)*. Similarly, cardiac ET production or expression is increased under pathological conditions such as hypertension *(16)*, myocardial ischemia/reperfusion *(17–19)*, cardiac hypertrophy *(20)*, coronary artery disease *(21)*, percutaneous trans-luminal coronary angioplasty (PTCA) *(22)*, and cardiac transplantation *(23)*.

CARDIAC ENDOTHELIN RECEPTORS

Both ET_A and ET_B receptors are present in atrial and ventricular tissue, the atrial and ventricular myocardium, and the coronary vasculature *(24,25)*. Both receptors have also been demonstrated on cardiac myocytes *(26)* and in normal rat hearts. The ET_A receptor mRNA levels were similar in the atria and ventricles *(20)*; however, under conditions of cardiac hypertrophy induced by an aortovenocaval fistula, the prevalence of the ET_B receptor increased in all chambers *(20)*. Changes in cardiac ET binding have also been reported under other pathological conditions, such as streptozotocin-induced diabetes *(27)*.

ET receptor-mediated cardiac effects involve multiple signaling pathways, including phosphoinositide hydrolysis *(28)*, increased intracellular calcium *(29–31)*, inhibition of adenylate cyclase *(28)*, regulation of L-type calcium channels *(32)*, voltage-dependent K channels *(33)*, protein kinase C *(34)*, mitogen-activated protein kinase *(35)*, and the Na^+/H^+ antiporter *(36,37)*. ET-induced Na^+/H^+ exchange appears to be impaired in hypertrophied hearts *(37)*.

CARDIAC ACTIONS OF ENDOTHELIN

In addition to being one of the most potent constrictors of the systemic vasculature, ET has significant effects on cardiac vessels and cardiac tissue. ET contracts isolated coronary arteries, as well as causing coronary vasoconstriction in Langendorff heart preparations *(38)*. At low doses, however, ET produces an initial coronary vasodilation in isolated hearts *(39,40)*. The mechanisms involved in the dilator response are unclear, because methylene blue, superoxidase dismutase, flurbiprofen, and BW 755C failed to alter this response *(39)*; however, there is one report that the dilator response can be blocked in part by indomethacin *(41)*. Intracoronary infusion of low doses of ET cause vasodilation in intact dogs *(42)*, but, high doses result in a profound reduction in coronary blood flow. This contractile activity leads to impaired ventricular function, delayed filling of distal coronary branches, and, in some cases, total occlusion of vessels in the epicardium, thus leading to profound disturbances in cardiac function, and ultimately ventricular fibrillation *(42–47)*. A study in neonatal pigs has demonstrated that ET-1-induced coronary vasoconstriction is enhanced by ischemia reperfusion, and by norepinephrine at concentrations typically near those observed following neonatal cardiopulmonary bypass *(48)*. ET may also mediate the coronary vasoconstriction mediated by cytokines such as tumor necrosis factor-alpha (TNFα) *(49)*. There is also evidence that ET will cause coronary artery vasoconstriction in humans. Thus, iv infusion of ET into healthy volunteers, at a dose that increased arterial plasma ET 35-fold, reduced coronary sinus blood flow maximally by 23%, and increased coronary vascular resistance by 48% *(50)*. Other investigators have demonstrated that systemic infusion of ET can cause significant impairment of left and right ventricular diastolic filling, even at a low dose that had no pulmonary or systemic pressor effects *(51)*.

ET also contracts isolated papillary muscle, and is a potent positive inotropic agent in paced left atria *(32,52,53)*. ET may also have a positive chronotropic effect in spontaneously beating right atria, but, this response is less robust *(38,54,55)*. Although ET-1 is released by the endocardial endothelium, it exhibits characteristics that make it distinct from the putative cardiotonic molecule, endocardin. ET also increases the amplitude and duration of the plateau phase of the cardiac action potential in guinea pig left atrium *(32)*.

ET can induce cardiomyocyte hypertrophy, as measured by protein synthesis, cell surface area, or tritiated leucine incorporation *(13,56)*, a response that is mediated by ET_A receptors *(13)*. There is also evidence that ET may mediate the cardiac hypertrophy induced by angiotensin II *(13)*.

ENDOTHELIN AND CARDIAC DISEASE

Congestive Heart Failure

Congestive heart failure (CHF) is a progressive disease involving progressive cardiac failure following myocardial damage. The increasing failure is a result of attempts to maintain cardiac output, which are accompanied by increased peripheral vasoconstriction and neurohumoral activation. Furthermore, there is impaired relaxation of the peripheral and coronary vasculatures and cardiac remodeling. Evidence that ET may be involved in the pathogenesis of CHF is growing. Numerous studies have demonstrated that circulating ET is increased in patients with heart failure (HF) *(57–65)*. It has also been reported that circulating big ET is increased in patients with HF and that this correlated with the magnitude of alterations of cardiac hemodynamics, functional class, and survival *(66,67)*. Circulating ET levels may also be increased in the acute phase of myocardial infarction (MI), and in CHF, and these levels correlate closely with indices of disease, such as capillary wedge pressure, left ventricular ejection fraction, cardiac index, New York Heart Association class, and 12-month survival *(68,69)*. Spontaneous release of ET from circulating mononuclear cells has also been reported in patients with HF *(70)*, and there is evidence to suggest that ET levels may increase transiently during physical activity by patients with HF *(71)*.

In experimental models of HF, circulating ET is increased *(72)*, and increase in systemic ET correlates with ventricular mass *(73–75)*. Enhanced preproET-1 mRNA and ET immunoreactivity *(76,77)*, and increased cardiac ET binding *(78)*, have been observed in various models of HF. In a dog model of chronic low cardiac output, circulating ET was increased, and there was evidence for enhanced ET-1 mRNA expression and immunostaining in atrial myocytes and pulmonary ECs *(79)*. A direct effect of ET to promote cardiac hypertrophy *(80)*, including mechanical stress-induced cardiomyocyte hypertrophy *(81–83)*, has been suggested.

A number of ET receptor antagonists have been studied in models of HF, and data suggests that they can reduce left ventricular mass *(84)* and lower blood pressure *(85)*. Inhibition of ET with BQ123 in rats with MI-induced HF resulted in increased survival and amelioration of left ventricular dysfunction and ventricular remodeling *(86)*. Furthermore, bosentan treatment has been shown to cause a marked increase in survival in rats with HF induced by coronary artery ligation *(80)*. Following 2 or 9 mo of treatment, bosentan reduced central venous pressure and left ventricular end diastolic pressure, as well as plasma catecholamines, urinary cyclic guanine monophosphate and left ventricular collagen density. ET receptor antagonists have also been shown to have beneficial effects in various dog and rat models of HF *(87–89)*.

Measurement of plasma ET levels in patients with HF following drug treatment have provided further evidence of a potential role of ET. Treatment of HF patients with angiotensin-converting enzyme inhibitors has been reported to produce a reduction in plasma ET levels *(90,91)*, but this observation has not been consistent *(92)*. The novel vasodilating beta blocker, carvedilol, also results in a decrease in circulating ET levels, and the change in ET was an independent, noninvasive predictor of the functional and hemodynamic responses to carvedilol *(93)*. Trials with the ET receptor antagonist, bosentan, indicate that it has beneficial effects when administered intravenously, reducing mean arterial blood pressure, pulmonary artery pressure, right atrial pressure, and pulmonary artery wedge pressure, and increasing cardiac index *(94)*. The beneficial effects of ET antagonists in patients with HF are of interest, because they may be occurring under conditions in which there is a decreased responsiveness to the vasoconstrictor effects of ET *(95)*.

Myocardial Ischemia

ET results in coronary artery vasoconstriction and, as such, its involvement in the pathogenesis of coronary artery vasospasm, angina pectoris, and MI has been suggested. Administration of ET to dogs results in myocardial ischemia *(46)*, and the primary cause of death caused by the venom of the burrowing asp, Atractaspis Engaddensis, has been shown to be coronary vasospasm *(96)*. The venom of this snake contains the ET isopeptide, sarafotoxin 6c, a potent ET_B receptor agonist.

Circulating ET levels are increased in patients with coronary vasospasm and following MI *(97–105)*. It has also been reported that arterial ET levels following MI correlates significantly with pulmonary artery pressure, central venous pressure, and pulmonary vascular resistance, and that the increased levels also correlated significantly with peak creatinine kinase and creatinine kinase isozyme myocardial band *(106)*. The authors of this study concluded that the increased plasma ET concentration at the early stages of MI might reflect higher pulmonary artery pressure and pulmonary vascular resistance; in later stages, the elevated plasma ET may be related to infarct size *(106)*. ET expression measured in hearts from pigs that had undergone myocardial ischemia increased twofold and *in situ* hybridization demonstrated a considerable increase in ET mRNA in ischemic myocytes *(19)*.

Evaluation of ET levels in noninfarct states, such as angina pectoris, have not provided consistent data, but there is evidence that ET levels are increased in acute unstable angina *(99,103,105,107–109)*. One study also reported that sympathetic stimulation induced during the cold pressor test increased plasma ET in patients with stable angina, but not in healthy subjects *(110)*. Furthermore, plasma ET increases in patients with effort angina, indicating that exercise-induced ischemia correlates with enhanced ET-1 production *(111)*. There is evidence that ET levels are increased following coronary angioplasty, but it is unclear whether the increased ET levels are related to myocardial injury or EC damage *(22,112)*.

Early studies using the ECE inhibitor, phosphoramidon, or ET antibodies, demonstrated that blockade of ET could reduce left ventricular infarct size following coronary artery ischemia/reperfusion in rats and rabbits *(113–115)*. Studies with selective ET_A and mixed ET_A/ET_B receptor antagonists have provided conflicting data, with some reports demonstrating a reduction in infarct size in both rabbits, and other reports demonstrating no effect *(116–118)*. In rabbits, FR139317 had no effect on infarct size following coronary artery occlusion *(119,120)*. Similar observations were made with this antagonist in dogs *(121)*, and with PD156707 in pigs *(122)*. In contrast, a number of ET receptor antagonists have been shown to reduce infarct size, including bosentan in rats and pigs *(118,123)*, BQ123 in dogs *(124)*, PD145065 and FR13917 in rabbits *(120,125)*, and TAK044 in rats *(126,127)*. Furthermore, BQ610 preserved mechanical function and energy metabolism during ischemia/reperfusion injury in isolated perfused hearts *(128)*, and inhibition of ET synthesis with phosphoramidon or ET receptor blockade with bosentan during prolonged hypothermic arrest has been shown to improve postischemic coronary flow *(129)*. In addition, it has been reported that BQ123 can prevent ET-induced exacerbation of ischemic arrythmias in rats *(130)*.

Although the experimental data indicating a role for ET in myocardial ischemia is not conclusive, it is nonetheless intriguing that long-term mortality of patients following acute MI appears to be related to circulating ET levels *(131)*.

Coronary Remodeling During Atherosclerosis and Angioplasty-Induced Restenosis

Coronary vasospasm and cardiac remodeling are important complications associated with vascular restenosis, such as that observed following percutaneous transluminal balloon angioplasty.

Vasospasm and abnormal vascular smooth muscle proliferation are important complications of both atherosclerosis and vascular wall trauma, as is seen following PTCA. Although the precise molecular and cellular mechanisms involved in experimental and clinical restenosis have not yet been defined, it is widely accepted that cellular proliferation/migration and matrix deposition are important factors. Since ET-1 has been shown to promote cellular proliferation/migration and matrix synthesis, the potential involvement of ET in coronary artery restenosis and cardiac remodeling has been studied *(see* following).

Oxidized low-density lipoprotein, a well-established atherogenic risk factor, stimulates ET-1 biosynthesis in human and porcine macrophage and EC cultures *(132–134)*. Indeed, both atherosclerosis and balloon angioplasty augment the contractile actions of ET-1 in blood vessels isolated from primates, rabbits, and rats *(135–137)*. In human atherosclerotic blood vessels, several groups have reported that, in addition to ECs, both macrophages and intimal smooth muscle cells are immunoreactive for ET-1 *(138,139)*. Systemic administration of (^{125}I)ET-1 accumulates within the atherosclerotic plaques of hypercholesterolemic rabbits *(140)*, and enhanced (^{125}I)ET-1 binding has been detected in hyperplastic lesions induced in pig femoral arteries, and in atheromatous regions of human saphenous veins and coronary arteries *(141)*. Based on the sensitivity of responses to ET-1 in atherosclerotic human coronary artery specimens to inhibition by an ET_A-selective antagonist, it has been suggested that this tissue expresses both ET_A receptors and "non-ET_A" receptors *(141,142)*.

Both acute and chronic administration of exogenous ET-1 to rats augments, in a dose-dependent manner, the degree of neointima formation associated with carotid artery balloon angioplasty *(137)*. Using quantitative reverse transcription and polymerase chain reaction, Wang et al. *(143)* have examined the temporal expression of mRNAs encoding ECE-1, preproET-1, and $ET_{A/B}$ receptors in the rat carotid artery balloon angioplasty model. A significant increase in ECE-1 and prepro-ET-1 mRNA is not observed until 6–24 h and 3–7 d, respectively, when levels are doubled. In contrast, both ET_A and ET_B receptor mRNAs are elevated by approx 20-fold, 3–7 and 1–3 d, respectively, following angioplasty. Furthermore, immunohistochemical studies clearly demonstrate a time-dependent increase in ET-immunoactivity as a consequence of balloon angioplasty *(143)*. Indeed, immunoreactive expression of this mitogenic protein closely mimics that of proliferating cell nuclear antigen, a marker of cellular proliferation.

The first report of an ET receptor antagonist exhibiting vasculoprotective efficacy in an animal model of restenosis resulted from the chronic administration of the nonpeptide-mixed $ET_{A/B}$ receptor antagonist, SB 209670, in the rat carotid artery model *(137)*. Subsequent studies also reported a protective effect of both peptidic and nonpeptidic $ET_{A/B}$ antagonists (Ro 46-2005 and TAK-044) in the rabbit iliac and rat carotid artery models, respectively *(144)*. In contrast, the ET_A-selective peptidic antagonist, BQ-123, was devoid of any vasculoprotective efficacy in either the rat or the rabbit *(145,146)*, leading to the postulation that inhibition of the ET_A receptor alone is insufficient to produce significant inhibition of neointima formation. However, more recent data indicates that the contribution made by the ET_A receptor to ET-induced neointima formation may show regional and/or species differences. Using a rat thoracic aorta model, Hele et al. *(147)* reported that oral administration of the $ET_{A/B}$ receptor antagonist, bosentan, and the ET_A-selective antagonist, BMS 182874, reduced the degree of (^3H)thymidine incorporation at the site of injury (but not in other rapidly proliferating tissues, such as testes) 2 d after injury, by 36 and 55%, respectively.

In models of hypercholestoremia-induced atherosclerosis, Kowala et al. *(148)* demonstrated that the ET_A-selective receptor antagonist, BMS-182874, significantly inhibited fatty streak formation in cholesterol-fed hamsters. These authors suggest that ET_A receptors may be involved in the early inflammatory phase of atherosclerosis.

Acute and chronic rejection are major obstacles in the successful application of organ transplantation. Complications are accompanied by intimal thickening, endothelial dysfunction, and graft arteriosclerosis, ultimately leading to graft vasculopathy and coronary artery disease. These cellular responses significantly limit the long-term survival of cardiac transplant patients, and frequently lead to death. It is of interest, therefore, that ET-1 expression is elevated in experimental allograft models of accelerated cardiac transplant atherosclerosis (expression predominantly associated with neointimal macrophages) *(23,149)*.

Thus, both experimental and clinical evidence exists to support a pathogenic role for ET in the phenomenon of atherosclerosis and restenosis.

SUMMARY

Since the discovery of ET a decade ago, considerable work has been conducted on its role in physiological and pathophysiological processes *(150)*. Of particular interest is the potential importance of ET in the heart and its role in cardiac disease.

ACKNOWLEDGMENTS

The authors are grateful to Sue Tirri for preparing this chapter.

REFERENCES

1. Yanagisawa M, Kurihara H, Kimura S, Tomobe Y, Kobayashi M, Mitsui Y, et al. Novel potent vasoconstrictor peptide produced by vascular endothelial cells. Nature (London) 1988;332:411–415.
2. Inoue A, Yanagisawa M, Kimura S. Human endothelin family: three structurally and pharmacologically distinct isopeptides predicted by three separate genes. Proc Natl Acad Sci USA 1989;86:2863–2867.
3. Wollberg Z, Shabo-Shina R, Intrator N, Bdolah N, Kochva E, Shavit G, et al. Novel cardiotoxic polypeptide from the venom of atractapisengaddensis (burrowing asp); cardiac effects in mice and isolated rat and human heart preparations. Toxicon 1988;26:525–534.
4. Bdolah A, Wollberg Z, Amber I, Kloog Y, Sokolovsky M, Kochava E. Disturbances in the cardiovascular system caused by endothelin and sarafotoxin. Biochem Pharmacol 1989;38:3145–3146.
5. Itoh Y, Yanagisawa M, Ohkubo S, Kimura C, Kosaka T, Inoue A, et al. Cloning and sequence analysis of cDNA encoding the precursor of a human endothelium-derived vasoconstrictor peptide, endothelin: identity of human and porcine endothelin. FEBS Lett 1988;23:440–444.
6. Ohnaka K, Takayanagi R, Nishikawa M, Haji M, Nawata H. Purification and characterization of a phosphoramidon-sensitive endothelin-converting enzyme in porcine aortic endothelium. J Biol Chem 1993;268:26,759–26,766.
7. Xu D, Emoto N, Giaid A, Slaughter C, Kaw S, Dewit D, Yanagisawa M. ECE-1: a membrane-bound metalloprotease that catalyzes the proteolytic activation of big endothelin-1. Cell 1994;78:473–485.

8. Arai H, Hori S, Aramori I, Ohkubo H, Nakanish S. Cloning and expression of a cDNA encoding an endothelin receptor. Nature (London) 1990;348:730–732.

9. Sakurai T, Yanagisawa M, Takuwa Y, Miyazaki H, Kimura S, Goto K, Masaki TE. Cloning of a cDNA encoding a nonisopeptide-selective subtype of an endothelin receptor. Nature (London) 1990; 348:732–735.

10. Kagamu H, Suzuki T, Arakawa M, Mitsui Y. Low oxygen enhances endothelin-1 (ET-1) production and responsiveness to ET-1 in cultured cardiac myocytes. Biochem Biophys Res Commun 1994;202: 1612–1618.

11. Mebazaa A, Mayoux E, Maeda K, Martin LD, Lakatta EG, Robotham JL, Shah AM. Paracrine effects of endocardial endothelial cells on myocyte contraction mediated via endothelin. Am J Physiol 1993; 265:H1841–H1846.

12. Eid H, deBold ML, Chen JH, Bold AJ. Epicardial mesothelial cells synthesize and release endothelin. J Cardiovasc Pharmacol 1994;24:715–720.

13. Ito H, Hirata Y, Adachi S, Tanaka M, Tsujino M, Koike A, et al. Endothelin-1 is an autocrine/paracrine factor in the mechanism of angiotensin II-induced hypertrophy in cultured rat cardiomyocytes. J Clin Invest 1993;92:398–403.

14. Arai M, Yoguchi A, Iso T, Takahashi T, Imai S, Murata K, Suzuki T. Endothelin-1 and its binding sites are upregulated in pressure overload cardiac hypertrophy. Am J Physiol 1995;268:H2084–H2091.

15. Giaid A, Saleh D, Yanagisawa M, Forbes RD. Endothelin-1 immunoreactivity and mRNA in the transplanted human heart. Transplantation 1995;59:1308–1313.

16. Feron O, Salomone S, Godfraind T. Influence of salt loading on the cardiac and renal preproendothelin-1 mRNA expression in stroke-prone spontaneously hypertensive rats. Biochem Biophys Res Commun 1995;209:161–166.

17. Brunner F, du Toit EF, Opie LH. Endothelin release during ischaemia and reperfusion of isolated perfused rat hearts. J Mol Cell Cardiol 1992;24:1291–1305.

18. Velasco CE, Jackson EK, Morrow JA, Vitola JV, Inagami T, Forman MB. Intravenous adenosine suppresses cardiac release of endothelin after myocardial ischaemia and reperfusion. Cardiovasc Res 1993;27:121–128.

19. Tonnessen T, Giaid A, Saleh D, Naess PA, Yanagisawa M, Christensen G. Increased in vivo expression and production of endothelin-1 by porcine cardiomyocytes subjected to ischemia. Circ Res 1995;76: 767–772.

20. Brown LA, Nunez DJ, Brookes CI, Wilkins MR. Selective increase in endothelin-1 and endothelin A receptor subtype in the hypertrophied myocardium of the aorto-venacaval fistula rat. Cardiovasc Res 1995;29:768–774.

21. Ravalli S, Szabolcs M, Albala A, Michler RE, Cannon PJ. Increased immunoreactive endothelin-1 in human transplant coronary artery disease. Circulation 1996;94:2096–2102.

22. Franco-Cereceda A, Grip LG, Moor E, Velander M, Liska J, Lundberg JM. Influence of percutaneous transluminal coronary angioplasty on cardiac release of endothelin neuropeptide Y and noradrenaline. Int J Cardiol 1995;48:231–233.

23. Watschinger B, Sayegh MH, Hancock WW, Russell ME. Upregulation of endothelin-1 mRNA and peptide expression in rat cardiac allografts with rejection and arteriosclerosis. Am J Pathol 1995; 146:1065–1072.

24. Molenaar P, O'Reilly G, Sharkey A, Kuc RE, Harding DP, Plumpton C, Gresham GA, Davenport AP. Characterization and localization of endothelin receptor subtypes in the human atrioventricular conducting system and myocardium. Circ Res 1993;72:526–538.

25. Godfraind T. Endothelin receptors in human coronary arteries. Trends Pharmacol Sci 1994;15:136–137.

26. Galron R, Bdolah A, Kloog Y, Sokolovsky M. Endothelin/sarafotoxin receptor induced phosphoinositide turnover: effects of pertussis and cholera toxins and of phorbol ester. Biochem Biophys Res Commun 1990;171:949–954.

27. Vesci L, Mattera GG, Tobia P, Corsico N, Calvani M. Cardiac and renal endothelin-1 binding sites in streptozotocin-induced diabetic rats. Pharmacol Res 1995;32:363–367.

28. Hilal-Dandan R, Urasawa K, Brunton LL. Endothelin inhibits adenylate cyclase and stimulates phosphoinositide hydrolysis in adult cardiac myocytes. J Biol Chem 1992;267:10,620–10,624.

29. Qiu Z, Wang J, Perreault CL, Meuse AJ, Grossman W, Morgan JP. Effects of endothelin on intracellular Ca^{2+} and contractility in single ventricular myocytes from the ferret and human. Eur J Pharmacol 1992;214:293–296.

30. Cheng TH, Chang CY, Wei J, Lin CI. Effects of endothelin 1 on calcium and sodium currents in isolated human cardiac myocytes. Can J Physiol Pharmacol 1995;73:1774–1783.

31. Touyz RM, Fareh J, Thibault G, Schiffrin EL. Intracellular Ca^{2+} modulation by angiotensin II and endothelin-1 in cardiomyocytes and fibroblasts from hypertrophied hearts of spontaneously hypertensive rats. Hypertension 1996;28:797–805.

32. Ishikawa T, Yanagisawa M, Kimura S, Goto K, Masaki T. Positive inotropic action of novel vasoconstrictor peptide endothelin on guinea pig atria. Am J Physiol 1988;255:H970–H973.

33. Kim D. Endothelin activation of an inwardly rectifying K+ current in atrial cells. Circ Res 1991;69: 250–255.

34. Suzuki T, Hoshi H, Mitsui Y. Endothelin stimulates hypertrophy and contractility of neonatal rat cardiac myocytes in a serum-free medium. FEBS Lett 1990;268:149–151.

35. Bogoyevitch MA, Glennon PE, Andersson MB, Clerk A, Lazou A, Marshall CJ, Parker PJ, Sugden PH. Endothelin-1 and fibroblast growth factors stimulate the mitogen-activated protein kinase signaling casade in cardiac myocytes. The potential role of the cascade in the integration of two signaling pathways leading to myocyte hypertrophy. J Biol Chem 1994;269:1110–1119.

36. Grinstein S, Rotin D, Mason MJ. Na+/H+ exchange and growth factor-induced cytosolic pH changes. Role in cellular proliferation. Biochim Biophys Acta 1989;988:73–97.

37. Ito N, Kagaya Y, Weinberg EO, Barry WH, Lorell BH. Endothelin and angiotensin II stimulation of Na+/H+ exchange is impaired in cardiac hypertrophy. J Clin Invest 1997;99:125–135.

38. Lembeck F, Decrinis M, Pertl C, Amann R, Donnerer J. Effects of endothelin on the cardiovascular system and on smooth muscle preparations in different species. Naunyn-Schmiedebergs Arch Pharmacol 1989;340:744–751.

39. Baydoun AR, Peers SH, Cirino G, Woodward B. Effects of endothelin-1 on the rat isolated heart. J Cardiovasc Pharmacol 1989;13(Suppl 5):S193–S196.

40. Folta A, Joshua IG, Webb RC. Dilator actions of endothelin in coronary resistance vessels and the abdominal aorta of the guinea pig. Life Sci 1989;45:2627–2635.

41. Neubauer S, Ertl G, Haas U, Pulzer F, Kochsiek K. Effects of endothelin-1 in isolated perfused rat heart. J Cardiovasc Pharmacol 1990;16:1–8.

42. Nichols AJ, Koster PF, Ohlstein EH. Effect of diltiazem on the coronary haemodynamic and cardiac functional effects produced by intracoronary administration of endothelin-1 in the anaesthetized dog. Br J Pharmacol 1990;99:597–601.

43. Clozel JP, Clozel M. Effects of endothelin on the coronary vascular bed in open-chest dogs. Circ Res 1989;65:1193–1200.

44. Ezra D, Goldstein RE, Czaja JF, Feuerstein GZ. Lethal ischemia due to intracoronary endothelin in pigs. Am J Physiol 1989;257:H339–H343.

45. Kurihara H, Yoshizumi M, Sugiyama T, Yamaoki K, Nagai R, Takaku F, et al. The possible role of endothelin-1 in the pathogenesis of coronary vasospasm. J Cardiovasc Pharmacol 1989;13(Suppl 5): S132–S137.

46. Larkin SW, Clarke JG, Keogh BE, Araujo L, Rhodes C, Davies GJ, Taylor KM, Maseri A. Intracoronary endothelin induces myocardial ischemia by small vessel constriction in the dog. Am J Cardiol 1989; 64:956–958.

47. Domenech R, Macho P, Gonzalez R, Huidobro-Toro JP. Effect of endothelin on total and regional coronary resistance and on myocardial contractility. Eur J Pharmacol 1991;192:409–416.

48. McGowan FX Jr, Davis PJ, Siewers RD, del Nido PJ. Coronary vasoconstriction mediated by endothelin-1 in neonates. Reversal by nitroglycerin. J Thorac Cardiovasc Surg 1995;109:88–97.

49. Klemm P, Warner TD, Hohlfield T, Corder R, Vane JR. Endothelin 1 mediates ex vivo coronary vasoconstriction caused by exogenous and endogenous cytokines. Proc Natl Acad Sci USA 1995; 92:2691–2695.

50. Pernow J, Ahlborg G, Lundberg JM, Kaijser L. Long-lasting coronary vasoconstrictor effects and myocardial uptake of endothelin-1 in humans. Acta Physiol Scand 1997;159:147–153.

51. Kiely DG, Cargill RI, Struthers AD, Lipworth BJ. Cardiopulmonary effects of endothelin-1 in man. Cardiovasc Res 1997;33:378–386.

52. Eglen RM, Michel AD, Sharif NA, Swank SR, Whiting RL. The pharmacological properties of the peptide, endothelin. Br J Pharmacol 1989;97:1297–1307.

53. Shah AM, Lewis MJ, Henderson AH. Inotropic effects of endothelin in ferret ventricular myocardium. Eur J Pharmacol 1989;163:365–367.

54. Hu JR, Berninger UG, Lang RE. Endothelin stimulates atrial natriuretic peptide (ANP) release from rat atria. Eur J Pharmacol 1988;158:177–178.

55. Vigne P, Lazdunski M, Frelin C. Inotropic effect of endothelin-1 on rat atria involves hydrolysis of phosphatidylinositol. FEBS Lett 1989;249:143–146.

56. Suzuki H, Sato S, Suzuki Y, Oka M, Tokihiko T, Iino I, et al. Endothelin immunoreactivity in cerebrospinal fluid of patients with subarachnoid haemorrhage. Ann Med 1990;22:233–236.

57. McMurray JJ, Ray SG, Abdullah I, Dargie HJ, Morton JJ. Plasma endothelin in chronic heart failure. Circulation 1992;85:1374–1379.

58. Cody RJ, Haas GJ, Binkley PF, Capers Q, Kelley R. Plasma endothelin correlates with the extent of pulmonary hypertension in patients with chronic congestive heart failure. Circulation 1992;85:504–509.

59. Lerman A, Kubo SH, Tschumperlin LK, Burnett JC, Jr. Plasma endothelin concentrations in humans with end-stage heart failure and after heart transplantation. J Am Coll Cardiol 1992;20:849–853.

60. Stewart DJ, Cernacek P, Costello KB, Rouleau JL. Elevated endothelin-1 in heart failure and loss of normal response to postural change. Circulation 1992;85:510–517.

61. Pacher R, Bergler-Klein J, Globits S, Teufelsbauer H, Schuller M, Krauter A, et al. Plasma big endothelin-1 concentrations in congestive heart failure patients with or without systemic hypertension. Am J Cardiol 1993;71:1293–1299.

62. Cacoub P, Dorent R, Nataf P, Carayon A, Maistre G, Piette JC, et al. Plasma endothelin and pulmonary pressures in patients with congestive heart failure. Am Heart J 1993;126:1484–1488.

63. Tomoda H. Plasma endothelin-1 in acute myocardial infarction with heart failure. Am Heart J 1993; 125:667–672.

64. de Groote P, Millaire A, Racadot A, Recoulx E, Ducloux G. Plasma levels of endothelin-1 at rest and after exercise in patients with moderate congestive heart failure. Int J Cardiol 1995;51:267–272.

65. Tsutamoto T, Hisanaga T, Fukai D, Wada A, Maeda Y, Maeda K, Kinoshita M. Prognostic value of plasma soluble intercellular adhesion molecule-1 and endothelin-1 concentration in patients with chronic congestive heart failure. Am J Cardiol 1995;76:803–808.

66. Wei CM, Lerman A, Rodeheffer RJ, McGregor CG, Brandt RR, Wright S, et al. Endothelin in human congestive heart failure. Circulation 1994;89:1580–1586.

67. Pacher R, Stanek B, Hulsmann M, Koller-Strametz J, Berger R, Schuller M, et al. Prognostic impact of big endothelin-1 plasma concentrations compared with invasive hemodynamic evaluation in severe heart failure. J Am Coll Cardiol 1996;27:633–641.

68. Omland T, Lie RT, Aakvaag A, Aarsland T, Dickstein K. Plasma endothelin determinations as a prognostic indication of one year mortality after acute myocardial infarction. Circulation 1994;89:1573–1579.

69. Pousset F, Isnard R, Lechat P, Kalotka H, Carayon A, Maistre G, et al. Prognostic value of plasma endothelin-1 in patients with chronic heart failure. Eur Heart J 1997;18:254–258.

70. Krum H, Itescu S. Spontaneous endothelin production by circulating mononuclear cells from patients with chronic heart failure but not from normal subjects. Clin Exp Pharmacol Physiol 1994;21:311–313.

71. Mangieri E, Tanzilli G, Barilla F, Ciavolella M, Serafini G, Nardi M, et al. Isometric handgrip exercise increases endothelin-1 plasma levels in patients with chronic congestive heart failure. Am J Cardiol 1997;79:1261–1263.

72. Gu X, Casley DJ, Cincotta M, Nayler WG. ^{125}I-endothelin-1 binding to brain and cardiac membranes from normotensive and spontaneously hypertensive rats. Eur J Pharmacol 1990;177:205–209.

73. Cavero PG, Miller WL, Heublein DM, Margulies KB, Burnett JC. Endothelin in experimental congestive heart failure in the anesthetized dog. Am J Physiol 1990;259:F312–F317.

74. Margulies KB, Hildebrand FL, Lerman A, Perrella MA, Burnett JC. Increased endothelin in experimental heart failure. Circulation 1990;82:2226–2230.

75. Loffler BM, Roux S, Kalina B, Clozel M, Clozel JP. Influence of congestive heart failure on endothelin levels and receptors in rabbits. J Mol Cell Cardiol 1993;25:407–416.

76. Yorikane R, Sakai S, Miyauchi T, Sakurai T, Sugishita Y, Goto K. Increased production of endothelin-1 in the hypertrophied rat heart due to pressure overload. FEBS Lett 1993;332:31–34.

77. Tonnessen T, Christensen G, Oie E, Holt E, Kjekshus H, Smiseth OA, Sejersted OM, Attramadal H. Increased cardiac expression of endothelin-1 mRNA in ischemic heart failure in rats. Cardiovasc Res 1997;33:601–610.

78. Miyauchi T, Sakai S, Ihara M, Kasuya Y, Yamaguchi I, Goto K, Sugishita Y. Increased endothelin-1 binding sites in the cardiac membranes in rats with chronic heart failure. J Cardiovasc Pharmacol 1995; 26:S448–S451.

79. Wei CM, Clavell AL, Burnett JC. Atrial and pulmonary endothelin mRNA is increased in a canine model of chronic low cardiac output. Am J Physiol 1997;273:R838–R844.

80. Mulder P, Richard V, Derumeaux G, Hogie M, Henry JP, Lallemand F, et al. Role of endogenous endothelin in chronic heart failure: effect of long-term treatment with an endothelin antagonist on survival, hemodynamics, and cardiac remodeling. Circulation 1997;96:1976–1982.

81. Shubeita HE, McDonough PM, Harris AN, Knowlton KU, Glembotski CC, Brown JH, Chien KR. Endothelin induction of inositol phospholipid hydrolysis, sarcomere assembly and cardiac gene expression in ventricular myocytes. A paracrine mechanism for myocardial cell hypertrophy. J Biol Chem 1990;265:20,555–20,562.

82. Guarda E, Katwa LC, Myers PR, Tyagi SC, Weber KT. Effects of endothelins on collagen turnover in cardiac fibroblasts. Cardiovasc Res 1993;27:2130–2134.

83. Luyken J, Hannan RD, Cheung JY, Rothblum LI. Regulation of rDNA transcription during endothelin-1-induced hypertrophy of neonatal cardiomyocytes. Circ Res 1996;78:354–361.

84. Ito H, Hiroe M, Hirata Y, Fujisaki H, Adachi S, Akimoto H, Ohta Y, Marumo F. Endothelin ET_A receptor antagonist blocks cardiac hypertrophy provoked by hemodynamic overload. Circulation 1994;89:2198–2203.

85. Teerlink JR, Loffler BM, Hess P, Maire JP, Clozel M, Clozel JP. Role of endothelin in the maintenance of blood pressure in conscious rats with chronic heart failure. Acute effects of the endothelin receptor antagonist Ro 47-0203 (bosentan). Circulation 1994;90:2510–2518.

86. Sakai S, Miyauchi T, Kobayashi M, Yamaguchi I, Goto K, Sugishita Y. Inhibition of myocardial endothelin pathway improves long-term survival in heart failure. Nature 1996;384:353–355.

87. Shimoyama H, Sabbah HN, Borzak S, Tanimura M, Shevlyagin S, Scicli G, Goldstein S. Short-term hemodynamic effects of endothelin receptor blockade in dogs with chronic heart failure. Circulation 1996;94:779–784.

88. Clavell AL, Mattingly MT, Stevens TL, Nir A, Wright S, Aarhus LL, Heublein DM, Burnett JC Jr. Angiotensin converting enzyme inhibition modulates endogenous endothelin in chronic canine thoracic inferior vena caval constriction. J Clin Invest 1996;97:1286–1292.

89. Spinale FG, Walker JD, Mukherjee R, Iannini JP, Keever AT, Gallagher KP. Concomitant endothelin receptor subtype-A blockade during the progression of pacing-induced congestive heart failure in rabbits. Beneficial effects on left ventricular and myocyte function. Circulation 1997;95:1918–1929.

90. Tohmo H, Karanko M, Klossner J, Scheinin M, Viinamaki O, Neuvonen P, Ruskoaha H. Enalaprilat decreases plasma endothelin and atrial natriuretic peptide levels and preload in patients with left ventricular dysfunction after cardiac surgery. J Cardiothorac Vasc Anesth 1997;11:585–590.

91. Davidson NC, Coutie WJ, Webb DJ, Struthers AD. Hormonal and renal differences between low dose and high dose angiotensin converting enzyme inhibitor treatment in patients with chronic heart failure. Heart 1996;75:576–581.

92. Grenier O, Pousset F, Isnard R, Kalotka H, Carayon A, Maistre G, et al. Captopril does not acutely modulate plasma endothelin-1 concentration in human congestive heart failure. Cardiovasc Drugs Ther 1996;10:561–565.

93. Krum H, Gu A, Wilshire-Clement M, Sackner-Bernstein J, Goldsmith R, Medina N, et al. Changes in plasma endothelin-1 levels reflect clinical response to beta-blockade in chronic heart failure. Am Heart J 1996;131:337–341.

94. Kiowski W, Sutsch G, Hunziker P, Muller P, Kim J, Oechslin E, et al. Evidence for endothelin-1-mediated vasoconstriction in severe chronic heart failure. Lancet 1995;346:732–736.

95. Katz SD, Krum H, Packer M. Blunted vasoconstriction response to administration of endothelin-1 in the peripheral circulation of patients with congestive heart failure. Circulation 1994;90:I546.

96. Lee S, Lee CY, Chen YM, Kochva E. Coronary vasospasm as the primary cause of death due to the venom of the burrowing asp, Atractaspis engaddensis. Toxicon 1986;24:285–291.

97. Miyauchi T, Yanagisawa M, Tomizawa T, Sugishata Y, Suzuki N, Fujino M, et al. Increased plasma concentrations of endothelin-1 and big endothelin-1 in acute myocardial infarction (letter to the editor). Lancet 1989;ii:53–54.

98. Matsuyama K, Saito Y, Nakao K, Jougasaki M, Okumura K, Yasue H, Imura H. Endothelin in myocardial ischaemia induced by coronary vasospasm. Circulation 1990;83:443.

99. Matsuyama K, Yasue H, Okumura K, Saito Y, Nakao K, Shirakami G, Imura H. Increased plasma level of endothelin-1-like immunoreactivity during coronary spasm in patients with coronary spastic angina. Am J Cardiol 1991;68:991–995.

100. Yasuda M, Kohno M, Tahara A, Itagane H, Toda I, Akioka K, et al. Circulating immunoreactive endothelin in ischemic heart disease. Am Heart J 1990;119:801–806.

101. Stewart DJ, Kubac G, Costello KB, Cernacek P. Increased plasma endothelin-1 in the early hours of acute myocardial infarction. J Am Coll Cardiol 1991;18:38–43.

102. Tsuji S, Sawamura A, Watanabe H, Takihara K, Park S, Azuma J. Plasma endothelin levels during myocardial ischemia and reperfusion. Life Sci 1991;48:1745–1749.

103. Ray SG, McMurray JJ, Morton JJ, Dargie HJ. Circulating endothelin in acute ischaemic syndromes. Br Heart J 1992;67:383–386.

104. Arendt RM, Wilbert-Lampen U, Heucke L, Schmoeckel M, Suhler K, Richter WO. Increased endothelin plasma concentrations in patients with coronary artery disease or hyperlipoproteinemia without coronary events. Res Exp Med 1993;193:225–230.

105. Artigou JY, Salloum J, Carayon A, Lechat P, Maistre G, Isnard R, et al. Variations in plasma endothelin concentrations during coronary spasm. Eur Heart J 1993;14:780–784.

106. Setsuta K, Seino Y, Tomita Y, Nejima J, Takano T, Hayakawa H. Origin and pathophysiological role of increased plasma endothelin-1 in patients with acute myocardial infarction. Angiology 1995;46: 557–565.

107. Nakao K, Saito Y, Matsuyama K, Okumura K, Jougasaki M, Yasue H. Implication of endothelin in variant angina. Circulation 1989;80:II586

108. Stewart JT, Nisbet JA, Davies MJ. Plasma endothelin in coronary venous blood from patients with either stable or unstable angina. Br Heart J 1991;66:7–9.

109. Qiu S, Theroux P, Marcil M, Solymoss BC. Plasma endothelin-1 levels in stable and unstable angina. Cardiology 1993;82:12–19.

110. Letizia C, Cerci S, Coscia M, Subioli S, Coassin S, D'Ambrosio C, Scavo D. Behavior of plasma levels of endothelin-1 and noradrenaline in patients with stable angina during the cold pressor test. Rec Prog Med 1997;88:312–316.

111. Fontana F, Tarsi G, Boschi S, De Iasio R, Monetti N, Bugiardini R. Relationship between plasma endothelin-1 levels and myocardial ischemia induced by exercise testing. Am J Cardiol 1997;79: 957–959.

112. Kyriakides ZS, Markianos M, Iiodromitis EK, Kremastinos DT. Vein plasma endothelin-1 and cyclic GMP increase during coronary angioplasty is related to myocardial ischaemia. Eur Heart J 1995; 16:894–898.

113. Watanabe T, Suzuki N, Shimamoto N, Fujino M, Imada A. Endothelin in myocardial infarction. Nature 1990;344:114.

114. Kusumoto K, Fujiwara S, Awane Y, Watanabe T. The role of endogenous endothelin in extension of rabbit myocardial infarction. J Cardiovasc Pharmacol 1993;22:S339–S342.

115. Grover GJ, Sleph PG, Fox M, Trippodo NC. Role of endothelin-1 and big endothelin-1 in modulating coronary vascular tone, contractile function and severity of ischemia in rat hearts. J Pharmacol Exp Ther 1992;263:1074–1082.

116. Nelson RA, Burke SE, Opgenorth T. Endothelin receptor antagonist FR 139317 reduces infarct size in a rabbit coronary artery occlusion model. FASEB J 1994;8:A854.

117. Lee JY, Warner RB, Adler AL, Opgenorth TJ. ET$_A$ receptor antagonist FR139317 reduces myocardial infarction induced by coronary artery occlusion and reperfusion in the rat. FASEB J 1994;8:A854.

118. Wang QD, Li X.S, Lundberg JM, Pernow J. Protective effects of nonpeptide endothelin receptor antagonist bosentan on myocardial ischaemic and reperfusion injury in the pig. Cardiovasc Res 1995; 29:805–812.

119. McMurdo L, Thiemermann C, Vane JR. Effects of the endothelin ETA receptor antagonist, FR 139317, on infarct size in a rabbit model of acute myocardial ischaemia and reperfusion. Br J Pharmacol 1994; 112:75–80.

120. Vitola JV, Forman MB, Holsinger JP, Kawana M, Atkinson JB, Quertermous T, Jackson EK, Murray JJ. Role of endothelin in a rabbit model of acute myocardial infarction—effects of receptor antagonists. J Cardiovasc Pharmacol 1996;28:774–783.

121. Erikson JM, Velasco CE. Endothelin-1 and myocardial preconditioning. Am Heart J 1996;132:84–90.

122. Mertz TE, McClanahan TB, Flynn MA, Juneau P, Reynolds EE, Hallak H, Bradford L, Gallagher KP. Endothelin-A receptor antagonism by PD156707 does not reduce infarct size after coronary artery occlusion/reperfusion in pigs. J Pharmacol Exp Ther 1996;278:42–49.

123. Wang QD, Li XS, Pernow J. Nonpeptide endothelin receptor antagonist bosentan enhances myocardial recovery and endothelial function during reperfusion of the ischemic rat heart. J Cardiovasc Pharmacol 1996;26(Suppl 3):S445–S447.

124. Grover GJ, Dzwonczyk S, Parham CS. Endothelin-1 receptor antagonist BQ123 reduces infarct size in a canine model of coronary occlusion and reperfusion. Cardiovasc Res 1993;27: 1613–1618.

125. Burke SE, Nelson RA. Endothelin receptor antagonist, FR 139317, reduces infarct size in a rabbit model when given before, but not after, coronary artery occlusion. J Cardiovasc Pharmacol 1997;29:87–92.

126. Kojima M, Kusumoto K, Fujiwara S, Watanabe T, Fujino M. Role of endogenous endothelin in the extension of myocardial infarct size studies with the endothelin receptor antagonist, TAK-044. J Cardiovasc Pharmacol 1995;26:S365–S368.

127. Watanabe T, Awane Y, Ikeda S, Fujiwara S, Kubo K, Kikuchi T, et al. Pharmacology of a non-selective ET_A and ET_B receptor antagonist TAK-044, and the inhibition of myocardial infarct size in rats. Br J Pharmacol 1995;114:949–954.

128. Illing B, Horn M, Han H, Hahn S, Bureik P, Ertl G, Neubauer S. Protective effect of the specific endothelin-1 antagonist BQ610 on mechanical function and energy metabolism during ischemia/reperfusion injury in isolated perfused rat hearts. J Cardiovasc Pharmacol 1996;27:487–494.

129. Goodwin AT, Amrani M, Gray CC, Chester AH, Yacoub MH. Inhibition of endogenous endothelin during cardioplegia improves low coronary reflow following prolonged hypothermic arrest. Eur J Cardio Thor Surg 1997;11:981–987.

130. Garjani A, Wainwright CL, Zeitlin IJ, Wilson C, Slee SJ. Effects of endothelin-1 and the ETA-receptor antagonist, BQ123:on ischemic arrhythmias in anesthetized rats. J Cardiovasc Pharmacol 1995;25:634–642.

131. Omland T, Bonarjee VV, Lie RT, Caidahl K. Neurohumoral measurements as indicators of long-term prognosis after acute myocardial infarction. Am J Cardiol 1995;76:230–235.

132. Ohlstein EH, Douglas SA. Endothelin-1 modulates vascular smooth muscle structure and vasomotion: implications in cardiovascular pathology. Drug Develop Res 1993;29:108–128.

133. Martin-Nizard F, Houssaini HS, Lestavel-Delattre S, Duriez P, Fruchart J. Modified low density lipoproteins activate human macrophages to secrete immunoreactive endothelin. FEBS Lett 1991;293:127–130.

134. Boulanger CM, Tanner FC, Beau M, Han AWA, Werner A, Luscher TF. Oxidized low density lipoproteins induce mRNA expression and release of endothelin from human and porcine endothelium. Circ Res 1992;70:1191–1197.

135. Lopez JAG, Armstrong ML, Piegors DJ, Heistad DD. Vascular responses to endothelin-1 in atherosclerotic primates. Artherosclerosis 1990;10:1113–1118.

136. Davies MG, Klyachkin ML, Kim JH, Hagen PO. Endothelin and vein bypass grafts in experimental atherosclerosis. J Cardiovasc Pharmacol 1993;22:S348–S351.

137. Douglas SA, Louden C, Vickery-Clark LM, Storer BL, Hart T, Feuerstein GZ, Elliott JD, Ohlstein EH. Role for endogenous endothelin-1 in neointimal formation after rat carotid artery balloon angioplasty. Protective effects of the novel nonpeptide endothelin receptor antagonist SB 209670. Circ Res 1994;75:190–197.

138. Lerman A, Edwards BS, Hallett JW, Heublein DM, Sandberg SM, Burnett JC, Jr. Circulating and tissue endothelin immunoreactivity in advanced atherosclerosis. N Engl J Med 1991;325:997–1001.

139. Zeiher AM, Goebel H, Schachinger V, Ihling C. Tissue endothelin-1 immunoreactivity in the active coronary atherosclerotic plaque. Circulation 1995;91:941–947.

140. Prat L, Carrio I, Roca M, Riambau V, Berne L, Estorch M, Ferrer I, Garcia C. Polyclonal ^{111}In-IgG, ^{125}I-LDL and ^{125}I-endothelin-1 accumulation in experimental arterial wall injury. Eur J Nucl Med 1993;20:1141–1145.

141. Dashwood M, Barker SGE, Muddle JR, Yacoub MH, Martin JF. [^{125}I] endothelin-1 binding to vasa vasorum and regions of neovascularization in human and porcine blood vessels: a possible role for endothelin in intimal hyperplasia and atherosclerosis. J Cardiovasc Pharmacol 1993;22:S343–S347.

142. Dashwood MR, Allen SP, Luu TN, Muddle JR. Effect of the ET_A receptor antagonist, FR 139317, on [^{125}I] ET-1 binding to the atherosclerotic human coronary artery. Br J Pharmacol 1994;112:386–389.

143. Wang X, Douglas SA, Ohlstein EH. Use of quantitative RT-PCR to demonstrate the increased expression of endothelin-related mRNAs following angioplasty-induced neointima formation in the rat. Circ Res 1996;78:322–328.

144. Tsujino M, Hirata Y, Eguchi S, Watanabe T, Chatani F, Marumoi F. Nonselective ETA/ETB receptor antagonists block proliferation of rat vascular smooth muscle cells after balloon angioplasty. Life Sci 1995;56:PL449–PL454.

145. Azuma H, Hamasaki H, Niimi Y, Terada T, Matsubara O. Role of endothelin-1 in neointima formation after endothelial removal in rabbit carotid arteries. Am J Physiol 1994;267:H2259–H2267.

146. Douglas SA, Vickery-Clark LM, Louden C, Elliott JD, Ohlstein EH. Endothelin receptor subtypes in the pathogenesis of angioplasty-induced neointima formation in the rat: a comparison of selective ETA receptor antagonism and dual ETA/ETB receptor antagonism using BQ-123 and SB 209670. J Cardiovasc Pharmacol 1996;26(Suppl 3):S186–S189.

147. Hele DJ, Birrell M, Bush RC, Flynn DA, Brown TJ, Roach DJ. Selective ETA and mixed ETA/ETB receptor antagonists inhibit balloon catheter-induced smooth muscle cell proliferation in the rat thoracic aorta. Br J Pharmacol 1995;114:199.

148. Kowala MC, Rose PM, Stein PD, Goller N, Recce R, Beyer S, et al. Selective blockade of the endothelin subtype A receptor decreases early atherosclerosis in hamsters fed cholesterol. Am J Pathol 1995;146: 819–826.

149. Clarke Forbes RD, Cernacek P, Zheng S, Gomersall M, Guttmann RD. Increased endothelin expression in a rat cardiac allograft model of chronic vascular rejection. Transplantation 1996;61:791–797.

150. Brooks DP, Jorkasky DK, Freed MI, Ohlstein EH. Pathophysiological role of endothelin and potential therapeutic targets for receptor antagonists. In: Highsmith RF, ed. Endothelin: Molecular Biology Physiology and Pathology. Humana, Totowa, NJ, 1997, pp. 223–268.

11

Nitric Oxide and the Heart

Robert D. Bernstein, Fabio A. Recchia,
Gabor Kaley, and Thomas H. Hintze

CONTENTS

INTRODUCTION

Nitric oxide (NO) is traditionally known as a molecule released from the vascular endothelium that plays an important role in regulating vascular tone *(1)*. However, in the heart, NO released from the vascular endothelium is involved in a number of important paracrine functions independent of vascular tone, as shown in Fig. 1. This chapter discusses the influence of NO on myocardial blood flow, substrate utilization, and oxygen consumption. The degree to which NO influences the contractility of the heart will also be discussed. NO has also been implicated in the control of apoptosis *(2)*, which may have important clinical implications *(3)* in terms of the pathogenesis of heart failure (HF). As will be demonstrated in this chapter, NO has many more roles in the heart than simply dilating blood vessels.

SOURCES OF NITRIC OXIDE

Nitric Oxide Synthases

NO is a gas produced by the enzyme nitric oxide synthase (NOS). This enzyme combines molecular oxygen with arginine to make NO *(1,4)*. There are three main isoforms of this enzyme. Isoform I is a constitutive enzyme, and is located primarily in neuronal and epithelial cells (also known as bNOS) *(5)*, but has also been isolated in human skeletal muscle *(6)*. Isoform II is the inducible form (also known as iNOS).

From: *Contemporary Endocrinology: Hormones and the Heart in Health and Disease*
Edited by: L. Share © Humana Press Inc., Totowa, NJ

Paracrine Actions of NO

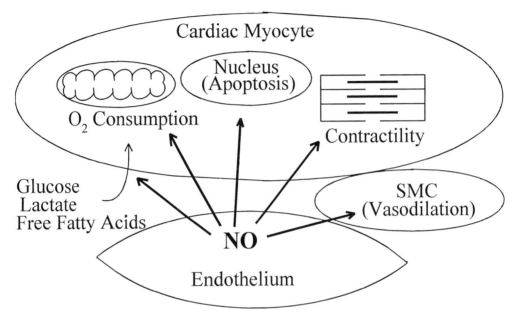

Fig. 1. Diagram of a capillary endothelial cell, a vascular smooth muscle cell, and a cardiac myocyte, which depicts the actions of endogenously released NO. NO can diffuse from the vascular endothelial cell and effect functions in both the vascular smooth muscle and the myocardial cells.

Expression of this enzyme requires pre-exposure to a combination of bacterial lipopolysaccharide (LPS) and cytokines *(7)*, and iNOS is found primarily in activated macrophages and leukocytes, but can be expressed in almost any tissue, including the heart, with the appropriate stimulation *(8)*. Isoform III is also constitutively expressed, and is found chiefly in vascular endothelial cells (thus known as ecNOS or just eNOS) *(9)*, including capillary endothelium (Fig. 2). In the normal heart, eNOS is the primary NOS enzyme, and is located mostly in the vascular endothelium *(10,11)*. Immunohistochemical staining has also shown a significant presence of bNOS in the atria *(12)*, and in a portion of the perivascular nerve fibers in the myocardium of the ventricle *(13)*. In certain disease states, and/or following exposure to cytokines or LPS, there may be an expression of NOS in cardiac myocytes *(14)*, or in activated macrophages *(15)*.

Synthesis of Nitric Oxide

All three isoforms of NOS function in a similar manner: either of the terminal guanidino nitrogens of arginine are combined with molecular oxygen to make NO and citrulline *(16)*. This reaction involves two successive mono-oxygenation reactions, with N^{ω}-hydroxy-L-arginine as an intermediate step in the formation of NO *(17)*. This reaction requires the presence of calmodulin, tetrahydrobiopterin, flavin mononucleotide, flavin adenine dinucleotide, and a nicotinamide adenine dinucleotide phosphate. Additionally, the catalytic site of the enzyme is an iron (Fe) protoporphyrin heme. Activation of the two constitutive enzymes requires an increase in intracellular calcium (Ca) that will bind to the associated calmodulin, leading to a conformational shift in the enzyme *(1)*. This conformational change allows an electron flux from the flavins to the heme moiety,

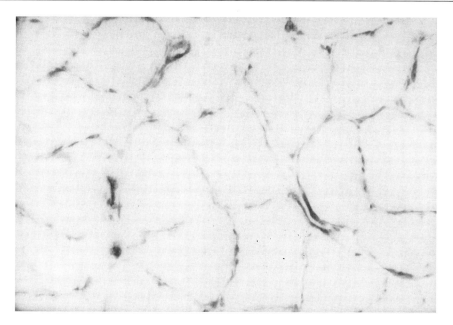

Fig. 2. eNOS staining in the capillary endothelium in rat skeletal muscle. Brown staining represents the presence of eNOS. Note that there is no significant distance between the edge of the capillary and the adjoining skeletal muscle cell. A similar relationship between the myocyte and the capillary endothelium would be expected in the heart.

enabling the synthesis of NO *(18)*. This increase in intracellular Ca can occur either through receptor activation with agonists like bradykinin or acetylcholine *(1,19)* or through physical alterations in the vessel wall induced by shear stress *(20,21)*. These intracellular fluxes of Ca result in small puffs of NO being released, usually in the picomolar concentration *(1)*. In the inducible NO synthesis, the calmodulin is closely associated with the enzyme, keeping the enzyme in the active state *(22)*. This tonically active iNOS produces nanomoles of NO *(1)*.

Nitric Oxide Activity

The NO that is made by any of the isoforms is a freely diffusible gas. Although rapidly degraded to nitrite and nitrate in aqueous solutions, NO has a diffusion distance of approximately 100 μm under physiologic conditions *(1)*, and may even be as far as 600 μm *(23)*. NO has a high affinity for Fe^{2+}-hemoproteins, and will interact with the heme moiety at low concentrations. Depending on the target enzyme, this interaction with NO may be either inhibitory or excitatory. For soluble guanylyl cyclase, the formation of the NO–heme complex activates the enzyme, and this activation leads to an increase in the cellular content of cyclic guanine monophosphate (cGMP) *(24,25)*. In terms of vascular control, this elevated cGMP will lead to a relaxation in vascular smooth muscle, thereby producing the vasodilatory effects of NO *(1)*. In addition to activation of guanylyl cyclase, NO also appears to activate both cyclo-oxygenase-1 and cyclo-oxygenase-2 through a similar interaction with the Fe^{2+}-heme centers of these enzymes *(26)*. The activation of these enzymes occurs at relatively low concentrations of NO, as would be produced by either bNOS or eNOS. Activated macrophages produce much higher levels of NO, which can lead to metabolic inhibition *(15,27,28)*. However, it has recently been shown that physi-

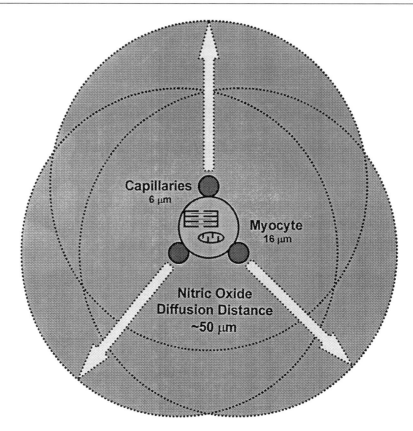

Fig. 3. Schematic diagram of a cardiac myocyte and the associated capillaries demonstrating the diffusion distance of NO. NO that is produced by the vascular endothelium can freely diffuse into the myocyte. Diffusion distance, myocyte, and capillaries are all drawn to scale.

ological levels of NO (as would be released by eNOS) are capable of influencing metabolism *(29)*. This has important implications for myocardial function and metabolism, because the physiologic levels of NO released from the vascular endothelium would bathe the adjacent myocytes in NO (Fig. 3). The metabolic aspects of NO will be discussed in more detail later, but, as Figs. 2 and 3 demonstrate, the presence of NO in the vascular endothelium is in close enough proximity to the myocytes to have the potential to influence both the metabolic apparatus (mitochondria) and the contractile apparatus of cardiac myocytes. The authors assumed the capillary endothelium is the primary source of NO for control of parenchymal cell metabolism. Capillary endothelium is the largest cross-section of endothelium, being 1000 times greater than all of the blood vessels combined. However, NO from both pre- and postcapillary vessels could contribute to the NO diffusing into the parenchymal cell, if the diffusion distance for NO is not limiting.

REGULATION OF BLOOD FLOW AND RESISTANCE

Role of Nitric Oxide in Regulation of Blood Flow in the Periphery

In terms of the peripheral circulation, NO plays an important role in the regulation of blood flow and vascular resistance. A majority of the studies demonstrating the role of

NO in the regulation of blood flow and resistance were performed using inhibitors of NO synthesis *(30)*. Systemic blockade of NO synthesis was first tested in anesthetized rabbits *(31)*. Inhibition of NO synthesis led to a significant elevation of blood pressure and resistance in the peripheral circulation, demonstrating a tonic release of NO by the endothelium. This increase in arterial pressure occurs in a variety of species, including guinea pigs *(32)*, rats *(33)*, dogs *(34,35)*, and humans *(36)*.

The increase in pressure caused by inhibition of NO synthesis is not uniform across all vascular beds. In a study in conscious dogs from this laboratory, using radioactive microspheres, systemic inhibition of NO synthesis led to an increased vascular resistance and a reduction in blood flow to the kidney, stomach, ileum, colon, pancreas, and resting skeletal muscle, without affecting the liver or spleen *(35)*. NO does not appear to be involved in the increase in skeletal muscle blood flow associated with acute exercise, because the level of skeletal muscle blood flow at a set level of exercise was not different before or after inhibition of NO synthesis *(35,37)*.

In terms of myocardial perfusion, systemic inhibition of NO synthesis with nitro-L-arginine (NLA) resulted in a significant increase in resistance in all layers of the myocardium, but there was only a reduction in blood flow to the left ventricular epicardium, septum, and right ventricle *(35)*. This resulted in an elevation in the ratio of endocardial to epicardial blood flow, which may be caused by the alterations in arterial pressure and ventricular work, and not the loss of NO *(35)*. Indeed, in further studies in conscious dogs, inhibition of NO synthesis does not have clear-cut effects on coronary blood flow *(38–40)*. Blockade of NO synthesis in conscious dogs not receiving any other medication (such as aspirin or sedatives) either has no effect *(35,39,40)* or results in a slight increase in baseline coronary blood flow *(38)*. In all of these studies, inhibition of NO synthesis was associated with significant changes in some of the major determinants of myocardial oxygen consumption, which will have indirect influences on coronary blood flow.

Traditional Mechanisms of Coronary Vascular Regulation

Before discussing the role of NO in the coronary circulation, there will be a brief examination of the traditional mechanisms of coronary vascular regulation. The coronary circulation has been thought to be primarily controlled by local factors related to the level of myocardial metabolism *(41,42)*. These local factors include adenosine, prostaglandins, potassium, oxygen, and carbon dioxide. Changes in carbon dioxide and adenosine are probably the primary links that help match myocardial blood flow to myocardial metabolism. Increases in metabolism will lead to elevations in both carbon dioxide and adenosine metabolites, both of which are potent vasodilators *(42)*. Although there is a neural input to the coronary circulation, it plays a modulatory role in blood flow regulation *(42)*. All of these metabolites work in a complementary fashion to coordinate the tight regulation of coronary blood flow, so that oxygen and substrate supply matches demand.

Nitric Oxide and Control of Coronary Blood Flow and Resistance

In isolated-heart preparations, interruption of the NO pathway will have significant effects on myocardial perfusion. In saline-perfused Langendorff heart preparations, scavenging NO with hemoglobin results in an increase in coronary resistance and a reduction in coronary blood flow *(43)*. Coronary blood flow was also reduced when inhibitors of NO synthesis were used in isolated-heart preparations *(44,45)*. These results are consistent with studies in open-chest anesthetized dogs *(46)* or pigs *(47)*, or in closed-chest, sedated *(48)* canines, in which inhibition of NO synthesis led to reductions in coronary blood flow. These *in situ* studies of the coronary circulation do not always agree with studies in conscious animals. Systemic or local (intracoronary) inhibition NOS in whole animals does not always result in reductions in coronary blood flow *(35,38-40,49)*. In fact, most studies using conscious animals and inhibitors of NO synthesis report either no change *(35,39,40,49)* or increases in coronary blood flow *(38)*. A study using an inhibitor of NO synthesis in humans suggests that blockade of NO synthesis reduces coronary blood flow *(50)*. However, closer examination of this study reveals another possible explanation. The study in humans demonstrated a significant reduction in coronary artery diameter and a fall in the oxygen content of the coronary venous blood. This fall in coronary venous oxygen content was assumed to be equivalent to a reduction in blood flow *(50)*, but coronary blood flow was not directly measured. Coronary venous oxygen content is a product of myocardial metabolism and coronary blood flow: If coronary venous oxygen content falls, then either coronary blood flow must have decreased or myocardial metabolism must have increased. In the study in humans, there was no change in the hemodynamic determinants of myocardial metabolism (no change in heart rate or blood pressure); therefore, the authors reasoned that coronary flow must have decreased *(50)*. However, reductions in coronary venous oxygen content could be a result of alterations in metabolism that occur in the absence of hemodynamic alterations. Blockade of NO synthesis may have important consequences for myocardial metabolism, which will be discussed in greater detail later. Briefly, if blockade of NO synthesis leads to an elevation in myocardial metabolism in the absence of hemodynamic alterations, coronary venous oxygen content would fall. This is exactly what is seen in the study by Lefroy et al. *(50)*; the reduction in the coronary venous oxygen content could simply be a result of a removal of the tonic inhibition of oxygen consumption by NO. Therefore, inhibition of NO synthesis might alter coronary blood flow by directly influencing myocardial metabolism, not through a direct action on vascular smooth muscle. With that caveat, inhibition of NO synthesis has, at best, a minor impact on coronary blood flow. However, all studies, whether reporting an increase *(38)*, no change *(35,39,40,49)*, or a decrease *(43–48)* in coronary blood flow following inhibition of NO synthesis, have shown an increase in coronary vascular resistance and/or a reduction in the diameter of large coronary arteries. Although the effects of NO on coronary blood flow are not clear, NO clearly influences coronary arterial tone.

Significant production of NO by the coronary circulation has been demonstrated both in vitro *(51–53)* and in vivo *(40)*, yet this NO does not appear to be important in the regulation of coronary blood flow in vivo. In a study using conscious dogs exercising on a treadmill, Bernstein et al. demonstrated the relative independence of the coronary circulation from NO *(40)*; Fig. 4 represents a replotting and recalculation of data from that study. Dogs were instrumented for the measurement of cardiovascular hemodynamics, and trained to run on a treadmill. NO synthesis was blocked with NLA, a potent inhibitor of NO synthesis *(1)*. As shown in Fig. 4A, coronary blood flow increases with acute exercise. When the same animals were run on the treadmill after NO synthesis had been blocked with NLA, there was no difference in coronary blood flow at each level of exercise. Because inhibition of NO synthesis will have a significant effect on the hemodynamic determinants of myocardial oxygen consumption, the levels of coronary blood flow were compared with the levels of cardiac work (Fig. 4B). Myocardial oxygen

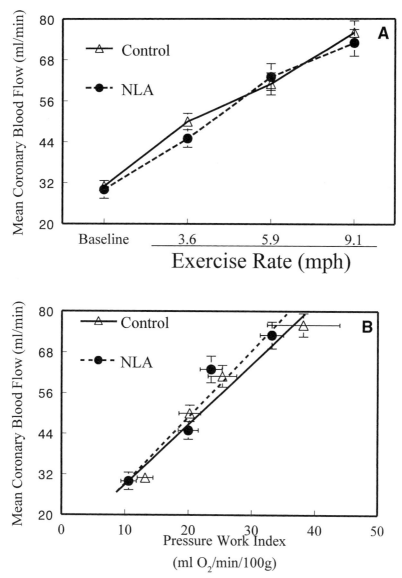

Fig. 4. Levels of coronary blood flow and myocardial work during acute exercise in the conscious dog. Exercise produced an increase in coronary blood flow that was not effected by blockade of NO synthesis with NLA. Additionally, blockade of NO synthesis did not alter the relationships between coronary blood flow and myocardial work (B). Adopted with permission from ref. *40*.

consumption is directly related to myocardial work, and is the major controlling factor in coronary blood flow *(41,42)*. To normalize any hemodynamic alterations caused by NLA, cardiac work was estimated using the pressure–work index developed by Rooke and Feigl *(54)*, and compared to the measured coronary blood flow. Although the levels of cardiac work were slightly different before and after NLA, there was no difference in the ratios of coronary blood flow to cardiac work before (Control) or after blockade of NO synthesis with NLA. It should be noted that lactate levels were measured across the heart, and there was never any net lactate production in any of the animals tested, suggesting that there was never an insufficient blood flow to the working myocardium.

These data demonstrate that NO is not necessary for the physiologic regulation of coronary blood flow in the normal working heart in vivo. However, in disease states or ischemia, NO may play a role in blood flow regulation.

The presence of multiple, redundant mechanisms that control coronary blood flow could explain why it has been difficult to demonstrate in vivo a role for NO in controlling the coronary circulation. Inhibition of NO synthesis may change coronary blood flow in vitro or in vivo, but this will occur only when one of the many factors controlling coronary blood flow has been compromised. The intact coronary circulation relies chiefly on metabolic vasodilators to regulate myocardial perfusion (41,42). Substances such as adenosine, prostaglandins, potassium, oxygen, and carbon dioxide all work in conjunction to regulate myocardial perfusion. The control of the coronary circulation can be explained completely (and has been historically) without a reference to NO (41,42), with the exception of flow-induced dilation (55,56). The role of NO in flow-induced dilation in the coronary circulation was established either through removal of the endothelium from a large coronary artery (57), or through the use of inhibitors of NO synthesis (34,58). These studies showed that increases in coronary blood flow/diameter as a result of rapid increases in coronary blood flow were dependent on NO. As discussed earlier, NO plays a minor role in the regulation of basal blood flow, or during physiological increases in blood flow during exercise in the normal heart (38–40). Although NO plays a minor role in the regulation of blood flow in the normal heart, studies have demonstrated both the presence of eNOS enzyme (10,11) and the production of NO by the coronary circulation (40,51–53). The ability of NO to dilate larger vessels may indicate a role in the control of capillary perfusion pressure and filtration. Thus, by dilating primarily large coronary vessels, the perfusion pressure is transmitted to the endocardium to increase both filtration and blood flow. However, because the NO that is being produced does not play a major role in the control coronary blood flow in the normal heart, the function of this NO may be to regulate myocardial metabolism.

NITRIC OXIDE AND METABOLISM

Activated macrophages were known to produce a substance that suppressed oxygen consumption (28). This substance was identified as NO (27). Through its ability to bind to the iron in Fe–sulfur centers, for instance, in complex I and II, or to compete with the oxygen-binding site on cytochrome-c oxidase, NO appears to modify oxygen consumption by binding to, and inactivating, specific enzymes in the electron transport chain (29,59,60). Evidence from this laboratory (37) and others (61) has shown that physiological levels of NO also play a role in the regulation of skeletal muscle metabolism in vivo. Work by King et al. (61) and Shen et al. (37) demonstrated that endogenously released NO can also function as a physiological mediator to modulate oxygen consumption in resting skeletal muscle and the whole body, respectively. That NO suppresses oxygen consumption at the mitochondrial level was demonstrated using isolated mitochondrial preparations (59,60,62–64). Because the effect of NO is increased at low oxygen tensions (64), and, because the myocardium has an extremely low oxygen tension (65), the heart must be more susceptible to the effects of NO to influence metabolism. Additionally, cardiac myocytes are in close proximity to the capillary endothelium (66), providing an abundant source for NO that could interact with the myocytes. However, NO may not even need to diffuse from the vascular endothelium to influence metabolism: A recent study using immunocytochemical staining has demonstrated the presence of eNOS in mitochondria isolated from rat heart *(67)*. Functional measurements of NO production were not performed in that study, Bates et al. *(67)* have demonstrated that there is a potential source of NO in direct proximity to the metabolic apparatus.

Regardless of the source of NO, whether it diffuses from the vascular endothelium or directly from the NOS in the mitochondria, there is evidence demonstrating that endogenous NO can reduce myocardial respiration, in vitro *(68,69)*, as well as in the conscious dog in vivo *(38,40)*. Although myocardial oxygen consumption was not measured in the study using inhibitors of NO in the human coronary circulation *(50)*, the reduction in coronary venous oxygen content would seem to support this role of NO in regulating oxygen consumption. In the absence of hemodynamic alterations that would change myocardial oxygen consumption, there was a significant reduction in the coronary venous oxygen content after blockade of NO synthesis. If endogenous NO were reducing oxygen consumption, then blockade of endogenous NO synthesis would lead to an increase in myocardial metabolism, independent of the work being performed by the heart. There is some controversy on this subject, because studies either in the *in situ* heart of anesthetized, open chest dogs *(46)* or pigs *(47)*, or in a model in which the heart is studied in the sedated canine *(48)*, have produced conflicting results. This conflict could arise from the presence of anesthetics, some of which interfere with cellular respiration at the same sites as NO *(70)*. The in vivo effects of NO on myocardial oxygen consumption remain to be elucidated, but this molecule clearly plays a role in regulating the respiration of isolated mitochondria *(64)*, cultured cells *(28,71)*, and isolated skeletal *(72)* and cardiac muscle *(68,69)*. NO reduces oxygen consumption, most likely through its ability to interfere with the transfer of electrons from cytochrome oxidase to oxygen *(29,59,62)*.

A potential reason for the lack of clarity on the role of NO is that there is an alteration in the substrate metabolism that occurs after blockade of NO synthesis *(40)*. After inhibition of NO synthesis, the myocardium consumes less free fatty acids and more lactate *(40,73,74*; Fig. 5). There was no evidence of glucose uptake in the normal canine heart in any of these studies *(40,73,74)*. Switching from fats to lactate could result in a reduction in oxygen consumption, because lactate is a more efficient fuel *(75,76)*. It is theoretically possible, simply switching from fats to lactate, to reduce oxygen consumption by approx 10% *(76)*. Switching to a more efficient fuel would either mask or attenuate the increase in oxygen consumption associated with blockade of NO synthesis. This shift in substrates could be a potential explanation for the differences in the various studies on NO and myocardial oxygen consumption in whole animals *(38–40,46–48)*.

HEART FAILURE AND NITRIC OXIDE

Alterations in Nitric Oxide Production During Heart Failure

There is some confusion as to the state of NO production and NO synthesis during heart failure (HF). A study of human patients with HF revealed an elevation in the plasma levels of nitrates, the stable breakdown products of NO *(77)*. Because HF is associated with elevated levels of tumor necrosis factor *(78)*, this increase in plasma nitrates was thought to be caused by an increase in basal NO production *(79)*. This increase in basal NO production was believed to result either from the presence of iNOS or from continuous stimulation of the constitutive form of NOS in patients with HF *(77)*. However, most experimental evidence, in dogs *(80–83)*, rats *(84)*, and humans *(85–87)*, suggests that

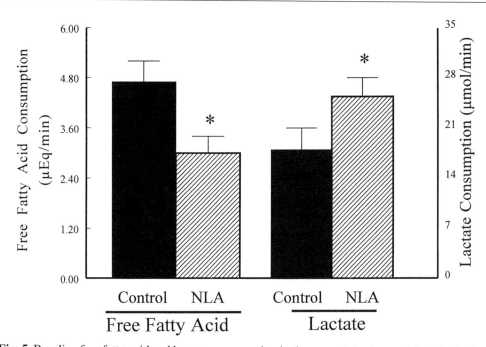

Fig. 5. Baseline free fatty acid and lactate consumption in the normal dog heart. After blockade of NO synthesis with NLA, there was a significant reduction in free fatty acid consumption, with an increase in lactate consumption. There was no measurable glucose uptake by the myocardium. $n = 15$; $*p < 0.05$.

there is a reduction in the ability of the blood vessels to synthesize NO in HF. Indeed, in a study that examined both the mRNA and the protein for the constitutive NO, both the message and the protein for eNOS virtually disappeared after the development of severe congestive HF in dogs *(88)*. And yet, the source for this confusion is that plasma nitrates are consistently elevated in HF *(77,79,83)*, and isolated tissue studies have revealed the presence of iNOS in cultured cells from failing hearts *(79,89,90)*. High levels of NO produced from this iNOS could explain the reduced contractility seen in HF, as high concentrations of NO have been shown to have a negative inotropic effect in vitro *(91,92)*. However, the presence of the message for iNOS does not necessarily mean that the protein is being expressed *(93)*. In addition to the canine studies demonstrating a reduction in the level of NOS expression after HF *(88,94)*, in experimental HF in rats, there is a selective reduction in aortic eNOS, with no evidence of iNOS in either the aorta or skeletal muscle vascular beds *(95)*. The explanation for the high circulating levels of nitrates during HF appears to come from a reduction in the clearance of nitrates, not an increased production of NO *(83,96)*. Nitrates are cleared from the plasma primarily by the kidneys *(97,98)*, and both experimental and clinical HF are associated with a reduction in renal function, and, presumably, renal clearance of nitrates *(83,96)*. Additionally, when NO production was actually measured across the heart, HF was associated with a net uptake of NO by the myocardium in humans *(96)* and in dogs *(99,100)*. Therefore, even if there is iNOS present in the myocardium in HF, it cannot be responsible for the elevated plasma nitrates seen in HF. Additionally, if there were an appreciable production of NO in cardiac myocytes during HF, it would have to show up as a positive difference in NO across the heart. This is clearly not the case either in animal models of

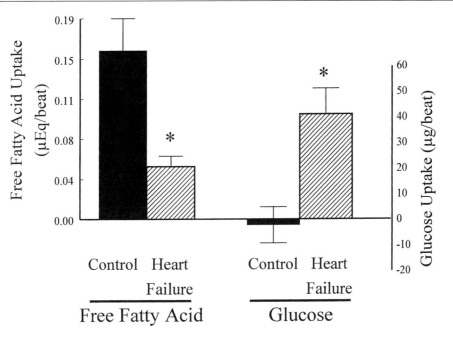

Fig. 6. Free fatty acid and glucose uptake at baseline and after the development of severe congestive HF. Similar to blockade of NO synthesis with NLA, there was a significant reduction in free fatty acid uptake and an increase in carbohydrate metabolism. $n = 8$, $*p < 0.05$. Data from ref. *100*.

HF *(99,100)* or in humans with end-stage HF *(96)*. HF is associated with a reduction in NO production by the coronary circulation *(96,99,100)*, and a reduction in the peripheral production of NO *(80–88)*.

Heart Failure, Nitric Oxide, and Substrate Metabolism

In the normal heart, the inhibition of NO synthesis is associated with a shift in the metabolic substrate utilized, from free fatty acids to carbohydrate-based fuels *(40,73,74)*. HF is a low NO state that may have similarities to inhibition of NO synthesis in normal hearts. When the metabolic substrates were analyzed in canine hearts with pacing induced failure, a similar shift in metabolites was seen (Fig. 6). The onset of HF, associated with a loss of NO production by the coronary circulation *(99,100)*, resulted in a shift in substrate utilization by the myocardium. As in the normal myocardium, this could represent a potential saving in oxygen consumption *(75,76)*, and would attenuate the changes that may be occurring through the direct action of NO on cellular respiration. Consistent with the role of NO in reducing oxygen consumption, in studies of isolated working canine hearts and in human hearts, after HF there was an elevation in myocardial oxygen consumption at given levels of work *(101,102)*.

Clinical *(85–87,96)* and experimental *(80–83,94,99,100)* evidence points toward a loss of NO after the development of HF. If endogenous NO reduces myocardial oxygen consumption *(29,59)*, the loss of NO has the potential to result in an increase in tissue oxygen consumption, independent of any alterations in myocardial work. Similar to blockade of NO synthesis in normal animals *(40,73,74)*, loss of NO in HF is associated with a shift in myocardial substrate utilization *(99,100*; Fig. 6).

Apoptosis and Nitric Oxide

In addition to the metabolic alterations associated with the loss of NO during HF, there appears to be an increase in myocyte apoptosis after HF *(3)*, which may be caused by the loss of NO *(2)*. In hepatocytes, NO has been demonstrated to inhibit apoptosis by inhibiting the caspase-3-like enzymes *(2,103)*. Activations of caspase-3 enzymes are key events in the progression of apoptosis *(104,105)*, because these enzymes cleave important components of the cellular repair system. This is relevant to the study of the heart, because, as previously discussed, HF is a low-NO state *(80–83,85–87,94,96,99,100)*. If NO can prevent apoptosis, then disease states with a loss of NO should display an increase in apoptosis. This is exactly what is seen, both in experimental models of HF *(3,106,107)* and in failing human hearts *(108)*. In fact, this increase in apoptosis in conjunction with the loss of NO may be an important step in the transition from a compensated to a decompensated HF *(108)*. Adding NO to prevent apoptosis in the liver has been shown to be effective in preventing certain types of liver damage *(109)*. Although this has yet to be tested in the heart, adding or maintaining NO synthesis in the myocardium could delay the transition from a compensated to a decompensated HF.

EXERCISE AND NITRIC OXIDE

Inotropic Effects of Nitric Oxide

There is some evidence that endogenous NO will have a significant effect on the inotropic state of the heart. NO was proposed to be a negative inotropic agent, based on evidence of an increase in the positive inotropic response to isoproterenol after blockade of NO synthesis *(110)*. Thus, it was postulated that the presence of endogenous NO was a negative inotropic agent. However, this negative inotropic effect appears to be limited to β-adrenergic stimulation only *(110–112)*. The inotropic effect can be observed as an augmentation of the positive inotropic effect of β-adrenergic stimulation following blockade of NO synthesis, both in experimental animals *(110,111)* and in humans *(113)*. Addition of exogenous NO will attenuate the positive inotropic effect of β-adrenergic, but not α-adrenergic, stimulation in isolated hearts *(112)*. This effect can be demonstrated by stimulating the vagus nerve in intact dogs, and observing an attenuation of the positive inotropic response to both dobutamine and isoproterenol, which can be blocked by inhibition of endogenous NO synthesis *(114)*. This antagonism may be the result of an interaction between cyclic adenosine monophosphate (cAMP) and cGMP, the intracellular signaling pathways for the β-adrenergic receptors and NO, respectively, because cGMP has been shown to attenuate the increase in inotropic state only when that increase is from β-adrenergic stimulation *(115,116)*. The physiologic increases in myocardial contractility was not augmented after blockade of NO synthesis in conscious exercising dogs *(38–40)*, supporting the premise of an interaction between NO and pure β-adrenergic receptor stimulation. NO clearly attenuates the positive inotropic response to pure β-adrenergic receptor stimulation; the in vivo effects of NO on the inotropic state appear to be minimal.

There is some evidence suggesting that NO is a negative inotropic agent independent of β-adrenergic receptor stimulation *(91,92)*, but this effect may be a result of the metabolic effect of NO on the heart *(117)*. In a study using exogenous NO in isolated guinea pig hearts, Kelm et al. *(117)* demonstrated that the direct negative inotropic effect of NO is associated with significant reductions in myocardial oxygen consumption, myocardial phosphocreatine and adenosine triphosphate levels, and a 70-fold increase in free adenosine release into the coronary circulation. In conjunction with the known inhibitory effects of NO on the metabolic pathway, it would follow that the negative inotropic effects of high levels of NO are probably caused by a reduction in the myocardial energy status, not a direct effect on the contractile apparatus.

Acute Exercise

As discussed earlier, NO does not appear to be important in controlling the physiologic increases in coronary blood flow associated with exercise. Blockade of NO synthesis during acute exercise either slightly augments (38) or has no effect on the exercise-induced increases in coronary blood flow (39,40). There is increased NO production from the coronary circulation during exercise (40) and systemically (118), which is probably caused by flow-mediated release of NO from the vascular endothelium (20,21). These effects in the coronary circulation are in sharp contrast to studies in the peripheral circulation, where blockade of NO synthesis significantly attenuates the exercise-induced increases in forearm blood flow (119). Additionally, studies have demonstrated that there is a potential for sympathetic vasoconstriction of the coronary circulation (120), which could occur during exercise. However, it appears that endogenous NO also functions to counterbalance any sympathetic vasoconstriction, because stimulation of the α_2-adrenergic receptors will also lead to a release of NO (121,122). So, although NO may not directly regulate coronary blood flow, it may function as a counterbalance to the increased sympathetic stimulation to the coronary circulation during exercise.

Exercise Training

Although HF is a condition with low NO, both short- and long-term exercise training are associated with an increase in NO-dependent responses (123–126). This increase in endothelium-dependent responses probably results from an upregulation of the gene for NOS (127). If the disappearance of NO is an important step in the progression of HF, exercise-induced upregulation of the eNOS gene (127) could be an explanation for the beneficial effects of exercise during HF. Indeed, in humans with HF, exercise training is associated with an increase in endothelium dependent responses (128). In a canine model of HF, long-term exercise prevented the loss of eNOS gene associated with HF (94). In addition to simply preserving eNOS gene expression and the endothelium-dependent responses, exercise training prevented the decompensation in cardiac function associated with this model of HF (94).

CONCLUSIONS

Although there is significant production of NO from the coronary circulation, NO has a minor influence on coronary blood flow in the normal heart, because of multiple redundant mechanisms. The major role of NO appears to be in regulating both oxygen consumption and substrate utilization of the myocardium. This regulation occurs in both the normal and failing heart. The NO that is produced by the coronary circulation disappears during HF, which may have important implications for the development of apoptosis and the transition from a compensated state to a decompensated HF. Conversely, the beneficial effects of exercise may result, in part, from an upregulation of both NOS and NO production by the coronary circulation.

REFERENCES

1. Moncada S, Palmer RMJ, Higgs EA. Nitric oxide: physiology, pathophysiology and pharmacology. Pharm Rev 1991;43:109–142.
2. Kim YM, Talanian RV, Billiar TR. Nitric oxide inhibits apoptosis by preventing increases in caspase-3-like activity via two distinct mechanisms. J Biol Chem 1997;272:31,138–31,148
3. Liu Y, Cigola E, Cheng W, Kajstura J, Olivetti G, Hintze TH, Anversa P. Myocyte nuclear mitotic division and programmed myocyte cell death characterize the cardiac myopathy induced by rapid ventricular pacing in dogs. Lab Invest 1997;73:771–787.
4. Palmer RMJ, Moncada S. Novel citrulline-forming enzyme implicated in the formation of nitric oxide by vascular endotehlial cells. Biochem Biophys Res Commun 1989;158:348–352.
5. Bredt DS, Snyder SH. Isolation of nitric oxide synthase, a calmodulin-requiring enzyme. Proc Natl Acad Sci USA 1990;87:682–685.
6. Nakane M, Schmidt HH, Pollock JS, Forstermann U, Murad F. Cloned human brain nitric oxide synthase is highly expressed in skeletal muscle. FEBS Lett 1993;316:17–180.
7. Stuehr DJ, Cho HJ, Kwon NS, Weise MF, Nathan CF. Purification and characterization of the cytokine-induced macrophage nitric oxide synthase: an FAD- and FMN-containing flavoprotein. Proc Natl Acad Sci USA 1991;88:7773–7777.
8. Bandaletova T, Brouet I, Bartsch H, Sugimura T, Esumi H, Ohshima H. Immunohistochemical localization of an inducible form of nitric oxide synthase in various organs of rats treated with propioni-bacterium-acnes and lipopolysaccharide. Apmis 1993;101:330–336.
9. Pollock JS, Nakane M, Buttery LK, Martinez A, Springall D, Polak JM, Forstermann U, Murad F. Characterization and localization of endothelial nitric oxide synthase using specific monoclonal antibodies. Am J Physiol 1993;265:C1379–C1387.
10. Ursell PC, Mayes M. Anatomic distribution of nitric oxide synthase in the heart. Int J Cardiol 1995;50: 217–223.
11. Andries LJ, Brutsaert DL, Sys SU. Nonuniformity of endothelial constitutive nitric oxide synthase distribution in cardiac endothelium. Circ Res 1998;82:195–203.
12. Tanaka K, Hassall CJ, Burnstock G. Distribution of intracardiac neurons and nerve terminals that contain a marker for nitric oxide, NADPH-diaphorase, in the guinea-pig heart. Cell Tissue Res 1993; 273:293–300.
13. Ursell PC, Mayes M. Majority of nitric oxide synthase in pig heart is vascular and not neural. Cardiovasc Res 1993;27:1920–1924.
14. Ballignad J-L, Ungureanu D, Kelly RA, Kobzik L, Pimental D, Michel T, Smith TW. Abnormal contractile function due to induction of nitric oxide synthesis in rat cardiac myocytes follows exposure to activated macrophage-conditioned medium. J Clin Invest 1993;91:2314–2319.
15. Hibbs JB, Vavrin Z, Taintor RR. L-arginine is required for expression of the activated macrophage effector mechanism causing selective metabolic inhibition in target cells. J Immunol 1987;138:550–565.
16. Stuehr DJ, Griffith OW. Mammalian nitric oxide synthases. Adv Enzymol 1992;65:287–346.
17. Stuehr DJ, Kwon NS, Nathan CF, Griffith OW, Feldman PL, Wiseman J. N$^\omega$-hydrohy-L-arginine is an intermediate in the biosynthesis of nitric oxide from L-arginine. J Biol Chem 1991;266:6259–6263.
18. Abu-soud HM, Stuehr DJ. Nitric oxide synthesis reveals a role for calmodulin in controlling electron transfer. Proc Natl Acad Sci USA 1993;90:10,769–10,772.
19. Knowles RG, Moncada S. Nitric oxide synthases in mammals. Biochem J 1994;298:249–258.
20. Koller A, Kaley G. Endothelial regulation of wall shear stress and blood flow in skeletal muscle microcirculation. Am J Physiol 1991;260(Heart Circ Physiol 29):H862–H868.
21. Lamontagne D, Pohl U, Busse R. Mechanical deformation of vessel wall and shear stress determine the basal release of endothelium-derived relaxing factor in the intact rabbit coronary vascular bed. Circ Res 1992;70:123–130.
22. Cho HJ, Xie QW, Calaycay J, Mumford RA, Swiderek KM, Lee TD, Nathan C. Calmodulin as a tightly bound subunit of calcium-, calmodulin-independent nitric oxide synthase. J Exp Med 1992;176:599–604.
23. Knowles RG, Moncada S. Nitric oxide as a signal in blood vessels. Trends Biochem Sci 1992;17: 399–402.
24. Arnold WP, Mittal CK, Katsuki S, Murad F. Nitric oxide activates guanylate cyclase and increases guanosine 3':5'-cyclic monophosphate level in various tissue preparations. Proc Natl Acac Sci USA 1977;74:3203–3207.

25. Ignarro LJ, Degnan JN, Baricos WH, Kadowitz PJ, Wolin MS. Activation of purified guanylate cyclase by nitric oxide requires heme: comparison of the heme-deficient, heme-reconstituted and heme-containing forms of soluble enzyme from bovine lung. Biochem Biophys Acta 1982;718:49–59.

26. Salvemini D, Misko TP, Masferrer JL, Seibert K, Currie MG, Needleman P. Nitric oxide activates cyclooxygenase enzymes. Proc Natl Acad Sci USA 1993;90:7240–7244.

27. Stuehr DJ, Nathan CF. Nitric oxide: a macrophage product responsible for cytostasis and respiratory inhibition in tumor target cells. J Exp Med 1989;169:1543–1555.

28. Granger DL, Lehninger AL. Sites of inhibition of mitochondrial electron transport in macrophage-injured neoplastic cells. J Cell Biol 1982;95:527–535.

29. Brown GC, Cooper CE. Nanomolar concentrations of nitric oxide reversibly inhibit synaptosomal respiration by competing with oxygen at cytochrome oxidase. FEBS Lett 1994;356:295–298.

30. Rees DD, Palmer RMJ, Schulz R, Hodson HF, Moncada S. Characterization of three inhibitors of endothelial nitric oxide synthase in vitro and in vivo. Br J Pharmacol 1990;101:746–752.

31. Rees DD, Palmer RMJ, Moncada S. Role of endothelium-derived nitric oxide in the regulation of blood pressure. Proc Natl Acad Sci USA 1989;86:3375–3378.

32. Aisaka K, Gross SS, Griffith OW, Levi R. N^G-methylarginine, an inhibitor of endothelium-derived nitric oxide synthesis, is a potent pressor agent in the guinea pig: does nitric oxide regulate blood pressure in vivo? Biochem Biophys Res Commun 1989;160:881–886.

33. Whittle BJR, Lopez-Belemonte J, Rees DD. Modulation of the vasodepressor actions of acetylcholine, bradykinin, substance P, and endothelin in the rat by a specific inhibitor of nitric oxide formation. Br J Pharmacol 1989;98:646–652.

34. Chu A, Lin CC, Chanbers DE, Moncada S, Cobb FE. Effects of inhibition of nitric oxide on basal formation and endothelium dependent responses of coronary arteries in awake dogs. J Clin Invest 1991;87:1964–1968.

35. Shen W, Lundborg M, Wang J, Stewart JM, Xu X, Ochoa M, Hintze TH. Role of EDRF in the regulation of regional blood flow and vascular resistance at rest and during exercise in conscious dogs. J Appl Physiol 1994;77:165–172.

36. Vallance P, Collier J, Moncada S. Effects of endothelium-derived nitric oxide on peripheral arteriolar tone in man. Lancet 1989;334:997–1000.

37. Shen W, Xu X, Ochoa M, Zhao G, Wolin MS, Hintze TH. Role of nitric oxide in the regulation of oxygen consumption in conscious dogs. Circ Res 1994;75:1086–1095.

38. Altman JD, Kinn J, Duncker DJ, Bache RJ. Effect of inhibition of nitric oxide formation on coronary blood flow during exercise in the dog. Cardiovasc Res 1994;28:119–124.

39. Duncker DJ, Bache RJ. Inhibition of nitric oxide production aggravates myocardial hypoperfusion during exercise in the presence of a coronary artery stenosis. Circ Res 1994;74:629–640.

40. Bernstein RD, Ochoa FY, Xu X, Forfia P, Shen W, Thompson CI, Hintze TH. Function and production of nitric oxide in the coronary circulation of the conscious dog during exercise. Circ Res 1996;79:840–848.

41. Belloni FL. Local control of coronary blood flow. Cardiovasc Res 1979;13:63–85.

42. Feigl EO. Coronary physiology. Phys Rev 1983;63:1–205.

43. Stewart DJ, Münzel T, Bassenge E. Reversal of acetylcholine-induced coronary resistance vessel dilation by hemoglobin. Eur J Pharmacol 1987;136:239–242.

44. Amezcua JL, Palmer RMJ, De Souza BM, Moncada S. Nitric oxide synthesized from L-arginine regulates vascular tone in the coronary circulation of the rabbit. Br J Pharmacol 1989;97:1119–1124.

45. Amrani M, O'Shea J, Allen NJ, Harding SE, Jayakumar J, Pepper JR, Moncada S, Yacoub MH. Role of basal release of nitric oxide on coronary flow and mechanical performance of the isolated rat heart. J Physiol (London) 1992;456:681–687.

46. Sadoff JD, Scholz PM, Weiss HR. Endogenous basal nitric oxide production does not control myocardial oxygen consumption or function. Proc Soc Exp Biol Med 1996;211:332–338.

47. Kirkebøen KA, Naess PA, Offstad J, Ilebekk A. Effects of regional inhibition of nitric oxide synthesis in intact porcine hearts. Am J Physiol 1994;266(Heart Circ Physiol 35):H1516–H1527.

48. Sherman AJ, Davis CA III, Klocke FJ, Harris KR, Srinivadan G, Yaacoub AS, et al. Blockade of nitric oxide synthesis reduces myocardial oxygen consumption in vivo. Circulation 1997;95:1328–1334.

49. Deussen A, Sonntag M, Flesche CW, Vogel RM. Minimal effects of nitric oxide on spatial blood flow heterogeneity of the dog heart. Pflugers Arch 1997;433:727–734.

50. Lefroy DC, Crake T, Uren NG, Davies GJ, Maseri A. Effect of inhibition of nitric oxide synthesis on epicardial coronary artery caliber and coronary blood flow in humans. Circulation 1993;88:43–54.

51. Kelm M, Schrader J. Nitric oxide release from the isolated guinea pig heart. Eur J Pharmacol 1988;155:317–321.
52. Pohl U, Busse R. EDRF increases cyclic GMP in platelets during passage through the coronary vascular bed. Circ Res 1989;65:1798–1803.
53. Kelm M, Schrader J. Control of coronary vascular tone by nitric oxide. Circ Res 1990;66:1561–1575.
54. Rooke GA, Feigl EO. Work as a correlate of canine left ventricular oxygen consumption, and the problem of catecholamine oxygen wasting. Circ Res 1982;50:273–286.
55. Hintze TH, Vatner SF. Reactive dilation of large coronary arteries in conscious dogs. Circ Res 1984; 54:50–57.
56. Holtz J, Forestermann U, Pohl U, Geisler M, Bassange E. Flow-dependent, endothelium mediated dilation of epicardial coronary artery in conscious dogs: effects of cyclo-oxygenase inhibition. J Cardiovasc Pharm 1984;6:1161–1169.
57. Inoue T, Tomoike H, Hasano K, Nakamura M. Endothelium determines flow-dependent dilation of epicardial coronary artery in dogs. J Am Coll Cardiol 1988;11:187–191.
58. Wang J, Kaley G, Wolin MS, Hintze TH. Nitro-L-arginine specifically inhibits flow velocity induced dilation of large coronary arteries by the L-arginine pathway in conscious dogs. FASEB J 1991;5:A660.
59. Borutaité V, Brown GC. Rapid reduction of nitric oxide by mitochondria, and reversible inhibition of mitochondrial respiration by nitric oxide. Biochem J 1996;315:259–299.
60. Cleeter MWJ, Cooper JM, Darley-Usmar VM, Moncada S, Schapira AVH. Reversible inhibition of cytochrome c oxidase, the terminal enzyme of the mitochondrial respiratory chain, by nitric oxide. FEBS Lett 1994;345:50–54.
61. King CE, Melinshyn MJ, Mewburn JD, Curtis SE, Winn ME, Cain SM, Chapler CK. Canine hindlimb blood flow and oxygen uptake after inhibition of EDRF/NO synthesis. J Appl Physiol 1994;76: 1166–1171.
62. Brown GC. Nitric oxide regulates mitochondrial respiration and cell function by inhibiting cytochrome oxidase. FEBS Lett 1995;369:136–139.
63. Okada S, Takehara Y, Yabuki M, Yoshioka T, Yasuda T, Inoue M, Utsumi K. Nitric oxide, a physiological modulator of mitochondrial function. Physiol Chem Phys Med NMR 1996;28:69–82.
64. Takehara Y, Nakahara H, Inai Y, Yabuki M, Hamazaki K, Yoshioka T, et al. Oxygen-dependent reversible inhibition of mitochondrial respiration by nitric oxide. Cell Struct Funct 1996;21:251–258.
65. Heinemann FW, Balaban RS. Control of mitochondrial respiration in the heart in vivo. Annu Rev Physiol 1990;52:523–542.
66. Berne RM, Rubio R. Coronary circulation. In: Handbook of Physiology. The Cardiovascular System. The Heart, American Physiological Society, Bethesda, MD, 1979, pp. 873–952.
67. Bates TE, Loesch A, Burnstock G, Clark JB. Mitochondrial nitric oxide synthase: a ubiquitous regulator of oxidative phosphorylation? Biochem Biophys Res Commun 1996;218:40–44.
68. Xie YW, Shen W, Zhao G, Xu X, Wolin MS, Hintze TH. Role of endothelium-derived nitric oxide in the modulation of canine myocardial mitochondrial respiration in vitro. Implications for the development of heart failure. Circ Res 1996;79:381–387.
69. Zhang X, Xie YW, Nasjletti A, Xu X, Wolin MS, Hintze TH. ACE inhibitors promote nitric oxide accumulation to modulate myocardial oxygen consumption. Circulation 1997;95:176–182.
70. Palmer G, Horgan DJ, Tisdale H, Singer TP, Beinert H. Studies on the respiratory chain-linked reduced nicotinamide adenine dinueleotide dehydrogenase: XIV Location of the sites of inhibition of rotenone, barbiturates, and piericidin by means of electron paramagnetic resonance spectroscopy. J Biol Chem 1968;243:844–847.
71. Granger DL, Taintor RR, Cook JL, Hibbs JB Jr. Injury of neoplastic cells by murine macrophages leads to inhibition of mitochondrial respiration. J Clin Invest 1980;65:357–370.
72. Shen W, Hintze TH, Wolin MS. Nitric oxide: an important signaling mechanism between vascular endothelium and parenchymal cells in the regulation of oxygen consumption. Circulation 1995;92: 1086–1095.
73. McConnell PI, Bernstein RD, Recchia FA, Xu X, Vogel T, Curran C, Hintze TH. Chronic inhibition of nitric oxide synthase alters cardiac substrate handling-underestimating changes in metabolism. Circulation 1997;96:I-314 (abstract).
74. Bernstein RD, Forfia PR, Xu X, Ochoa M, Hintze TH. Nitric oxide regulates myocardial oxygen consumption and substrate utilization in the conscious dog. Circulation 1997;96:I-381 (abstract).
75. Randle PJ, England PJ, Denton RM. Control of the tricarboxylic acid cycle and its interactions with glycolysis during acetate utilization in rat heart. Biochem J 1970;117:677–695.

76. Opie LH. Myocardial energy metabolism. Adv Cardiol 1974;12:70–83.
77. Winlaw DS, Smythe GA, Keogh AM, Schyvens CG, Spratt PM, Macdonald PS. Increased nitric oxide production in heart failure. Lancet 1994;344:373–374.
78. Levine B, Kalman J, Mayer L, Fillit HM, Packer M. Elevated circulating levels of tumor necrosis factor in severe chronic heart failure. N Engl J Med 1990;323:236–241.
79. Drexler H, Hayoz D, Munzel T, Horing B, Just H, Brunner HR, Zelis R. Endothelial function in chronic congestive heart failure. Am J Cardiol 1992;69:1596–1601.
80. Wang J, Seyedi N, Xu X, Wolin MS, Hintze TH. Defective endothelium-mediated control of coronary circulation in conscious dogs after heart failure. Am J Physiol 1994;266(Heart Circ Physiol 35): H670–H680.
81. Zhao G, Shen W, Xu X, Ochoa M, Bernstein R, Hintze TH. Selective impairment of vagally mediated, nitric oxide-dependent coronary vasodilation in conscious dogs after pacing-induced heart failure. Circulation 1995;91:2655–2663.
82. Kaiser L, Spickard RC, Olivier NB. Heart failure depresses endothelium-dependent responses in canine femoral artery. Am J Physiol 1989;256(Heart Circ Physiol 25):H962–H967.
83. Bernstein RD, Zhang X, Zhao G, Forfia PR, Tuzman J, Ochoa M, Vogel T, Hintze TH. Mechanisms of nitrate accumulation in plasma during pacing induced heart failure in conscious dogs. Nitric Oxide: Biol Chem 1997;1:386–396.
84. Ontkean M, Gay R, Greenberg B. Diminished endothelium-derived relaxing factor activity in an experimental model of chronic heart failure. Circ Res 1991;69:1088–1096.
85. Kichuk MR, Seyedi N, Zhang X, Marboe CC, Michler RE, Addonizio LJ, et al. Regulation of nitric oxide production in human coronary microvessels and the contribution of local kinin formation. Circulation 1996;94:44–51.
86. Kubo SH, Rector TS, Bank AJ, Williams RE, Heifetz SM. Endothelium-dependent vasodilation is attenuated in patients with heart failure. Circulation 1991;84:1589–1596.
87. Hirooka Y, Imaizumi T, Harada S, Masaki H, Momohara M, Tagawa T, Takeshita A. Endothelium-dependent forearm vasodilation to acetylcholine but not to substance P is impaired in patients with heart failure. J Cardiovasc Pharm1992;20(Suppl 12):S221–S225.
88. Smith CJ, Sun D, Hoegler C, Roth BS, Zhang X, Zhao G, et al. Reduced gene expression of vascular endothelial NO synthase and cyclooxygenase-1 in heart failure. Circ Res 1996;78:58–64.
89. DeBelder AJ, Radomski MW, Why HJF, Richardson PJ, Bucknall CA, Salas E, Mertin JF, Moncada S. Nitric oxide synthase activities in human myocardium. Lancet 1993;341:84–85.
90. Ungureanu-Longrois D, Ballingand JL, Kelly RA, Smith TW. Myocardial contractile disfunction in the systemic inflammatory response syndrome: role of a cytokine-inducible nitric oxide synthase in cardiac myocytes. J Mol Cell Cardiol 1995;27:155–167.
91. Brady AJ, Warren JB, Poole-Wilson PA, Williams TJ, Harding SE. Nitric oxide attenuates cardiac myocyte contraction. Am J Physiol 1993;265:H176–H182.
92. Weyrich AS, Ma X-L, Buerke M, Murohara T, Armstead VE, Lefer AM, et al. Physiological concentrations of nitric oxide do not elicit an acute negative inotropic effect in unstimulated cardiac muscle. Circ Res 1994;75:692–700.
93. Luss H, Li RK, Shapiro RA, Tzeng E, McGowan FX, Yoneyama T, et al. Dedifferentiated human ventricular cardiac myocytes express inducible nitric oxide synthase mRNA but not protein in response to IL-1, TNF, IFN gamma, and LPS. J Mol Cell Cardiol 1997;29:1153–1165.
94. Wang J, Yi G-H, Knecht M, Cai B-L, Poposkis S, Packer M, Burkhoff D. Physical training alters the pathogenesis of pacing-induced heart failure through endothelium mediated mechanisms in awake dogs. Circulation 1997;96:2683–2692.
95. Comini L, Bachetti T, Gaia G, Pasini E, Agnoletti L, Pepi P, et al. Aorta and skeletal muscle NO synthase expression in experimental heart failure. J Mol Cell Cardiol 1996;28:2241–2248.
96. Kaye DM, Chin-Dusting J, Esler MD, Jennings GL. The failing human heart does not release nitrogen oxides. Life Sci 1998;62:883–887.
97. Radomski JL, Palmiri C, Hearn WL. Concentrations of nitrate in normal human urine and the effects of nitrate ingestion. Toxicol Appl Pharmacol 1978;45:63–68.
98. Wennmalm A, Benthin G, Edlund A, Jungersten L, Kieler-Jensen N, Lundin S, et al. Metabolism and excretion of nitric oxide in Humans: an experimental and clinical study. Circ Res 1993;73: 1121–1127.
99. Recchia FA, Bernstein RD, Vogel T, Xu X, Hintze TH. Reduced cardiac NO production during pacing-induced heart failure. J Mol Cell Cardiol 1997;29:A168 (abstract).

100. Recchia FA, Bernstein RD, McConnell PI, Xu X, Vogel T, Hintze TH. Relationship between reduced NO production and altered myocardial metabolism during cardiac decompensation in conscious dogs. Circulation 1997;96:I–571 (abstract).

101. Wolff MR, de Tombe PP, Harasawa Y, Burkhoff D, Bier S, Hunter WC, Gerstenblith G, Kass DA. Alterations in left ventricular mechanics, energetics, and contractile reserve in experimental heart failure. Circ Res 1992;70:516–529.

102. Hayashi Y, Takeuchi M, Takaoka H, Hata K, Mori Yokoyama M. Alteration in energetics in patients with left ventricular dysfunction after myocardial infarction. Circulation 1996;93:932–939.

103. Li J, Billiar TR, Talanian RV, Kim YM. Nitric oxide inhibits seven members of the caspase family via S-nitrosylation. Biochem Biophys Res Commun 1997;240:419–424.

104. Tewari M, Quan LT, O'Rourke K, Desnoyers S, Zeng Z, Beidler DR, et al. Yama/CPP32 beta a mammalian homolog of CED-3, is a CrmA-inhibitable protease that cleaves the death substrate poly (ADP-ribose) polymerase. Cell 1995;81:810–809.

105. Casciola-Rosen L, Nicholson DW, Chong T, Rowan KR, Thornberry NA, Miller DK, Rosen A. Apopain/CPP32 cleaves proteins that are essential for cellular repair: a fundamental principle of apoptotic death. J Exp Med 1996;183:1957–1964.

106. Kajstura J, Zhang X, Liu Y, Szoke E, Cheng W, Olivetti G, Hintze TH, Anversa P. Cellular basis of pacing-induced dilated cardiomyopathy: myocyte cell loss and myocyte cellular reactive hypertrophy. Circulation 1995;92:2306–2317.

107. Cheng W, Li B, Kajstura J, Li P,Wolin MS, Sonnenblick EH, et al. Stretch-induced programmed myocyte cell death. J Clin Invest 1995;96:2247–2259.

108. Narula J, Haider N, Virmani R, DiSalvo TG, Kolodgie FD, Hajjar RJ, et al. Apoptosis in myocytes in end-stage heart failure. N Engl J Med 1996;335:1182–1189.

109. Saavedra JE, Billiar TR, Williams DL, Kim YM, Watkins SC, Keefer LK. Targeting nitric oxide (NO) delivery in vivo. Design of a liver-selective NO donor prodrug that blocks tumor necrosis factor-alpha-induced apoptosis and toxicity in the liver. J Med Chem 1997;40:1947–1954.

110. Balligand JL, Kelly RA, Marsden PA, Smith TW, Michel T. Control of cardiac muscle cell function by an endogenous nitric oxide signaling system. Proc Natl Acad Sci USA 1993;90:347–351.

111. Keaney JF Jr, Hare JM, Balligand JL, Loscalzo J, Smith TW, Colucci WS. Inhibition of nitric oxide synthase augments myocardial contractile responses to beta-adrenergic stimulation. Am J Physiol 1996;271(Heart Circ Physiol 40):H2646–H2652.

112. Ebihara Y, Karmazyn M. Inhibition of beta- but not alpha 1-mediated adrenergic responses in isolated hearts and cardiomyocytes by nitric oxide and 8-bromo cyclic GMP. Cardiovasc Res 1996;32:622–629.

113. Hare JM, Loh E, Creager MA, Colucci WS. Nitric oxide inhibits the positive inotropic response to beta-adrenergic stimulation in humans with left ventricular dysfunction. Circulation 1995;92:2198–2203.

114. Hare JM, Keaney JF, Balligand JL, Loscalzo J, Smith TW, Colucci WS. Role of nitric oxide in parasympathetic modulation of beta-adrenergic myocardial contractility in normal dogs. J Clin Invest 1995;95:360–366.

115. Molinoff PB. Alpha- and beta-adrenergic receptor subtype properties, distribution, and regulation. Drugs 1984;28:1–15.

116. Watanabe A, Besch HR. Interaction between cyclic adenosine monophosphate and cyclic guanosine monophosphate in guinea pig ventricular myocardium. Circ Res 1975;37:309–317.

117. Kelm M, Schafer S, Dahmann R, Dolu B, Perings S, Decking UK, Schrader J, Strauer BE. Nitric oxide induced contractile dysfunction is related to a reduction in myocardial energy generation. Cardiovasc Res 1997;36:185–194.

118. Bode-Böger SM, Böger RH, Schröder EP, Frölich JC. Exercise increases systemic nitric oxide production in men. J Cardiovasc Risk 1994;1:173–178.

119. Gilligan DM, Panza JA, Kilcoyne CM, Waclawiw MA, Casino PR, Quyyumi AA. Contribution of endothelium-derived nitric oxide to exercise induced vasodilation. Circulation 1994;90:2853–2858.

120. Ishibashi Y, Duncker DJ, Bache RJ. Endogenous nitric oxide masks alpha 2-adrenergic coronary vasoconstriction during exercise in the ischemic heart. Circ Res 1997;80:196–207.

121. Cocks TM, Angus JA. Endothelium-dependent relaxation of coronary arteries by noradrenaline and serotonin. Nature 1983;1305:627–630.

122. Vanhoutte PM, Miller VM. Alpha2-adrenoceptors and endothelium-derived relaxing factor. Am J Med 1989;87(Suppl 3C):1S–5S.

123. Delp MD, McAllister RM, Laughlin MH. Exercise training alters endothelium dependent vasoreactivity of rat abdominal aorta. J Appl Physiol 1993;75:1354–1363.

124. Muller JM, Myers PR, Laughlin MH. Vasodilator responses of coronary resistance arteries of exercise-trained pigs. Circulation 1994;89:2308–2314.

125. Wang J, Wolin MS, Hintze TH. Chronic exercise enhances endothelium-mediated dilation of epicardial coronary artery in conscious dogs. Circ Res 1993;73:829–838.

126. Zhao G, Zhang X, Xu X, Ochoa M, Hintze TH. Short-term exercise training enhances reflex cholinergic nitric oxide-dependent coronary vasodilation in conscious dogs. Circ Res 1997;80:868–867.

127. Sessa WC, Pritchard K, Seyedi N, Wang J, Hintze TH. Chronic exercise in dogs increases coronary vascular nitric oxide production and endothelial nitric oxide synthase gene expression. Circ Res 1994;74:349–353.

128. Horing B, Maier V, Drexler H. Physical training improves endothelial function in patients with chronic heart failure. Circulation 1996;93:210–214.

12

Contribution of Eicosanoids in the Heart

Kafait U. Malik

INTRODUCTION

Over the past three decades, considerable progress has been made in the knowledge of synthesis and metabolism of eicosanoids, and their physiological and pathophysiological roles in various tissues and organs, including those of the cardiovascular and renal systems *(1–5)*. This chapter will briefly review the present state of knowledge of the neurohumoral mechanisms regulating the production of eicosanoids and their physiological and pathophysiological role in the heart. Exhaustive coverage of the field is not intended, and only pertinent references have been cited. The reader is referred to other excellent reviews on eicosanoids in the cardiovascular system *(1,2,6–10)*.

Eicosanoids are products of the metabolism of arachidonic acid (5,8,11,14-*cis*-eicosatetraenoic acid; AA), which is released from the Sn-2 position of tissue phospholipids in response to neurohumoral stimuli after activation of one or more phosphohydrolases (Fig. 1), chiefly calcium-dependent phospholipase A_2 (PLA$_2$) *(3–6)*. A less common pathway for the release of AA is through activation of phospholipase C (PLC), which promotes breakdown of polyphosphoinositides and generates diacyglycerol (DAG), which in turn is hydrolyzed by diacylglycerol lipase to AA and monoacyglycerol *(11)*. DAG may also be phosphorylated by DAG kinase to phosphatiditic acid, which can be hydrolyzed by PLA$_2$ to release AA *(12)*. Activation of phospholipase D (PLD) can also result

From: *Contemporary Endocrinology: Hormones and the Heart in Health and Disease*
Edited by: L. Share © Humana Press Inc., Totowa, NJ

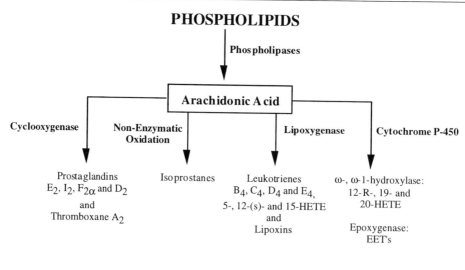

Fig. 1. Pathways of arachidonic acid metabolism.

in generation of phosphatidic acid from phosphatidylcholine, which can then be hydrolyzed either by PLA_2 or by phosphatidate hydrolase to DAG, and subsequently by DAG
lipase, to release AA *(13)*.

AA is metabolized to various biologically active eicosanoids by cyclo-oxygenase
(COX), lipoxygenases (LO), and cytochrome-P450 (CYP-450) mono-oxygenases *(3–6;*
Fig. 1). In addition, AA can also undergo nonenzymatic free-radical-mediated peroxidation to isoprostanes, which also possess potent biological activity *(14,15)*. COX exists
in two isoforms. COX1 is widely distributed and constitutively expressed, and is associated with the nucleus *(16)*; COX2 has a narrower distribution, but it is induced by inflammatory stimuli, including endotoxins and cytokines *(17)*. It is localized in the endoplasmic
reticulum. Prostaglandin (PG) cyclo-oxgenases (PGG/H synthases), which possess both
COX and peroxidase activity, metabolize AA into the unstable cyclic endoperoxide
PGG_2, the precursor of PGH_2 *(18)*. The latter is metabolized by various enzymes to the
prostanoids PGI_2, PGE_2, $PGF_{2\alpha}$, or PGD_2, or by thromboxane (TX) synthase to TXA_2 *(4)*.
PGs are not stored, and their increased release in response to a stimulus represents
enhanced synthesis *(2)*.

LOs, which are cytosolic enzymes, convert AA to hydroperoxyeicosatetraenoic acids
(HEPETEs), which are further metabolized to leukotrienes (LTs) and hydroxyeicosatetraenoic acids (HETEs) (3,6,19). LOs also convert AA to another class of biologically active eicosanoids, lipoxins *(6)*. The third pathway of AA metabolism, catalyzed
by membrane-bound nicotinamide adenine dinucleotide phosphate-dependent CYP-450
mono-oxygenases, results in the formation of four regioisomers of epoxyeicosatetra-
enoic acids (EETs) and 12(R)-, 19-, and 20-HETEs *(5,19–22)*. The EETs are hydrolyzed
to vic-dihydroxyeicosatetraenoic acids by the cytosolic epoxide hydrolases *(19,23,24)*.
The enzymes that convert AA into EETs are referred as epoxygenases, and those that
convert it into HETEs are referred as ω- and ω-1 hydroxylases *(19,24)*. In contrast to PGs,
CYP-450–AA metabolites can be stored in tissues and can act on both intra- and intercellular sites *(20)*.

Eicosanoid Synthesis in the Heart

Biologically active eicosanoids are formed from AA in the heart by COX, LO, and CYP-450. PGI_2 is the major AA metabolite generated by the COX pathway in the mammalian heart, accompanied by smaller amounts of other prostanoids (1,25). Hseuh and Needleman (26) and Wennmalm (27), using different techniques, demonstrated that the coronary vasculature is the major site of cardiac PG synthesis. Coronary endothelial cells (CECs) appear to be primarily responsible, although smooth muscle cells contribute to PG release (28,29). In addition, pericardium (30) and endocardial endothelial cells (ECs) (31) synthesize substantial amounts of PGI_2, and cardiac myocytes and fibroblasts are also capable of synthesizing PGs (32–34). Cardiac myocytes convert exogenous AA to PGI_2, PGE_2, $PGF_{2\alpha}$, and PGD_2 (33); PGE_2 is the major product formed in fibroblasts and smooth muscle cells (34). The heart synthesizes very little TXA_2 under normoxic conditions, but its levels are increased during ischemia and during platelet activation (35,36).

Products of the LO pathway in the heart include 12- and 15-HETE and LTCs (37,38). LO in both cultured cardiac myocytes and CECs converts AA to 12(S)-HETE and 15(S)-HETE (38–40). CECs also convert AA to CYP-450 products, 12(R)-HETE and 5,6-, 8,9-, 11,12-, and 14,15-EETs (40). Production of 20-HETE, an ω-, ω-1 hydroxylase (CYP-450) product, has been demonstrated in the smooth muscle cells (41). Moreover, CYP2J2, a human CYP-450 AA epoxygenase, is highly expressed in cardiac cells (42).

INFLUENCE OF NEUROHUMORAL STIMULI ON EICOSANOID SYNTHESIS IN THE HEART

Effect of Adrenergic and Cholinergic Nervous System

Stimulation of both adrenergic and cholinergic cardiac nerves, or administration of norepinephrine (NE) and acetylcholine (ACh), stimulates synthesis of eicosanoids (43–47). PGI_2 is the principal product released in response to either adrenergic or cholineric stimuli, although small amounts of other prostanoids can also be detected (45–47). Several other circulating and locally generated vasoactive agents also stimulate PG synthesis in the heart (47–50).

Adrenergic and cholinergic transmitters stimulate PG synthesis through specific receptors. Studies in isolated, Krebs-perfused rabbit heart showed that sympathetic nerve stimulation or administration of NE enhances PGI_2 synthesis by activating β_1 adrenergic receptors (45). β-adrenergic receptors, coupled to PG synthesis, are located in cardiac myocytes, CECs, and, to a very small degree, in smooth muscle cells (51,52). Prostanoid synthesis in the heart, elicited by parasympathetic nerve stimulation or administration of ACh, is mediated by muscarinic receptors, because it is selectively blocked by atropine (46,47). Studies using selective cholinergic agonists and antagonists in the isolated rabbit heart have shown that the muscarinic ACh receptors linked to PGI_2 synthesis are of the M_2 and M_3 subtypes: M_2 and M_3 receptors in ventricular myocytes, and M_3 receptors in CECs (54).

Alterations in the mechanical function of various tissues, including the heart, through activation of β-adrenergic receptors or muscarinic receptors, are known to involve distinct signaling mechanisms (55,56). Therefore, it is possible that β-adrenergic and muscarinic receptor stimulated cardiac PG synthesis is also mediated by different mechanisms. Activation of all subtypes of β-adrenergic receptors is associated with increased levels of cyclic adenosine 3', 5' monophosphate (cAMP) *(57)*. In the isolated rabbit heart, infusion, of the stable cAMP analog 8-(4-cholorophenylthio)-cAMP, or agents that increase or decrease cAMP levels, does not alter the basal output of 6-keto-PGF$_{1\alpha}$, and reduces and enhances isoproterenol-induced 6-keto-PGF$_{1\alpha}$ production, respectively. This suggests that cAMP does not mediate cardiac PG synthesis elicited by stimulation of β-adrenergic receptors, but rather acts as an inhibitory modulator *(59)*. In contrast, although activation of M$_2$ muscarinic receptors in the heart is associated with decreased cAMP levels, agents that alter cAMP levels do not affect ACh-stimulated PG synthesis *(51)*; this points to a difference in the mechanism by which synthesis of cardiac PGs is elicited by NE and ACh.

β-adrenergic receptor-stimulated cardiac PG synthesis is positively correlated with extracellular Ca^{2+} concentration, and is inhibited by voltage-operated Ca^{2+} channel blockers, diltiazem and nifidipine, and by the intracellular Ca^{2+} channel antagonist, ryanodine, but not by calmodulin inhibitors *(58)*. These findings led to the proposal that stimulation of β-adrenergic receptors increases extracellular Ca^{2+} influx via voltage-sensitive Ca^{2+} channels, which, in turn, promotes further release of intracellular Ca^{2+} that increases the activity of Ca^{2+}-sensitive, but calmodulin-independent, lipases, and releases AA from tissue lipids for PGI$_2$ synthesis *(58)*.

Muscarinic-receptor-stimulated PGI$_2$ in the heart is also dependent on extracellular Ca^{2+} concentration, but is not altered by voltage operated Ca^{2+} channel antagonists or calmodulin inhibitors *(60)*. Therefore, it appears that ACh in the heart increases influx of Ca^{2+} via voltage-independent channels, most likely receptor-operated Ca^{2+} channels, which in turn liberate AA from tissue lipids by activating a lipase independent of calmodulin. In CEC, PGI$_2$ synthesis elicited by activation of M$_3$ muscarinic receptors has been demonstrated to be mediated by a pertussis-toxin-sensitive G protein, through increased influx of extracellular Ca^{2+} through a G-protein-independent, receptor-operated Ca^{2+} channel *(61)*.

Extracellular Ca^{2+}, by activating one or more lipases, promotes AA release in response to NE and ACh *(58)*. The demonstration that inhibitors of PLA$_2$ reduced muscarinic-receptor-induced PGI$_2$ synthesis in CEC, but not that stimulated by β-adrenergic receptors *(58)*, suggests that a different lipase is involved in AA release for PG synthesis in the latter case. The recent demonstration that β-adrenergic-receptor-stimulated PGI$_2$ synthesis in rabbit CEC is attenuated by the PLD inhibitor C-2 ceramide, and by the diacylglycerol lipase inhibitor RHC-80267, but not by the PLC inhibitor D609, suggests that AA released for β-adrenergic-receptor-stimulated PG synthesis is released via activation of PLD *(52)*. Supporting this conclusion, it was shown that the β-adrenergic-receptor agonist isoproterenol increases PLD, but not PLA$_2$, activity in CEC. On the other hand, ACh increased both PLA$_2$ and PLD activity, and inhibition of both PLD and PLA$_2$ activity reduced ACh-induced 6-keto-PGF$_{1\alpha}$ synthesis in CEC *(52)*. Activation of muscarinic receptors with carbachol has also been reported to increase PLD activity in the chicken heart *(63)*. The type of PLD linked to muscarinic and β-adrenergic receptors in CEC appears to be distinct, because β-adrenergic-, but not muscarinic, receptor-induced increase in PLD activity is inhibited by cAMP *(52)*. Several types of PLD have been described, and two isoforms, cytosolic (PLD$_1$) and membrane-bound (PLD$_2$) have been cloned *(64,65)*. It is possible that β-adrenergic and muscarinic receptors are selectively linked to these, or to some other isoform of PLD *(66)*. The mechanism by which activation of β-adrenergic and muscarinic receptors stimulates PLD activity remains to be established.

Effect of Humoral Agents

Several humoral agents, including angiotensin II (ANG II), vasopressin, endothelin, bradykinin, and adenosine, stimulate PG synthesis in the intact heart, cardiac myocytes, CECs or fibroblasts *(39,45,48–50,67–70)*. Some agents, such as ANG II and bradykinin, also stimulate the production of AA metabolites derived through LO or CYP-450 pathways in cardiac cells or CEC *(39,71)*. AA release for eicosanoid synthesis, stimulated by these agents in the heart, cardiac myocytes, or CECs, may involve activation of PLA_2, PLC, and/or PLD *(72,73–75)*. The contribution of each of these lipases to the release of AA for eicosanoid synthesis, and the underlying mechanism of their activation by humoral agents, has not yet been established. PLA_2, PLC, and PLD may be activated simultaneously or sequentially by distinct mechanisms. ANG II has been reported to activate PLC and PLD through AT_1 receptors and PLA_2 via AT_2 receptors in cardiac myocytes *(72)*. It is well established that the PLD activity is regulated by protein kinase C (PKC) in several cell types *(66)*. It is possible that 1,2 DAG, generated through breakdown of phosphoinositides consequent to PLC activation, increases PKC, and consequently, PLD activity *(66)*. Bradykinin and endothelin have been shown to stimulate PLD activity in cardiomyocytes through activation of PKC *(73)*. These humoral agents may also activate PLD and other lipases by increasing levels of cell Ca^{2+}, or by stimulating one or more serine and/or tyrosine kinases *(66)*.

Actions of Eicosanoids and Their Physiological Role in the Heart

PGs, depending upon the type (PGI_2, PGE_2, $PGF_{2\alpha}$, PGD_2), concentration, animal species, and experimental conditions (in vivo or in vitro), have been reported to increase or decrease cardiac contractility, heart rate, coronary vascular tone, and electrical activity in the heart *(9,10,75)*. PGI_2, the principal product of AA generated by COX in the heart, produces coronary vasodilation *(1)*, although lower concentrations have also been reported to cause constriction of coronary vessels in some species *(9,76)*. PGI_2 increases myocardial contractility, but not heart rate *(9,75)*. PGI_2 in doses that reduce blood pressure (BP) in vivo, causes a decrease in heart rate that is abolished by vagotomy *(77,78)*. PGI_2 also inhibits platelet aggregation *(1)*. On the other hand, TXA_2, a principal product of COX generated in platelets, and whose level increases in the heart during ischemia, promotes platelet aggregation and causes coronary vasoconstriction *(79,80)*.

The products of AA generated via the LO pathway include LTs, generated primarily by neutrophils and macrophages, and which produce coronary vasoconstriction *(81)*, and 15- and 12(S)-HETE, which are formed in CECs *(39)*, and could also alter coronary vascular tone. The products of AA generated through the CYP-450 pathway, which include mostly EETs, produce coronary vasodilation, and are thought to be the hyperpolarizing factor generated in blood vessels in response to some vasodilators *(82,83)*. Another CYP-450 product of AA formed in smooth muscle cells, 20-HETE, is a potent vasoconstrictor, and inhibits Na^+-K^+ ATPase *(2,41)*.

The basal concentrations of eicosanoids prevailing in the heart in the absence of neurohumoral factors have minimal effects on cardiac function. However, during activation of neurohumoral systems, the concentration of eicosanoids increases to levels that exert cardioprotective effects by modulating neuroeffector events, inhibiting platelet aggregation, increasing coronary blood flow, and inhibiting free radical production and lipid peroxidation and lipolysis.

Modulation of Cardiac Adrenergic and Cholinergic Transmission

The products of AA formed via COX in the heart, in response to adrenergic nerve stimulation, PGI_2 and PGE_2, inhibit the release of NE elicited by sympathetic nerve stimulation, potassium , or nicotine, in different species *(43,84,87)*. These observations, and the demonstration that inhibition of PG synthesis augments the release of NE and the positive inotropic and chronotropic effects elicited by cardiac sympathetic nerves, has led to the suggestion that PGs synthesized in postsynaptic effector cells act as negative feedback inhibitory modulators of adrenergic transmission in the heart *(87)*. In addition to their effect on prejunctional sites, PGs also act at postjunctional sites to reduce the myocardial contractile response to NE *(87)*. PGs do not appear to uniformly exert inhibitory effects on adrenergic neuroeffector junctions in all structures of the heart of different animal species. For example, PGs do not modulate the positive inotropic or chronotropic response to sympathetic nerve stimulation in the isolated blood-perfused canine atrium *(88)*. However, both PGI_2 and PGE_2 inhibit, and indomethacin, an inhibitor of PG synthesis, enhances the increase in ventricular contractility in response to left cardiac sympathetic nerve stimulation in the dog *(87)*. On the other hand, in guinea pig atria, the inhibitory effect of PGs on muscle contraction in response to sympathetic nerve stimulation was much greater than in the ventricles *(89)*. PGs also do not appear to inhibit the positive chronotropic response in all animal species. Thus, PGI_2, PGE_2, or indomethacin do not alter the positive chronotropic response to sympathetic nerve stimulation in the dog heart, or to transmural stimulation in the blood-perfused atrium, and in the isolated guinea pig SA node *(87,90)*. On the other hand, PGE_2 inhibits the positive chronotropic response to sympathetic nerve stimulation in the isolated heart, and to transmural stimulation in the SA node of rabbit *(84,90)*.

The effect of prostanoids in inhibiting adrenergic transmission may serve as a cardioprotective mechanism against the deleterious effects of increased activity of the sympathetic nervous system in the heart, such as alterations in the electricophysiological events leading to arrhythmias *(91)*. For example, pericardial application of AA, which increases pericardial concentrations of both PGI_2 and PGE_2, inhibits the effect of stimulation of bilateral efferent ansae subclavia, induced shortening of sinus cycle length, atrio-His interval, and effective refractory period of the right and left ventricular myocardium; these effects of AA were abolished by indomethacin *(91)*. TXA_2, a COX product of AA that produces coronary vasoconstriction, has also been shown to attenuate the effect of sympathetic nerve stimulation in guinea pig atria *(92)*. The significance of this effect of TXA_2, and the contribution of AA metabolites formed via LO and CYP-450 pathways to adrenergic transmission, remain to be determined.

Cardiac PGs may also modulate the metabolic effect of the sympathetic nervous system and of catecholamines in the heart. PGI_2 and PGE_2 and exogenous AA inhibit, and sodium meclofenamate enhances, β-adrenergic-receptor-stimulated lipolysis, measured by glycerol output in the rabbit heart *(92)*.

Prostanoids have been shown to modulate the effect of humoral agents influencing the activity of the adrenergic nervous system. For example, PGI_2 and PGE_2 attenuate, and COX inhibitors enhance, the facilitatory effect of ANG II on release of NE elicited by sympathetic nerve stimulation in the rat and dog heart *(94,95)*. Increase in PG levels in the pericardial fluid in the dog also inhibits the facilitatory effect of ANG II on cardiac electrophysiological responses elicited by sympathetic nerve stimulation *(91)*.

The effect of eicosanoids on cholinergic transmission and its functional significance have not yet been thoroughly investigated. PGE_1 has been shown to attenuate the effect of vagal nerve stimulation and ACh release in isolated guinea pig atria (96). Whether PGI_2, the major prostanoid synthesized in the heart, and the products of AA formed through the LO and CYP-450 pathways, affect cholinergic transmission in the heart, remains to be determined. AA, in concentrations that increase PGI_2 and PGE_2 levels in the pericardium, does not alter vagal nerve stimulation-induced lengthening of the effective refractory period or the duration of sinus arrest (91). However, it is possible that PGI_2 synthesized in response to cholinergic nerve stimulation complements the cardioprotective effect of nitric oxide (NO) synthesized in response to ACh in the coronary vasculature (97).

Modulation of Cardiac Reflexes

Spinal sympathetic afferent fibers with their endings in the heart are excited by mechanical stretch, as well by chemical agents generated in the heart, especially bradykinin, during ischemia. Application of bradykinin to the ventricular surface of the dog heart produces a reflex increase in BP, tachycardia, renal vasoconstriction, vasodilation in the muscles, and pain via activation of B_2 receptors (98). Epicardial application of PGI_2 and PGE_2 in low concentrations does not cause any reflexogenic effect, but potentiates the bradykinin-induced reflex pressor response and tachycardia (98,99). It has been proposed that PGI_2 and PGE_2 selectively sensitize sympathetic chemosensitive nerve endings that are involved in nociception (99). These observations, and the finding that indomethacin attenuates the reflexogenic effects of bradykinin, suggest that PGs generated in the heart by this peptide act as positive modulators of its reflexogenic effect (99). The finding that aspirin, a COX inhibitor, reduces the activity of A and C sympathetic fibers elicited by epicardial application of bradykinin (100) supports this view. However, the effects of intracoronary administration of bradykinin, which also produces tachycardia accompanied by a depressor (not pressor) response, are not affected by prostanoids in the dog heart (91). The reflex tachycardia and the rise in BP produced by application to the epicardium of capsaicin, the active principle of hot peppers, is also not modified by PGs (98). The inability of PGs to modulate the reflexogenic effects of intracoronarily administered bradykinin and epicardially applied capsaicin could be caused by differences in the mechanisms and/or structures involved in the cardiovascular reflexogenic effects of bradykinin and capsaicin. Similarly, epicardial application of nicotine, which produces bradycardia and a depressor response, is not modulated by PGs in the heart (99). This has been attributed to the ability of nicotine to stimulate mechanoreceptors and not chemoreceptors involved in nociception caused by bradykinin (99).

Eicosanoid Contribution to Coronary Circulation

Prostanoids have been implicated in coronary autoregulation, hypoxia-induced coronary vasodilation, and reactive hyperemia (9,10). Studies conducted by Moretti et al. (101) and Moretti and Abraham (102) showed that coronary autoregulation in the isolated rabbit heart perfused with blood plasma, but not with saline buffer, was inhibited by indomethacin. However, Rubio and Berne (103) failed to show any effect of indomethacin on coronary autoregulation in the dog. Kalsner (104) has shown that, in isolated bovine coronary arteries, hypoxia causes relaxation that is associated with increased output of PGs, and that anoxia causes contraction of the arteries and decreased PG output.

These observations, and the demonstration that, in the dog, the COX inhibitor, indometha-cin, minimizes coronary vasodilation, suggest that PGs contribute to hypoxia-induced coronary vasodilation *(104)*.

Eicosanoids as Mediators of Action of Other Humoral Agents

Atrial natriuretic peptide (ANP) is released from the heart in response to myocardial stretch, and to vasoactive agents such as catecholamines, vasopressin, and ANG II *(105)*. The increase in the release of ANP in response to these agents has been shown to be mediated by PGs via generation of cAMP (catecholamines; *106*) or activation of PKC (vasopressin, ANG II; *107,108*). Supporting this view, it has been demonstrated that PGE_2 and PGI_2 stimulate ANP secretion from atrial slices or cardiac myocytes *(106,107)*; activation of PKC with 4 β-phorbol 12-myristate 13-acetate stimulates PGI_2 levels in ventricular myocytes *(109)*, and COX inhibitors attenuate vasopressin, ANG II, isopro-terenol, or PKC-activated ANP release from cardiomyocytes *(105,106,109)*.

Eicosanoids also mediate the coronary vascular effects of bradykinin in the heart. Although bradykinin stimulates the production of NO and PGI_2 in the coronary endo-thelium, the vasodilator effect of the peptide is mediated by an endothelial-derived hyperpolarizing factor that appears to be an EET metabolite of AA, and that acts by stim-ulating Ca^{2+}-activated K^+ channels *(110)*. The EETs and their diol products dihydroxy-eicosatetraenoic acids (DHETs), which are taken up by the ECs and incorporated into tissue phospholipids, have also been reported to potentiate bradykinin-induced relax-ation in porcine coronary arteries *(83)*.

Modulation by Eicosanoids
of Plasma Membrane Ion Channels in the Heart

A number of cell-surface receptors are coupled to ion channels via specific hetero-trimeric G proteins. The function of the cardiac inwardly rectifying K^+ channel, coupled to the M_2 acetylcholine receptor (IK.ACh) and the A_1-adenosine receptor, is regulated by a pertussis-toxin-sensitive G protein (Gk) *(111)*. Fatty acids can directly modulate the activity of some types of ion channels, including K^+ and Ca^+ channels in the heart *(117)*. However, AA has been shown to modulate the activity of IK.ACh through conversion to LO (and not COX) products *(112)*. LO metabolites, including 5-HETE, LTB_4 and LTC_4, increase the activity of IK.ACh in neonatal rat atrial cell membranes *(112)*. Metabolites of AA generated through the 5-LO pathway have also been shown to mediate activation of IK.ACh by α-adrenergic and platelet-activating protein receptors in atrial myocytes *(113,114)*. Although the site of action and the underlying mechanism of LO metabolites have not been established, it appears that eicosanoids modulate IK.ACh channel activity through the G protein Gk *(111,113,115,116)*. IK.ACh activity in the heart can be regu-lated by both Gα- and βγ-subunits *(111,117)*. Gα has been found to be much less effective than the βγ-subunit of G on IK.ACh channel activity *(111,117)*. On the other hand, Gα, but not Gβγ, activates ATP-sensitive K^+ channels (K^+-ATP) in atrial cells *(111)*. Activa-tion of IK.ACh by Gβγ is modulated by 5-LO products of AA, resulting from activation of PLA_2 *(117)*. Because the direct effects of 5-LO metabolites on the IK.ACh channel are 6–16 times less than that of the Gβγ-subunit, it appears that it is Gβγ that activates IK.ACh channel activity independent of AA release; the LO products act indirectly by modifying the kinetic properties of Gk (turn-on reaction) *(111,117)*.

Although products of AA generated by the COX pathway have some minimal inhibitory effect on IK.ACh activity in atrial cells *(111)*, they may activate adenosine triphosphate-activated potassium channel (KATP) channels in the myocardium and coronary vessels *(118,119)*. The effect of the KATP channel blocker, glibenclamide, to attenuate the coronary vasodilator effects of AA, PGI_2, PGE_2, and PGD_2, and of PGE_1 and PGE_0, on myocardial infarct size caused by coronary artery occlusion has been attributed to activation of KATP channels *(120)*.

AA has also been reported to increase the amplitude and duration of Ca^{2+} transients and myocyte shortening *(121,122)*. CYP-450 products of AA may also regulate ion channel activity in the heart. Recently, it has been reported that the inhibitors of PLA_2 and CYP-450, and intracellular dialysis with the P-450 antibody antirat CYP1A2, reduced, and AA and its CYP-450 metabolite, 11,12-EET, increased L-type Ca^{2+} current (ICa) and cell shortening in the rat single ventricular myocytes *(123)*. These effects of AA and its metabolites were mediated by cAMP *(123)*.

PATHOPHYSIOLOGICAL ROLE OF EICOSANOIDS

Eicosanoids have also been shown to be involved in a number of cardiovascular disorders, including myocardial ischemia/reperfusion injury, arrhythmias, congestive heart failure (CHF), coronary arteriosclerosis, and cardiac hypertrophy.

Eicosanoids and Ischemia/Reperfusion

In cardiac ischemia/reperfusion, tissue levels of fatty acids, including AA, rise as a result of increased hydrolysis of membrane phospholipids and decreased reacylation. Although the degradation of membrane phospholipids has been attributed mostly to increased PLA_2 activity, PLC and PLD may also contribute *(11,13,125–127)*. Increased activities of these lipases during ischemia/reperfusion in the heart have been demonstrated *(124–128)*. The heart contains different types of PLA_2. Secretory PLA_2 is 14 kDa, and is related to group II PLA_2. In addition, there is a high molecular cytosolic PLA_2 (85-110 kDa) and a 40-kDa PLA_2 that are localized both in the membrane and the cytosol *(129)*. The secretory PLA_2 requires millimolar concentrations of Ca^{2+}, and exhibits no selectivity among fatty acids esterified at the Sn-2 position of phospholipids *(129)*. Although the physiological significance of this PLA_2 in the heart is not known, it may contribute to the release of AA during restoration of flow to ischemic areas, when the intracellular Ca^{2+} concentration is increased *(129)*. The high-mol-wt cytosolic PLA_2, which selectively hydrolyzes phospholipids containing AA at the Sn-2 position, is activated by translocation to intracellular membranes in the presence of micromolar concentrations of Ca^{2+} *(129)*. Activation of cytosolic PLA_2, which provides AA for eicosanoid synthesis in response to agonist receptor interaction under physiological conditions, may also contribute to the release of AA during ischemia/reperfusion in the myocardium *(128,129)*. The 40-kDa PLA_2, which preferentially hydrolyzes Sn-2 arachidonoyl plasmalogens, does not require Ca^{2+}. Its activity is modulated by ATP, and it migrates to cellular membranes, along with phosphofructokinase, during states of energy depletion *(130,131)*. This enzyme does not appear to play an important role in the accumulation of AA in the ischemic myocardium *(132)*.

In the dog heart, the level of AA increases slowly, by about 10-fold during 120 min of ischemia; further increase occurs during reperfusion *(133)*. The degree of AA accumulation and of ischemia/reperfusion-induced myocardial damage (as indicated by accumulation of lactate dehydrogenase) appears to be correlated *(134)*. AA, like other fatty acids accumulated in the ischemic/reperfused myocardium, could influence cardiac function directly, as well as indirectly, by its conversion to eicosanoids. There is a substantial increase in the amount of PGs during the initial reperfusion phase *(135)*. PGs have been reported to produce both protective and deleterious effects in the ischemic/reperfused heart, depending on concentration *(10)*. The principal product of AA generated in the heart, PGI_2, in low concentrations, promotes ischemic insult and produces coronary vasoconstriction and arrhythmias; higher concentrations of PGI_2 or its stable analog, iloprost, produce cardioprotective effects, viz. coronary vasodilation and antiarrhythmic actions *(9,10)*. Experiments using inhibitors of COX to determine the influence of endogenous PGs on cardiac function in response to ischemia/reperfusion have led to conflicting results *(10,130–136)*. The nonsteriodal anti-inflammatory COX inhibitors have been shown to both improve *(137,138)* and reduce *(139)* postischemic ventricular recovery. Because, in the latter study in the isolated guinea pig heart during reperfusion, the tissue content and the release of isoprostane 8-iso-$PGF_{2\alpha}$ from the heart during reperfusion was increased 15-fold over that in the control group, it has been suggested that increased synthesis of isoprostanes promotes coronary vasoconstriction and causes myocardial oxygen deprivation *(139)*.

On the other hand, beneficial effects in studies of COX inhibitors in ischemia/reperfusion could result from decreased production of TXA_2, a coronary vasoconstrictor and promoter of platelet aggregation *(137,138,140,141)*. Under resting normoxic conditions, the heart synthesizes PGI_2, but not TXA_2 *(36)*. However, the production of TXA_2 is increased in myocardial ischemia and following reperfusion in the heart of experimental animals, as well as in patients with angina pectoris and after cardiopulmonary bypass *(36,142–144)*. Levels of TXB_2 (the stable hydrolysis product of TXA_2) are also correlated with the infarct size after ischemia/reperfusion in dogs *(36)*. These observations, and the demonstration that myocardial ischemia, early phase of transmural myocardial infarction (MI), and coronary artery ligation are associated with increased platelet aggregability, has led to the suggestion that increased platelet aggregation could promote regional myocardial ischemia *(145)*. Atherosclerotic lesions with reduced coronary production of PGI_2 may also aggravate ischemia because of unopposed coronary constrictor and proaggregatory actions of TXA_2 *(1,146)*. Evidence supporting the role of TXA_2 in myocardial ischemia/reperfusion has been provided by the demonstration that inhibitors of TXA_2 synthesis and TXA_2 receptor antagonists promote preservation of myocardial function and decrease infarct size as indicated by decreased release of creatinine kinase from the myocardial tissue *(145)*. Because TXA_2 receptor antagonists also block the action of PG endoperoxides (PGG_2 and PGH_2), which produce vasoconstrictor and platelet proaggregatory effects, the latter may also contribute to ischemic myocardial injury. Mullane and Fornabaio *(147)* proposed that the protective effect of TX synthesis inhibitors could also be caused by shunting of PG endoperoxides from platelets to PG synthesis in blood vessels.

Because administration of TX synthesis inhibitors also results in a decrease in accumulation of neutrophils in the myocardium, it was proposed that increased PG synthesis preserves myocardial function by reducing neutrophil accumulation *(147)*. Neutrophils are a source of 12-HETE and LTs that cause coronary constriction and decrease in myocardial contractility (LTC_4 and LTD_4). The beneficial effects of TXA_2 synthesis and receptor antagonists on postischemic abnormalities does not appear to be the result of decrease in TX synthesis, but rather because of shunting of PG endoperoxides to PGI_2 synthase, and subsequent increase in PGI_2 production in the myocardium (148,149). PGI_2 has been shown to reduce infarct size in ischemic myocardium by a direct flow-independent mechanism (150). The ability of PGI_2 to inhibit free oxygen radical production (151), NE release from sympathetic fibers (84,85,87), lipid peroxidation (152), and LTC_4 production, and to suppress arrhythmias (153), may also contribute to its beneficial effects in preserving myocardial damage in ischemia/reperfusion.

The products of AA generated by LO may also contribute to ischemia/reperfusion-induced myocardial injury. The levels of LO products 5-, and 12-HETE are markedly increased in ischemic myocardial tissue, which is in proportion to infiltration of neutrophils (145). LTs have been shown to be formed in the heart, and an increase in LTC_4, LTD_4, or LTE_4 has been documented in myocardial ischemia produced by activated complement C5a in pigs (156). Moreover, inhibition of leukotriene synthesis or leukotriene receptor antagonists minimize the coronary vasoconstriction and decrease in myocardial contractility produced by complement C5a (156). These observations, and the demonstration that inhibitors of LO decrease neutrophil infiltration and arrhythmias, and promote preservation of myocardial function in ischemia/reperfusion, suggest that AA products generated via LO by neutrophils, and, within the heart, contribute to the deleterious effect of ischemia/ reperfusion on the myocardium (157). However, O'Neill et al. (158) failed to demonstrate any protective effect in dogs of the LO inhibitor, nafazatrom, at a dose that decreased neutrophil infiltration, during reperfusion following ischemia by coronary artery occlusion. The reason for the discrepancy between this study and those conducted by other investigators is not known.

The contribution of AA metabolites formed through the CYP-450 pathway in myocardial injury induced by ischemia/reperfusion is not known. A recent study conducted by Moffat et al. (159) indicates that 5,6- or 11,12-EET, which caused an increase in intracelluar levels of Ca^{2+} and shortening of ventricular myocytes, produced a delay of 10 min in the recovery of cardiac function in the isolated guinea pig heart subjected to low-flow ischemia. Further studies using selective inhibitors of the ω- and ω-1 hydroxylase and epoxygenase functions of CYP-450 should clarify the contribution of AA metabolites generated via this pathway in myocardial ischemia/reperfusion.

Eicosanoids and Cardiac Arrhythmias

PGs, depending on the concentration, produce both antiarrhythmic and proarrhythmogenic effects in the heart (153). Both PGE_1 and PGE_2 and high concentrations of PGI_2 inhibit cardiac arrythmias caused by ischemia or by various experimental interventions (160,161), and in patients with previous MI (162). However, low concentrations of PGI_2 produce arrhythmogenic effects (162). In cultured neonatal rat heart cells, PGE_2, PGD_2, and $PGF_{2\alpha}$, and the TXA_2 receptor agonist U-446619, also produce tachyarrythmias; PGI_2 was protective against $PGF_{2\alpha}$- and U-446619-induced arrhythmias (163). The demonstration that several COX inhibitors minimize ventricular tachycardia and fibrillation in cats and rats during ischemia/reperfusion suggests that PGs exert proarrhythmic actions in the heart (164–166). However, a study using ibuprofen failed to show modification of electrophysiological responses in the canine Purkinje fibers (167). Attenuation by COX inhibitors of cardiac arrhythmias caused by ischemia/reperfusion could be caused by decreased production of TXA_2, which exerts arrhythmogenic actions by causing coronary vasoconstriction and aggregation of platelets *(153,168)*. Arrhythmias can also be produced by TX analogs in the absence of ischemia *(169)*. Moreover, TX synthesis inhibitors and receptor antagonists suppress reperfusion-induced arrhythmias in various animal species *(168,170–172)*. The protective effect of these agents could be the result of shunting of endoperoxides to PGI_2 synthesis. Supporting this view is the finding that agents such as nafazatrom and defibrotide, which increase PGI_2 production, reduce arrhythmias and ventricular fibrillation *(172,173)*. The beneficial effect in ischemia/ reperfusion of low doses of aspirin has been attributed to its selective inhibition of TXA_2 synthesis and intact PGI_2 synthesis. Evidence supporting the protective effect of endogenous PGs, and of inhibiting TX synthesis against ischemia/reperfusion-induced arrhythmias, is strengthened by the finding that the TX-synthesis inhibitor, dezmegrel, loses its protective effect when given together with the COX inhibitor, sodium meclofenamate *(174)*. In anesthetized dogs, the antiarrhythmic effects of preconditioning, which is associated with increased PGI_2 production, is lost by prior administration of sodium meclofenamate *(175)*. In the canine model of myocardial reperfusion injury, PGI_2 appears to exert an antiarrhythmic effect that is independent of TXA_2 levels, because aspirin did not enhance the cardioprotective effect of iloprost, a PGI_2 analog *(175)*. PGs have also been reported to mediate, in part, the effect of bradykinin in suppressing epinephrine-induced arrhythmias in dogs *(177)*. The effect of captopril, a converting-enzyme inhibitor, to reduce the incidence of ischemia/reperfusion-induced ventricular fibrillation, has also been attributed to decreased catecholamine release, decrease in TXA_2, and increased PGI_2 production consequent to decreased ANG II production *(178)*.

The contribution of products of AA generated by LO and CYP-450 to cardiac arrhythmogenesis is not well studied. The effect of leukotrienes in producing coronary vasoconstriction, and promoting platelet aggregation, and in the accumulation of neutrophils by promoting chemotaxis (LTB_4), may contribute to arrhythmias associated with ischemia/ reperfusion. The leukotrienes alter sinus rhythm and elevate the ST segment, but do not produce ventricular fibrillation *(81,179,180)*. A few studies conducted with the inhibitors of LO and leukotriene receptor antagonists have been shown to attenuate or to have no effect on the pathogenesis of arrhythmias *(180–182)*. In the guinea pig isolated heart, digoxin-induced tachyarrhythmias were associated with increased levels of LTB_4 in the coronary effluent, but the lipoxygenase inhibitor, BW A4C, failed to suppress arrhythmias in response to digoxin *(183)*. Further studies are required to assess the contribution of leukotrienes, as well as other lipoxygenase and CYP-450 products of AA in cardiac arrhythmogenesis.

Eicosanoids and Congestive Heart Failure (CHF)

CHF is associated with alterations in neurohumoral balance, as indicated by increased activities of the sympathetic nervous and renin-ANG II–aldosterone systems, and increased levels of vasopressin, and, consequently, increased synthesis of PGs *(184)*. The enhanced PG production in CHF serves to protect cardiovascular and renal function *(184)*. PGI_2 has been shown to produce a significant improvement in contractile function in CHF, and also in myocardial stunning and ischemia *(185–188)*. The PGI_2 mimetic, iliprost, and PGE_1 also protect myocardial contractility of stunned myocardium. Intravenous low-dose home therapy with PGE_1 has been shown to produce sustained hemodynamic improvement in patients with severe CHF or in patients with refractory HF *(189,190)*. In addition, as reviewed above, PGI_2 produces coronary vasodilation, and also has antiarrhythmic effects. The principal prostanoids produced in the kidney, PGE_2 and

PGI_2, protect renal function in CHF by producing vasodilation, decreasing vascular reactivity to pressor agents, inhibiting NE release from sympathetic fibers, promoting diuresis and natriuresis, and by antagonizing the renal effect of vasopressin *(184)*. Evidence supporting a protective function of prostanoids in CHF is derived from the report that COX inhibitors produce a marked reduction in renal blood flow and glomerular filtration rate in this condition, and, in advanced cases, cause reversible oligouric renal failure *(191)*. COX inhibitors also decrease leg blood flow during exercise, and consequently decrease oxygen consumption and increase lactate levels *(192)*. They may also increase arterial BP and increase further cardiac work and deterioration of cardiac function in CHF *(191)*. Recently, it has been shown that, in patients with ischemic and valvular heart disease referred for cardiac surgery, the pericardial levels of coronary vasoconstrictor, 8-iso-$PGF_{2\alpha}$, a marker of oxidant stress, is increased, and significantly correlated with left ventricular end-diastolic and end-systolic diameters *(193)*. PGs have also been reported to contribute to the action of an angiotensin-converting enzyme inhibitor, enalapril, to cause functional improvement of alveolar capillary membranes, and, consequently to increase oxygen uptake in CHF in humans *(194)*. This effect of enalapril is probably mediated by accumulation of bradykinin, which in turn promotes PG synthesis, because aspirin inhibited the effect of enalapril, but not that of the ANG II receptor blocker, losartan, on oxygen uptake *(194)*. The use of nonsteriodal anti-inflammatory agents, along with angiotensin-converting enzyme inhibitors, can therefore produce harmful effects *(191,194)*.

The pathophysiological role of LO and CYP-450 products of AA in CHF is not well known. In a study conducted in dogs with heart failure caused by ventricular pacing, an LT receptor antagonist, FPL55712, increased systemic and renal vascular resistance and decreased cardiac output *(195)*. Whether this resulted from blockade of the vasodilator effect of endogenous LTs, or from the nonselective effect of this antagonist, remains to be determined; LTs decrease myocardial contractility.

Eicosanoids and Coronary Atherosclerosis

Endothelium-derived relaxing factors, including PGI_2 and NO, play an important role in the regulation of coronary vascular tone and blood flow *(196)*. It has been proposed that the balance between production of TXA_2 by platelets, which causes vasoconstriction and platelet aggregation, and of PGI_2 by blood vessels, which produces vasodilation and inhibits platelet aggregation, is critical in cardiovascular diseases such as atherosclerosis *(1,146)*. Hypercholesterolemia has been shown to reduce PGI_2 and NO production in coronary vessels *(197,198)*, and to impair endothelium-dependent relaxation and increase response of coronary vessels to some vasoconstrictor agents *(199,200)*. Endothelium-dependent vascular relaxation has also been shown to be impaired in genetically hyperlipidemic mice *(201)*. A bioactive peptide with PGI_2-stimulating properties has been has been reported to be decreased in atherosclerotic human coronary arteries *(202)*. The half-life of PGI_2 is decreased in acute MI and in unstable angina pectoris, which has been attributed to decreased molar ratio of apolipoprotein (Apo A-I) to Apo A-II and high-density lipoprotein-associated Apo A-I, required for the stabilization of PGI_2 *(203)*. The production of oxygen-free radicals during conversion of PGG_2 to PGH_2 may also promote oxidation of other lipids and fatty acids *(204)*. Oxidative modification of low-density lipoproteins (LDL) is believed to play an important role in atherogenesis *(205)*. Oxidized lipids in atherosclerotic lesions of high-cholesterol-fed rabbits and humans have been shown to contain esterified hydroxy and keto derivatives of linoleic acids *(206–208)*. More recently, peroxidation products of AA, isoprostane, 8-iso-PGF$_{2\alpha}$, with vasoconstrictor and vascular smooth muscle cell proliferating actions, has been found in increased amounts in human atherosclerotic lesions *(209)*. Increased urinary levels of 8-iso-PGF$_{2\alpha}$ have also been found in patients with hypercholestrolemia and other cardiovascular risk factors, including cigarette smoking and diabetes mellitus *(210)*. The levels of isoprostanes and other lipid peroxidation products in plasma and urine may serve as an index of lipid peroxidation and the efficacy of antioxidants in cardiovascular disease.

Eicosanoids and Cardiac Hypertrophy

The hypertrophic response to various stimuli in the heart is characterized by an increase in the size and protein content of individual cardiac muscle cells. Cardiac hypertrophy is a risk factor in the clinical course of heart failure (HF) *(211)*. Increased levels of neurohumoral factors, i.e., NE and ANG II, which are associated with HF, promote cardiac hypertrophy *(212)*. These agents also promote synthesis of prostanoids in the cardiovascular system *(212)*. Although the major prostanoid synthesized in the heart, PGI$_2$, has an antimitogenic effect in vascular smooth muscle cells *(213)*, it has no effect on cardiac cell growth *(214)*. On the other hand, a minor AA metabolite, PGF$_{2\alpha}$, the levels of which are elevated in the heart during compensatory growth, has been shown to stimulate hypertrophy of cardiac myocytes *(215)*. The increase in myocardial weight in response to pressure overload by coarctation of the abdominal aorta has been reported to correlate with the increase in the ratio of PGE/PGF$_{2\alpha}$ *(216)*. Whether the endogenous PGs influence cardiac cell growth is not clear. For example, in rats, both sulfinpyrazone and high doses of aspirin (50 mg/kg) suppressed plasma levels of PGs, but only the former reduced cardiac necrosis and hypertrophy induced by isoproterenol *(217)*. On the other hand, low doses of aspirin (25 mg/kg), which inhibited platelet TX synthesis without altering plasma levels of PGE$_2$ and PGI$_2$, decreased collagen deposition in noninfarcted myocardium during remodeling after coronary artery ligation in the rat *(218)*. A PGI$_2$ analog, beraprost, has been shown to decrease growth rate, DNA synthesis, and expression of collagen types I and III mRNA in cardiac fibroblasts; cells from spontaneously hypertensive rats (SHR) were less responsive than those from Wistar Kyoto (WKY) rat hearts *(219)*. Moreover, there was more PGI$_2$ production in cardiac fibroblasts from WKY than from SHR *(219)*. The increase in the number of fibroblasts and their capacity to produce a twofold increase in PGI$_2$ synthesis in the area of a healing myocardial infarct (MI), compared with cells from normal ventricles in the dog, suggests that they may contribute to healing after MI *(220)*.

SUMMARY AND CONCLUSION

This brief review summarizes developments over the past two decades in the knowledge of the participation of eicosanoids in physiological and pathophysiological aspects of cardiac function. It is clear that activation of both cholinergic and adrenergic nervous systems, and several circulating and locally generated humoral factors, promote breakdown of tissue phospholipids in the heart, and releases AA. AA is metabolized in various cell types in the heart through COX, LO, or CYP-450 pathways, generating products with potent biological activity. Metabolites of AA, including PGs, play an important role in modulating adrenergic and cholinergic transmission, cardiac reflexes, coronary vascular tone and blood flow, and the activity of plasma membrane ion channels, and mediating the cardiac action of other humoral agents, such as ANG II and bradykinin. Eicosanoids also participate in several pathophysiological processes, including ischemia/reperfusion, cardiac arrhythmias, HF, coronary atherosclerosis, and cardiac hypertrophy. The recent demonstration of the presence of LO and CYP-450 in the heart and the potent biological effects of AA metabolites generated through these enzymes, chiefly HETEs and EETs, significantly expands the possible physiological and pathophysiological roles of eicosanoids in the heart. More important, further studies on the cellular and molecular mechanisms of eicosanoids in the myocardium and coronary vasculature should allow development of rational approaches to the treatment of cardiovascular diseases.

ACKNOWLEDGMENTS

The author thanks Lauren Cagen for his kind assistance in editing this manuscript and Donna Jackett for typing the manuscript. The author also thanks former graduate students, postdoctoral fellows, and Ann Estes for their contributions to the work conducted in this laboratory, supported by National Institute of Health grant 19134-24, and cited in this chapter.

REFERENCES

1. Moncada S, Vane JR. Pharmacology and endogenous role of prostaglandin endoperoxides, thromboxane A_2 and prostacyclin. Pharmacol Rev 1978;30:243–331.
2. McGiff JC. Prostaglandins, prostacyclin and thromboxanes. Annu Rev Pharmacol Toxicol 1981;21: 479–509.
3. Samuelsson B. Leukotrienes: mediators of immediate hypersensitivity reactions and inflammation. Science 1983;220:568–575.
4. Needleman P, Turk J, Jakschik BA, Morrison AR, Lefkowith JB. Arachidonic acid metabolism. Annu Rev Biochem 1986;55:69–102.
5. Capdevila J, Marnett LJ, Chacos N, Prough RA, Estabrook RW. Cytochrome P-450 dependent oxygenation of arachidonic acid to hydroxyeicosatetraenoic acids. Proc Natl Acad Sci USA 1982;79:767–770.
6. Serhan CN. Lipoxins and novel aspirin-triggered 15-epi-lipoxins (ATL): a jungle of cell-cell interactions or a therapeutic opportunity? Prostaglandins 1997;53:107–137.
7. Needleman P, Kaley G. Cardiac and coronary prostaglandin synthesis and function. N Engl J Med 1978;298:1122–1128.
8. Nasjletti A, Malik KU. Interrelations between prostaglandins and vasoconstrictor hormones: contribution to blood pressure regulation. Fed Proc 1982;41:2394–2399.
9. Karmazyn M, Dhalla NS. Physiological and pathophysiological aspects of cardiac prostaglandins. Can J Physiol Pharmacol 1983;61:1207–1225.
10. Karmazyn M. Synthesis and relevance of cardiac eicosanoids with particular emphasis on ischemia and reperfusion. Can J Physiol Pharmacol 1989;67:912–921.
11. Balsinde J, Diez E, Mollinedo F. Arachidonic acid release from diacylglycerol in human neutrophils: translocation of diacylglycerol-decylating enzyme activities from an intracellular pool to plasma membrane upon cell activation. J Biol Chem 1991;256:15,638–15,643.
12. Lapetina EG, Billah MM, Cuatrecasas P. Initial action of thrombin on platelets. J Biol Chem 1981;256: 5037–5040.
13. Brindley DN. Intracellular translocation of phosphatidate phosphohydrolase and its possible role in the control of glycerolipid synthesis. Prog Lipid Res 1984;23:115–133.
14. Morrow JD, Hill KE, Burk RF, Nammour TM, Badr KF, Roberts LJ. Series of prostaglandin F_2-like compounds are produced in vivo in humans by a non-cyclooxygenase, free radical-catalyzed mechanism. Proc Natl Acad Sci USA 1990;87:9383–9387.
15. Morrow JD, Roberts LJ. Isoprostanes. Current knowledge and direction of future research. Biochem Pharmacol 1996;51:1–9.
16. Goetzl EJ, An S, Smith WL. Specificity of expression and effects of eicosanoid mediators in normal physiology and human diseases. FASEB J 1995;9:1051–1058.

17. Crofford LJ. Cox-1 and Cox-2 tissue expression: implications and predictions. J Rheumatol 1997; 24(Suppl 49):15–19.
18. Kulmaez RJ, Lands WEM. Prostaglandin H synthase stoichiometry of heme cofactor. J Biol Chem 1984;259:6358–6363.
19. Capdevila JH, Falck JR, Estabrook RW. Cytochrome P-450 and the arachidonate cascade. FASEB J 1992;6:731–736.
20. McGiff JC. Cytochrome P-450 metabolism of arachidonic acid. Annu Rev Pharmacol Toxicol 1991; 31:339–369.
21. Fitzpatrick FA, Murphy RC. Cytochrome P-450 metabolism of arachidonic acid: formation and biological actions of 'epoxygenase'-derived eicosanoids. Pharmacol Rev 1988;40:229–241.
22. Laniado-Schwartzman M, Davis KL, McGiff JC, Levere RD, Abraham NG. Purification and characterization of cytochrome P-450 dependent arachidonic acid epoxygenase from human liver. J Biol Chem 1988;263:2536–2542.
23. Falck JR, Manna S, Jacobson HR, Estabrook RW, Chacos N, Capdevilla J. Absolute configuration of epoxyeicosatrienoic acids (EETs) formed during catalytic oxygenation of arachidonic acid by purified rat liver microsomal cytochrome P-450. J Am Chem Soc 1984;106:3334–3336.
24. Karara A, Dishman E, Jacobson H, Falck JR, Capdevila JH. Arachidonic acid epoxygenase. Stereochemical analysis of the endogenous epoxyeicosatrienoic acids of human kidney cortex. FEBS Lett 1990;268:227–230.
25. De Decker EAM, Nugteren DH, Ten Hoor F. Prostacyclin is the major prostaglandin released from isolated perfused rabbit and rat heart. Nature 1977;268:163–168,
26. Hsueh W, Needleman P. Sites of lipase activation and prostaglandin synthesis in isolated, perfused rabbit hearts and hydronephrotic kidneys. Prostaglandins 1978;16:661–681.
27. Wennmalm A. Prostaglandin-mediated inhibition of noradrenaline release. VI. On the intra-cardiac source of prostaglandin released from isolated rabbit hearts. Acta Physiol Scand 1979;105:254–256.
28. Gerritsen ME, Cheli CD. Arachidonic acid and prostaglandin endoperoxide metabolism in isolated rabbit and coronary microvessels and isolated and cultivated coronary microvessel endothelial cells. J Clin Invest 1983;72:1658–1671.
29. Kan H, Ruan Y, Malik KU. Localization and characterization of the subtype(s) of muscarinic receptor involved in prostacyclin synthesis in rabbit heart. J Pharmacol Exp Ther 1996;276:934–941.
30. Dusting GJ, Nolan RD. Stimulation of prostacyclin release from the epicardium of anesthetized dogs. Br J Pharmacol 1981;74:553–652.
31. Mebazza A, Martin LD, Robotham JL, Maeda K, Gabrielson EU, Wetzel RC. Right and left ventricular cultured endocardial endothelium produces prostacyclin and PGE$_2$. J Mol Cell Cardiol 1993;25:245–248.
32. Ahumada GG, Sobel BE, Needleman P. Synthesis of prostaglandins by cultured rat heart myocytes and cardiac mesenchymal cells. J Mol Cell Cardiol 1980;12:685–700.
33. Bolton HS, Chanderbhan R, Bryant RW, Bailey JM, Weglicki WB, Vahouny GV. Prostaglandin synthesis by adult heart myocytes. J Mol Cell Cardiol 1980;12:1287–1298.
34. Cole OF, Fan TPD, Lewis GP. Release of eicosanoids from cultured rat aortic endothelial cells; studies with arachidonic acid and calcium ionophore A23187. Cell Biol Int Rep 1986;10:407–413.
35. Szczeklik A, Gryglewski RJ, Musial J, Grodzinska L, Serwonska M, Marcinkiewicz E. Thromboxane generation and platelet aggregation in survivals of myocardial infarction. Thromb Haemest 1978;40: 66–74.
36. Kuzuya T, Hoshida S, Nishida M, Kim Y, Kamada T, Tada M. Increased production of arachidonate metabolites in an occlusion-reperfusion model of canine myocardial infarction. Cardiovasc Res 1987; 21:551–558.
37. Breitbart E, Sofer Y, Shainberg A, Grossman S. Lipoxygenase activity in heart cells. FEBS Lett 1996; 395:148–152.
38. Garlick PB, Mashiter GD, Di-Marzo V, Tippins JR, Morris HR, Maisey MN. Synthesis, release and action of leukotrienes in the isolated, unstimulated, buffer-perfused rat heart. J Mol Cell Cardiol 1989; 21:1101–1110.
39. Revtyak GE, Johnson AR, Campbell WB. Cultured bovine coronary arterial endothelial cells synthesize HETEs and prostacyclin. Am J Physiol 1988;254:C8–C19.
40. Rosolowsky M, Campbell WB. Synthesis of hydroxyeicosatetraenoic (HETEs) and epoxyeicosatrienoic acids (EETs) by cultured bovine coronary artery endothelial cells. Biochem Biophys Acta 1996; 1299:267–277.

41. Harder DR, Campbell WB, Roman RJ. Role of cytochrome P-450 enzymes and metabolites of arachidohnic acid in the control of vascular tone. J Vasc Res 1995;32:79–92.

42. Wu S, Chen W, Murphy E, Gabel S, Tomer KB, Foley J, et al. Molecular cloning, expression, and functional significance of a cytochrome P-450 highly expressed in rat heart myocytes. J Biol Chem 1997;272:12,551–12,559.

43. Hedqvist P. Basic mechanism of prostaglandin actions on autonomic neurotransmission. Annu Rev Pharmacol Toxicol 1977;17:259–279.

44. Junstad M, Wennmalm A. On the release of prostaglandin E_2 from the rabbit heart following infusion of noradrenaline. Acta Physiol Scand 1973;87:573–574.

45. Shaffer JE, Malik KU. Enhancement of prostaglandin output during activation of beta-1 adrenoceptors in the isolated rabbit heart. J Pharmacol Exp Ther 1982;223:729–735.

46. Junstad M, Wennmalm A. Release of prostaglandin from the rabbit isolated heart following vagal nerve stimulation or acetylcholine infusion. Br J Pharmacol 1974;52:375–370.

47. Jaiswal N, Malik KU. Prostaglandin synthesis elicited by cholinergic stimuli is mediated by activation of M_2 muscarinic receptors in rabbit heart. J Pharmacol Exp Ther 1988;245:59–66.

48. Needleman P, Marshall GR, Sobel BE. Hormone interactions in the isolated rabbit heart, synthesis and coronary vasomotor effects of prostaglandins, angiotensin, and bradykinin. Circ Res 1975;37:802–808.

49. Weis MT, Malik KU. Uptake and hormonally-induced hydrolysis of [^{3}H]phosphatidylcholine in the isolated rabbit heart. J Pharmacol Exp Ther 1989;248:614–620.

50. Prasad MR. Endothelin stimulates degradation of phospholipids in isolated rat hearts. Biochem Biophys Res Commun 1991;174:952–957.

51. Ruan Y, Kan H, Malik KU. Modulation by cyclic AMP of beta-adrenergic receptor stimulated prostacyclin synthesis in rabbit ventricular myocytes. J Pharmacol Exp Ther 1996;278:482–489.

52. Ruan Y, Kan H, Malik KU. Beta-adrenergic receptor stimulated prostacyclin synthesis in rabbit coronary endothelial cells is mediated by selective activation of phospholipase D: inhibition by adenosine 3',5'-cyclic monophosphate. J Pharmacol Exp Ther 1997;281:1038–1046.

53. Jaiswal N, Lambrecht G, Mutschler E, Malik KU. Contribution of $M_{2\alpha}$ and $M_{2\beta}$ muscarinic receptors to the action of cholinergic stimuli on prostaglandin synthesis and mechanical function in the isolated rabbit heart. J Pharmacol Exp Ther 1988;247:104–113.

54. Kan H, Ruan Y, Malik KU. Localization and characterization of the subtype(s) of muscarinic receptor involved in prostacyclin synthesis in rabbit heart. J Pharmacol Exp Ther 1996;276:934–941.

55. Jones SV, Heilman CJ, Brann MR. Functional responses of cloned muscarinic receptors expressed in CHO-K1 cells. Mol Pharmacol 1991;40:242–247.

56. Ostrowski J, Kjelsberg MA, Caron MG, Lefkowitz RJ. Mutagenesis of β_2-adrenergic receptor: how structure elucidates function. Annu Rev Pharmacol Toxicol 1992;32:167–183.

57. Strader CD, Sigal IS, Dixon RAF. Structural basis of β-adrenergic receptor function. FASEB J 1989;3:1825–1832.

58. Weis MT, Malik KU. Beta-adrenergic receptor-stimulated prostaglandin synthesis in the isolated rabbit heart: relationhip to extra- and intracellular calcium. J Pharmacol Exp Ther 1985;235:178–185.

59. Schwartz DD, Williams JL, Malik KU. Contribution of calcium to isoproterenol-stimulated lipolysis in the isolated perfused rabbit heart. Am J Physiol 1993;265:E439–E445.

60. Malik KU, Weis MT, Jaiswal N. Mechanism of action of adrenergic and cholinergic stimuli on cardiac prostaglandin synthesis. In: Samuelsson B, Wong PY-K, Sun FF, eds. Advances in Prostaglandin, Thromboxane and Leukotriene Research. Raven, New York, vol. 19, 1989, pp. 327–330.

61. Kan H, Ruan Y, Malik KU. Signal transduction mechanism(s) involved in prostacyclin production elicited by acetylcholine in coronary endothelial cells of rabbit heart. J Pharmacol Exp Ther 1997;282:113–122.

62. Kan H, Ruan Y, Malik KU. Involvement of mitogen-activated protein kinase and translocation of cytosolic phospholipase A_2 to the nuclear envelope in acetylcholine-induced prostacyclin synthesis in rabbit coronary endothelial cells. Mol Pharmacol 1996;50:1139–1147.

63. Lindmar R, Löffelholz K, Sandman J. On the mechanism of muscarinic hydrolysis by choline phospholipids in the heart. Biochem Pharmacol 1988;37:4689–4695.

64. Hammond SM, Altshuller YM, Sung TC, Rudge SA, Rose K, Engebrecht J, Morris AJ, Frohman MA. Human ADP-ribosylation factor-activated phosphatidylcholine specific phospholipase D defines a new and highly conserved gene family. J Biol Chem 1995;270:29,640–29,643.

65. Colley WC, Sung TC, Roll R, Jenco J, Hammond SM, Altshuller Y, et al. Phospholipase D_2, a distinct phospholipase D isoform with novel regulatory properties that provokes cytoskeletal reorganization. Curr Biol 1997;7:191–201.

66. Exton JH. Phospholipase D: enzymology, mechanisms of regulation, and function. Physiol Rev 1997; 77:303–320.

67. Hecker M, Dambacher T, Busse R. Role of endothelium-derived bradykinin in the control of vascular tone. J Cardiovasc Pharmacol 1992;20(Suppl 9):S55–S61.

68. Gunther S, Cannon PJ. Modulation of angiotensin II coronary vasoconstriction by cardiac prostaglandin synthesis. Am J Physiol 1980;238:H895–H901.

69. Yu H, Gallagher AM, Garfin PM, Printz MP. Prostacyclin release by rat cardiac fibroblasts: inhibition of collagen expression. Hypertension 1997;30:1047–1053.

70. Ciabattoni C, Wennmalm A. Adenosine-induced coronary release of prostacyclin at normal and low pH in isolated heart of rabbit. Br J Pharmacol 1985;85:557–563.

71. Karwatowska-Prokopczuk E, Ciabattoni G, Wennmalm A. Effect of adenosine on the formation of prostacyclin in the rabbit isolated heart. Br J Pharmacol 1988;94:721–728.

72. Rogers TB, Lokuta AJ. Angiotensin II signal transduction pathways in the cardiovascular system. Trend Cardiovasc Med 1994;4:110–116.

73. Clerk A, Sugden PH. Regulation of phospholipases C and D in rat ventricular myocytes: stimulation by endothelin-1, bradykinin and phenylephrine. J Mol Cell Cardiol 1997;29:1593–1604.

74. Fulton D, McGiff JC, Quilley J. Role of phospholipase C and phospholipase A_2 in the nitric oxide-independent vasodilator effect of bradykinin in the rat perfused heart. J Pharmacol Exp Ther 1996; 278:518–526.

75. Malik KU, McGiff JC. Cardiovascular actions of prostaglandins. In: Kavim SMM, ed. Prostaglandins: Physiological, Pharmacological and Pathological Aspects. MTP, Lancaster, England, 1976, pp. 103–200.

76. Karmazyn M, Horrobin DF, Manku MS, Cunnane SC, Karamali RA, Ally AI, et al. Effects of prostacyclin on perfusion pressure, electrical activity, rate of force of contraction in isolated rat and rabbit hearts. Life Sci 1978;22:2079–2086.

77. Armstrong JM, Chapple D, Dusting GJ, Hughes R, Moncada S, Vane JR. Cardiovascular actions of prostacyclin in chloralose anesthetized dogs. Br J Pharmacol 1977;61:136P.

78. Chiba S, Malik KU. Mechanism of chronotropic effects of prostacyclin in the dog: Comparison with the actions of prostaglandin E_2. J Pharmacol Exp Ther 1980;213:261–266.

79. Svensen J, Hamberg M. Thromboxane A_2 and prostaglandin H_2: Potent stimulant of the swine coronary artery. Prostaglandins 1976;12:943–950.

80. Giannessi D, Lazzerini G, Sicari R, DeCaterina R. Vasoactive eicosanoids in the rat heart: clues to a contributory role of cardiac thromboxane to post-ischaemic hyperemia. Pharmacol Res 1992;26: 341–356.

81. Letts LG, Piper PJ. Actions of leukotriene C_4 and D_4 on guinea-pig isolated hearts. Br J Pharmacol 1982;76:169–176.

82. Campbell WB, Gebremedhin D, Pratt PF, Harder DR. Identification of epoxyeicosatrienoic acids as endothelium-derived hyperpolarizing factors. Circ Res 1996;78:415–423.

83. Weintraub NL, Fang X, Kaduce TL, Van Rollins M, Chatterjee P, Spector AA. Potentiation of endothelium-dependent relaxation by epoxy-eicosatrienoic acids. Circ Res 1997;81:258–267.

84. Wennmalm A. Studies on the mechanisms controlling the secretion of neurotransmitters in the rabbit heart. Acta Physiol Scand 1971;365(Suppl):1–32.

85. Khan MT, Malik KU. Modulation by prostaglandins of the release of [^{3}H]-noradrenaline evoked by potassium and nerve stimulation in the isolated rat heart. Eur J Pharmacol 1982;78:213–218.

86. Westfall TC, Brasted M. Inhibition by prostaglandins of adrenergic transmission in the left ventricular myocardium of anesthetized dogs. J Cardiovasc Pharmacol 1985;7:659–664.

87. Lanier SM, Malik KU. Inhibition by prostaglandins of adrenergic transmission in the left ventricular myocardium of anesthetized dogs. J Cardiovasc Pharmacol 1985;7:653–659.

88. Chiba S, Malik KU. Prostaglandins do not modulate the positive chronotropic and inotropic effects of sympathetic nerve stimulation and injected norepinephrine in the isolated blood perfused canine atrium. Life Sci 1981;28:687–695.

89. Mantelli L, Amerini S, Ledda F. Different effects of prostaglandins on adrenergic neurotransmission in atrial and ventricular preparations. Br J Pharmacol 1990;99:717–720.

90. Courtney KR, Colwell WT, Jensen RA. Prostaglandins and pacemaker activity in isolated guinea-pig SA node. Prostaglandins 1978;16:451–459.

91. Miyazaki T, Pride HP, Zipes DP. Prostaglandins in the pericardial fluid modulate neural regulation of cardiac electrophysiological properties. Circ Res 1990;66:163–175.

92. Amerini S, Mantelli L, Rubino A, Ledda F. On the presence of inhibitory prejunctional thromboxane receptors on the adrenergic nerve terminals of mammalian heart. Pharmacol Res 1990;22(Suppl 1):11–12.

93. Ruan Y, Hong K, Cano C, Malik KU. Modulation of β-adrenergic receptor-stimulated lipolysis in the heart by prostaglandins. Am J Physiol 1996;271:34:E556–E562.

94. Lanier SM, Malik KU. Attenuation by prostaglandins of the facilitatory effect of angiotensin II at adrenergic prejunctional sites in the isolated Krebs-perfused rat heart. Circ Res 1982;51:594–601.

95. Lanier SM, Malik KU. Facilitation of adrenergic transmission in the canine heart by intracoronary infusion of angiotensin II: effect of prostaglandin synthesis inhibition. J Pharmacol Exp Ther 1983; 227:676–682.

96. Hadhazy P, Illes P, Knoll J. The effect of PGE_1 on responses to cardiac vagus nerve stimulation and acetylcholine release. Eur J Pharmacol 1973;23:251–255.

97. Feigl EO. Neural control of coronary blood flow. J Vasc Res 1998;35:85–92.

98. Staszewska-Woolley J, Gray W. Cardiac nociceptive reflexes: Role of kinins, prostaglandins and capsaicin-sensitive afferents. Pol J Pharmacol Pharm 1990;42:237–247.

99. Staszewska-Barezak J, Dusting GJ, May DE, Nolan PN. Effect of prostacyclin on cardiovascular reflexes from the ventricular epicardium of the dog: comparison with the effects of prostaglandin E_2. Prostaglandins 1981;21:905–915.

100. Uchida Y, Murao S. Bradykinin-induced excitation of afferent cardiac sympathetic nerve fibers. Jpn Heart J 1974;15:84–91.

101. Moretti RL, Abraham S, Ecker RR. Stimulation of cardiac prostaglandin production by blood plasma and its relationship to the regulation of coronary flow in isolated rabbit hearts. Circ Res 1978;42:317–323.

102. Moretti RL, Abraham S. Stimulation of microsomal prostaglandin synthesis by a blood plasma constituent which augments auto-regulation and maintenance of vascular tone in isolated rabbit hearts. Circ Res 1978;42:317–323.

103. Rubio R, Berne RM. Regulation of coronary blood flow. Prog Cardiovasc Dis 1975;18:105–122.

104. Kalsner S. Endogenous prostaglandin release contributes directly to coronary artery tone. Can J Physiol Pharmacol 1975;53:560–565.

105. Melo LG, Sonnenberg H. Requirement for prostaglandin synthesis in secretion of atrial natriuretic factor from isolated rat heart. Regul Pept 1995;60:79–87.

106. Azizi C, Barthelemy C, Masson F, Maistre G, Eurin J, Carayon A. Myocardial production of prostaglandins: its role in atrial natriuretic release1. Eur J Endocrinol 1995;133:255–259.

107. Church DJ, Braconi S, Van der Bent V, Vallotton MP, Lang U. Protein kinase C-dependent prostaglandin production mediates angiotensin II-induced atrial-natriuretic peptide release. Biochem J 1994; 298:451–456.

108. Van der Bent V, Church DJ, Vallotton MB, Meda P, Kem DC, Capponi AM, Lang U. [Ca^{2+}]i and protein kinase C in vasopressin-induced prostacyclin and ANP release in rat cardiomyocytes. Am J Physiol 1994;266:H597–H605.

109. Church DJ, Van der Bent V, Vallotton MB, Lang U. Role of prostaglandin-mediated cyclic AMP formation in protein kinase C-dependent secretion of atrial natriuretic peptide in rat cardiomyocytes. Biochem J 1994;303:217–225.

110. Gebremedhin D, Harder DR, Pratt PF, Campbell WB. Bioassay of an endothelium-derived hyperpolarizing factor from bovine coronary arteries: role of a cytochrome P-450 metabolite. J Vasc Res 1998;35:274–284.

111. Yamada M, Terzic A, Kurachi Y. Regulation of potassium channels by G-protein subunits and arachidonic acid metabolites. Methods Enzymol 1994;238:344–422.

112. Kurachi Y, Ito H, Sugimoto T, Shimizu T, Miki I, Ui M. Arachidonic acid metabolites as intracellular modulators of the G protein-gated cardiac K^+ channel. Nature 1989;337:555–557.

113. Nakajima T, Sugimoto T, Kurachi Y. Platelet-activating factor activates cardiac GK via arachidonic acid metabolites. FEBS Lett 1991;289:239–243.

114. Kurachi Y, Ito H, Sugimoto T, Shimizu T, Miki I, Ui M. Alpha-adrenergic activation of the muscarinic K^+ channel is mediated by arachidonic acid metabolites. Pflügers Arch 1989;414:102–104.

115. Scherer RW, Lo CF, Breitwieser GE. Leukotriene C_4 modulation of muscarinic K+ current activation in bullfrog atrial myocytes. J Gen Physiol 1993;102:125–141.

116. Scherer RW, Breitwieser GE. Arachidonic acid metabolites alter G protein-mediated signal transduction in heart. Effects on muscarinic K^+ channels. J Gen Physiol 1990;96:735–755.

117. Kim D, Lewis DL, Graziadei L, Neer EJ, Bar-Sagi D, Clapham DE. G protein beta gamma-subunits activate the cardiac muscarinic K$^+$-channel via phospholipase A$_2$. Nature 1989;337:557–560.

118. Nakhostine N, Lamontagne D. Contribution of prostaglandins in hypoxia-induced vasodilation in isolated rabbit hearts. Relation to adenosine and KATP channels. Pflügers Arch 1994;428:526–532.

119. Bouchard JF, Dumont E, Lamontagne D. Evidence that prostaglandins I$_2$, E$_2$ and D$_2$ may activate ATP-sensitive potassium channels in the isolated rat heart. Cardiovasc Res 1994;28:901–905.

120. Hide EJ, Ney P, Piper J, Thiemermann C, Vane JR. Reduction by prostaglandin E$_1$ or porstaglandin E$_0$ of myocardial infarct size in the rabbit by activation of ATP-sensitive potassium channels. Br J Pharmacol 1995;116:2435–2440.

121. Kang JX, Leaf A. Effects of long-chain polyunsaturated fatty acids on the contraction of neonatal rat cardiac myocytes. Proc Natl Acad Sci USA 1994;91:9886–9890.

122. Hoffman P, Richards D, Heinroth-Hoffman T, Mathias P, Wey H, Toraason M. Arachidonic acid disrupts calcium dynamics in neonatal rat cardiac myocytes. Cardiovasc Res 1995;30:889–898.

123. Xiao YF, Huang L, Morgan JP. Cytochrome P-450:a novel system modulating Ca^{2+} channels and contraction in mammalian heart cells. J. Physiol (London) 1998;508:777–792.

124. Weiglicki WB, Owens K, Urshel CW, Seur JR, Sonnenblick EH. Hydrolysis of myocardial lipids during acidosis and ischemia. Recent Adv Stud Card Struct Metabo 1973;3:781–793.

125. Van der Vusse GJ, Glatz JF, Stam HC, Reneman RS. Fatty acid homeostasis in the normoxic and ischemia heart. Physiol Rev 1992;72:881–940.

126. Prasad RM, Popescu LM, Moraru II, Liu X, Maity S, Engelman RM, Das DK. Role of phospholipase A$_2$ and C in myocardial reperfusion injury. Am J Physiol 1991;260:H877–H883.

127. Eskildsen-Helmond YEG, Van Heugten HAA, Lamers JM. Regulation and functional significance of phospholipase D in myocardium. Mol Cell Biochem 1996;157:34–48.

128. Van der Vusse GH, Reneman RS, Van Bilsen M. Accumulation of arachidonic acid in ischemic/reperfused cardiac tissue: possible causes and consequences. Prostaglandins, Leukotrienes Essential Fatty Acids 1997;57:85–93.

129. Van Bilsen M, Van der Vusse GJ. Phospholipase A$_2$-dependent signalling in the heart. Cardiovasc Res 1995;30:518–529.

130. Hazen SL, Gross RW. ATP-dependent regulation of rabbit myocardial cytosolic calcium-dependent phospholipase A$_2$. J Biol Chem 1991;266:4526–4534.

131. Hazen SL, Wolf MJ, Ford DA, Gross RW. Rapid and reversible association of phosphofructokinase with myocardial membranes during myocardial ischemia. FEBS Lett 1994;339:213–216.

132. Davies NJ, Schulz R, Olley PN, Strydnadka KD, Panas DL, Lopaschuk GD. Lysoplasmenyletha-nolamine accumulation in ischemic/reperfused isolated fatty acid-perfused hearts. Circ Res 1992;70:1161–1168.

133. Van der Vusse GJ, Roemen THM, Prinzen FW, Coumans WA, Reneman RS. Uptake and tissue content of fatty acids in dog myocardium under normoxic and ischemic conditions. Circ Res 1982;50:538–546.

134. Van Bilsen M, Van der Vusse GJ, Willemsen PHM, Coumans WA, Roemen TH, Reneman RS. Lipid alterations in isolated, working rat heart during ischemia and reperfusion: its relation to myocardial damage. Circ Res 1989;64:304–314.

135. Engels W, Van Bilsen M, De Groot MJM, Lemmens PJ, Willemsen PH, Reneman RS, Van der Vusse GJ. Ischemia and reperfusion-induced formation of eicosanoids in isolated rat hearts. Am J Physiol 1990;258:H1865–H1871.

136. Ogletree ML, Lefer AM. Influence of non-steroidal anti-inflammatory agents on myocardial ischemia. J Pharmacol Exp Ther 1976;197:582–593.

137. Capurro NL, Marr KC, Aamodt R, Goldstein RE, Epstein S. Aspirin-induced increase in collateral flow after acute coronary occlusion in dogs. Circulation 1979;59:744–747.

138. Karmazyn M. Contribution of prostaglandins to reperfusion-induced ventricular failure in isolated rat hearts. Am J Physiol 1986;251:H133–H140.

139. Mobert J, Becker BF. Cyclooxygenase inhibition aggravates ischemia-reperfusion injury in the per-fused guinea-pig heart: involvement of isoprostanes. J Am Coll Cardiol 1998;31:1687–1694.

140. Ruf W, MacNnamara JJ, Suehiro A, Suehiro G, Wickline SA. Platelet trapping in myocardial infarct in baboons: therapeutic effect of aspirin. Am J Cardiol 1980;46:405–412.

141. Chierchia S, Patrono C. Role of platelet and vascular eicosanoids in the pathophysiology of ischemic heart disease. Fed Proc 1987;46:81–88.

142. Tada M, Kuzuya T, Inoue M, Kodana K, Mishima M, Yamada M, Inui M, Abe H. Elevation of thromboxane B_2 levels in patients with classical and variant angina pectoris. Circ Res 1981;64:1107–115.

143. Otani H, Engelman RM, Rausou JA, Breyer RH, Das DK. Enhanced prostaglandin synthesis due to phospholipid breakdown in ischemic-reperfused myocardium control of its production by a phospholipase inhibitor or free radical scavenger. J Mol Cell Cardiol 1986;18:953–961.

144. Teoh KH, Fremes SE, Weisel RD, Christakis GT, Teasdale SJ, Madonik MM, et al. Cardiac release of prostacyclin and thromboxane A_2 during coronary revascularization. J Thorac Cardiovasc Surg 1987;93:120–126.

145. Tada M, Kuzuya T, Hoshida S, Nishida M. Arachidonate metabolism in myocardial ischemia and reperfusion. J Mol Cell Cardiol 1988;20:135–143.

146. Dusting GJ, Moncada S, Vane JR. Prostaglandins, their intermediates and precursors: cardiovascular action and regulatory roles in normal and abnormal circulatory systems. Prog Cardiovasc Dis 1979; 21:405–430.

147. Mullane KM, Fornabaio D. Thromboxane synthetase inhibitors reduce infarct size by a platelet dependent, aspirin-sensitive mechanism. Circ Res 1988;62:668–678.

148. Farber NE, Pieper GM, Gross GJ. Lack of involvement of thromboxane A_2 in post-ischemic recovery of stunned canine myocardium. Circulation 1988;78:450–461.

149. Farber NE, Gross GJ. Prostaglandin redirection by thromboxane synthetase inhibition. Attenuation of myocardial stunning in canine heart. Circulation 1990;81:369–380.

150. Melin JA, Becker LC. Salvage of ischemic myocardium by prostacyclin during experimental myocardial infarction. J Am Coll Cardiol 1983;2:279–286.

151. Thiemermann C, Steinhagen-Thiessen E, Schrör K. Inhibition of oxygen-centered free radical formation by the stable prostacyclin-mimetic iloprost (ZK 36374) in acute myocardial ischemia. J Cardiovasc Pharmacol 1984;6:365–366.

152. Herbaczynsko-Cedro K, Gordon-Majszak W. Attenuation by prostacyclin of adrenaline-stimulated lipid peroxidation in the myocardium. Pharmacol Res Comm 1986;81:321–332.

153. Parratt JR. Endogenous myocardial protective (anti-arrhythmic) substances. Cardiovasc Res 1993;27: 693–702.

154. Rossoni G, Sala A, Buccellati C, Maclouf J, Falco GC, Berti F. Vasoconstriction to polymorphonuclear leukocytes in the isolated, perfused rabbit heart: inhibition by prostacyclin mimetics. J Cardiovasc Pharmacol 1996;27:680–685.

155. Garlick PB, Mashiter GD, Di Marzo V, Tippins JR, Morris HR, Maisey MN. Synthesis, release and action of leukotrienes in the isolated, unstimulated, buffer-perfused rat heart. J Mol Cell Cardiol 1989; 21:1101–1110.

156. Ito BR, Roth DM, Engler RL. Thromboxane A_2 and peptidoleukotrienes contribute to the myocardial ischemia and contractile dysfunction in response to intracoronary infusion of complement C5a in pigs. Circ Res 1990;66:596–607.

157. Mullane KM, Read N, Salmon JA, Moncada S. Role of leukocytes in acute myocardial infarction in anesthetized dogs: relationship to myocardial salvage by anti-inflammatory drugs. J Pharmacol Exp Ther 1984;228:510–522.

158. O'Neill PG, Charlat ML, Kim HS, Pocius J, Michael LH, Hartley CJ, et al. Lipoxygenase inhibitor nafazatrom fails to attenuate postischemic ventricular dysfunction. Cardiovasc Res 1987;21:755–760.

159. Moffat MP, Ward CA, Bend JR, Mock T, Farhangkhoee P, Karmazyn M. Effects of epoxyeicosatrienoic acids on isolated hearts and ventricular myocytes. Am J Physiol 1993;264:H154–H160.

160. Zijlstra WG, Brunsting JR, Ten Hoor P, Vergrosen AJ. Prostaglandin E_1 and cardiac arrhythmia. Eur J Pharmacol 1972;18:392–395.

161. Au TL-S, Collins GA, Harrie CJ, Walker MJA. Actions of prostaglandins I_2 and E_2 on arrhythmias produced by coronary occlusion in the rat and dog. Prostanglandins 1979;18:707–720.

162. Karmazyn M, Dhalla NS. Selective concentration-dependent dysrhythmogenic and antidysrhythmic action of prostaglandins E_2, $F_{2\alpha}$ and I_2 (prostacyclin) on isolated rat hearts. Experientia 1980;36: 996–998.

163. Li Y, Kang JX, Leaf A. Differential effects of various eicosanoids on the production or prevention of arrhythmias in cultured neonatal rat cardiac myocytes. Prostaglandins 1997;54:511–530.

164. Dix RK, Kelliher GJ, Furkiewicz N, Bryan-Smith J. Effect of sulfinpyrazone on ventricular arrhythmias. Prostaglandin synthesis and catecholamine release following coronary occlusion in the cat. J Cardiovasc Pharmacol 1982;4:1068–1076.

165. Karmazyn MA. Direct protective effect of sulphinpyrazone on ischaemic and reperfused rat hearts. Br J Pharmacol 1984;93:331–336.

166. Fagbemi SO. Effect of aspirin, indomethacin and sodium meclofenamate on coronary artery ligation arrhythmias in anesthetized rats. Eur J Pharmacol 1984;97:283–287.

167. Ellis EF, Oelz O, Roberts II, LJ. Coronary arterial smooth muscle contraction by a substance released from platelets: evidence that it is thromboxane A_2. Science 1976;193:1135–1137.

168. Curtis MJ, Pugsley MK, Walker MJA. Endogenous chemical mediators of ventricular arrhythmias in heart disease. Cardiovasc Res 1993;27:703–719.

169. Mehta J, Nichols W, Mehta P, Conti CR. Thromboxane and prostacyclin in systemic and coronary vascular beds following endoperoxide analog infusion. Am J Cardiol 1982;49:1014.

170. Coker SJ. Further evidence that thromboxane exacerbates arrhythmias: effects of UK 38485 during coronary artery occlusion and reperfusion in anesthetized greyhounds. J Mol Cell Cardiol 1984;16: 633–641.

171. O'Connor KM, Freihling TD, Kowey PR. Effect of thromboxane inhibition on vulnerability to ventricular fibrillation in the acute and chronic feline infarction models. Am Heart J 1989;117:848–853.

172. Coker SJ, Parratt JR. Effects of nafazatrom on arrhythmias and prostanoid release during coronary artery occlusion and reperfusion in anesthetized greyhounds. J Mol Cell Cardiol 1984;16:43–52.

173. Berti F, Rossini G, Omini C, Daffonchio L, Tondo C, Cali G. Defibrotide protects rabbit myocardium from ischemia: relationship with the eicosanoid system. Pol J Pharmacol Pharm 1987;39:657–665.

174. Wainwright CL, Parratt JR. Failure of cyclooxygenase inhibition to protect against arrhythmias induced by ischaemia and reperfusion: implications for the role of prostaglandins as endogenous myocardial protective substances. Cardiovasc Res 1991;25:93–101.

175. Vegh A, Szekeres L, Parratt JR. Protective effects of preconditioning of the ischaemic myocardium involve cyclooxygenase products. Cardiovasc Res 1990;24:1020–1023.

176. Maulik M, Seth SD, Manchanda SC, Maulik SK. Lack of any additional benefit in combining aspirin with iloprost in a canine model of myocardial reperfusion injury. Prostaglandins 1997;53:291–303.

177. Rajani V, Hussain Y, Bolla BS, de Guzman FQ, Montiague RR, Igic R, Rabito SF. Attenuation of epinephrine-induced dysrhythmias by bradykinin: role of nitric oxide and prostaglandins. Am J Cardiol 1997;80:153A–157A.

178. Birincioglu M, Olmez E, Aksoy T, Acet A. Role of prostaglandin synthesis stimulation in the protective effect of captopril on ischaemia-reperfusion arrhythmias in rats in vivo. Pharmacol Res 1997;36: 299–304.

179. Ezeamuzie IC, Assem ESK. Effects of leukotrienes C_4 and D_4 on guinea-pig heart and the participation of SRS-A in the manifestations of guinea-pig cardiac anaphylaxis. Agents Actions 1983;13:182–187.

180. Beatch GN, Courtice ID, Salari H. Comparative study of the antiarrhythmic properties of eicosanoid inhibitors, free radical scavangers and potassium channel blockers on reperfusion-induced arrhythmias in the rat. Proc Western Pharmacol Soc 1989;32:285–289.

181. Hahn RA, MacDonald BR, Simpson PJ, Potts BD, Parli CJ. Antagonism of leukotriene B_4 receptors does not limit canine myocardial infarct size. J Pharmacol Exp Ther 1990;253:58–66.

182. Ito T, Toki Y, Heida N, Okumura K, Hashimoto H, Ogawa K, Satake T. Protective effects of a thromboxane synthase inhibitor, a thromboxane antagonist, a lipoxygenase inhibitor, and a leukotriene C_4, D_4 antagonists on myocardial injury caused by acute myocardial infarction in the canine heart. Jpn Circ J 1989;53:1115–1121.

183. Gok S, Ulker S, Huseyinov A, Evinc A. Effects of lipoxygenase inhibitor on digoxin-induced cardiac arrhythmias in the isolated perfused guinea-pig heart. Gen Pharmacol 1997;29:789–792.

184. Cannon PJ. Prostaglandins in congestive heart failure and the effects fo nonsteroidal anti-inflammatory drugs. Am J Med 1986;81:123–132.

185. Awan NA, Evenson MK, Needham KE, Beattie JM, Amsterdam EA, Mason DT. Cardiocirculatory and myocardial energetic effects of prostaglandin E_1 in severe left ventricular failure due to chronic coronary heart disease. Am Heart J 1981;102:703–709.

186. Farber NE, Gross GJ. Prostanglandin E_1 attenuates post-ischemic contractile dysfunction after brief coronary occlusion and reperfusion. Am Heart J 1989;118:17–24.

187. Farber NE, Pieper GM, Thomas JP, Gross GJ. Beneficial effects of iloprost in the stunned canine myocardium. Circ Res 1988;62:204–215.

188. Hohlfeld T, Strobach H, Schrör K. Stimulation of prostacyclin synthesis by defibrotide: improved contractile recovery from myocardial 'stunning'. J Cardiovasc Pharmacol 1991;17:108–115.

189. Pacher R, Stanek B, Hulsmann M, Bojic A, Berger R, Frey B, et al. Prostaglandin E₁ infusion compared with prostacyclin infusion in patients with refractory heart failure: effects on hemodynamics and neurohumoral variables. J Heart Lung Transplant 1997;16:878–881.
190. Hulsmann M, Stanek B, Frey B, Berger R, Rodler S, Siegel A, et al. Hemodynamic and neurohumoral effects of long-term prostaglandin E₁ infusions in outpatients with severe congestive heart failure. J Heart Lung Transplant 1997;16:556–562.
191. Feenstra H, Grobbee DE, Mosterd A, Stricker BH-Ch. Adverse cardiovascular effects of NSAIDs in patients with congestive heart failure. Drug Safety 1997;17:166–180.
192. Lang CC, Chomsky DB, Butler J, Kapoor S, Wilson JR. Prostaglandin production contributes to exercise-induced vasodilation in heart failure. J Appl Physiol 1997;83:1933–1940.
193. Mallat Z, Philip I, Lebret M, Chatel D, Maclouf J, Tedgui A. Elevated levels of 8-iso-prostaglandin F2 alpha in pericardial fluid of patients with heart failure: a potential role in vivo oxidant stress in ventricular dilatation and progression to heart failure. Circulation 1998;97:1536–1539.
194. Guazzi M, Melzi G, Agostoni P. Comparison of changes in respiratory function and exercise oxygen uptake with losartan versus enalapril in congestive heart failure secondary to ischemia or idopathic dilated cardiomyopathy. Am J Cardiol 1997;80:1572–1576.
195. Pfeifer M, Muders F, Luchner A, Blumberg F, Riegger GA, Elsner D. Leukotriene receptor blockade in experimental heart failure. Res Exp Med 1997;197:177–187.
196. Fleming I, Bauersachs J, Busse R. Paracrine functions of the coronary vascular endothelium. Mol Cell Biochem 1996;157:137–145.
197. Dembinska-Kiec A, Gryglewski T, Zmuda A, Gryglewski J. The generation of prostacyclin by arteries and by the coronary vascular bed is reduced in experimental atherosclerosis in rabbits. Prostaglandins 1972;14:1025–1034.
198. Chester AH, O'Neil GS, Moncada S, Tadjkarimi S, Yacoub MH. Low basal and stimulated release of nitric oxide in atherosclerotic epicardial coronary arteries. Lancet 1990;336:897–900.
199. Cohen RA, Zitnay KM, Haudenschild CC, Cunningham LD. Loss of selective endothelial cell vasoactive functions caused by hypercholesterolemia in pig coronary arteries. Circ Res 1988;63:903–910.
200. Förstermann U, Mügge A, Alheid U, Haverich A, Frölich JC. Selective attenuation of endothelium-mediated vasodilation in atherosclerotic human coronary arteries. Circ Res 1988;62:185–190.
201. Bonthu S, Heistad DD, Chappell DA, Lamping KG, Faraci FM. Atherosclerosis, vascular remodeling, and impairment of endothelium-dependent relaxation in genetically altered hyperlipidemic mice. Arterioscler Thromb Vas Biol 1997;17:2333–2340.
202. Sekiguchi N, Umeda F, Masakado M, Ono Y, Hashimoto T, Nawata H. Immunohistochemical study of prostacyclin-stimulating factor (PSF) in the diabetic and atherosclerotic human coronary artery. Diabetes 1997;46:1627–1632.
203. Aoyama T, Yui Y, Marishita H, Kawai C. Prostaglandin I₂ half-life regulated by high density lipoprotein is decreased in acute myocardial infarction and unstable angina pectoris. Circulation 1990; 81:1784–1791.
204. Kuehl FA, Humes JL, Torchiana ML, Ham EA, Egan RW. Oxygen centered radicals in the inflammatory process. In: Weissman G, ed. Advances in Inflammation Research, vol. 1, Raven, New York, 1979, pp. 419–430.
205. Steinberg D, Parthasarathy S, Carew TE, Khoo JW, Witzum JL. Beyond cholesterol: modification of low density lipoprotein that increase its atherogenicity. N Engl J Med 1989;320:915–924.
206. Kühn H, Belkner J, Zaiss S, Fahrenklemper T, Wohlfeil S. Involvement of 15-LOX in early stages of aterogenesis. J Exp Med 1994;179:1903–1911.
207. Kühn H, Belkner J, Wiesner R, Schewe T, Lankin VZ, Tikhaze AK. Structure elucidation of oxygenated lipids in human atherosclerotic lesions. Eicosanoids 1992;5:17–22.
208. Folcik VA, Nivar-Aristy RA, Krajewski LP, Cathcarrt MK. Lipoxygenase contributes to the oxidation of lipids in human atherosclerotic plaques. J Clin Invest 1995;96:504–510.
209. Gniwotta C, Morrow JD, Roberts LJ II, Kühn H. Prostaglandin F₂α-like compounds, F₂-isoprostanes, are present in increased amounts in human atherosclerotic lesions. Arterioscler Thromb Vasc Biol 1997;17:3236–3241.
210. Patrono C, Fitzgerald GA. Isoprostanes: potential markers of oxidant stress in atherothrombotic disease. Arterioscler Thromb Vasc Biol 1997;17:2309–2315.
211. Katz AM. Scientific insights from clinical studies of converting enzyme inhibitors in the failing heart. Trends Cardiovasc Med 1995;5:37–44.

212. Susic D, Nunez E, Frolich ED. Reversal of hypertrophy: an active biological process. Curr Opin Cardiol 1995;10:466–472.
213. Schrör K, Weber AA. Roles of vasodilatory prostaglandins in mitogenesis of vascular smooth cells. Agents Actions 1997;48(Suppl):63–91.
214. Lai J, Jin H, Yang R, Winer J, Li W, Yen R, et al. Prostaglandin $F_{2\alpha}$ induces cardiac myocyte hypertrophy in vitro and cardiac growth in vivo. Am J Physiol 1996;271:H2197–H2208.
215. Adams JW, Migita DS, Yu MK, Young R, Hellickson MS, Castro-Vargas FE, et al. Prostaglandin $F_{2\alpha}$ stimulates hypertrophic growth of cultured neonatal rat ventricular myocytes. J Biol Chem 1996; 271:1179–1186.
216. Gelyng NG, Pomounetskii VD, Sanfirova VM. Prostaglandins, cyclic nucleotides and heart adaptation to acute and chronic pressure overload. Biull Eksp Biol Med. 1979;88:525–528.
217. Hashimoto H, Ogawa K. Effects of sulfinpyrazone, aspirin and propranolol on the isoproterenol-induced myocardial mecrosis. Jpn Heart J 1981;22:643–652.
218. Kalkman EA, Van Suylen RJ, Van Dijk JP, Saxena PR, Schoemaker RG. Chronic aspirin treatment affects collagen deposition in non-infarcted myocardium during remodeling after coronary artery ligation in the rat. J Mol Cell Cardiol 1995;27:2483–2494.
219. Yu H, Gallagher AM, Garfin PM, Printz MP. Prostacyclin release by rat cardiac fibroblasts: inhibition of collagen expression. Hypertension 1997;30:1047–1053.
220. Weber DR, Stroud ED, Prescott SM. Arachidonate metabolism in cultured fibroblasts derived from normal and infarcted canine heart. Circ Res 1989;65:671–683.

13 Estrogen and the Heart

Jay M. Sullivan

INTRODUCTION

Premenopausal women have far fewer heart attacks than comparably aged men, and the incidence of cardiovascular disease increases after menopause: These facts were first commented upon in the 1930s. Since then, over 35 observational studies have reported that the total mortality rate and cardiovascular events rates of postmenopausal women who chose to take estrogen replacement therapy (ERT) is about 40–50% lower than women who go without hormone replacement *(1)*.

Perhaps the most significant unanswered questions about estrogen replacement are two. First, is the apparent benefit concerning total mortality and cardiovascular mortality entirely, or in large part, the result of selection bias, i.e., do women who choose to take hormone replacement also choose a healthy lifestyle that improves their survival? In support of this viewpoint are the observations that women who use estrogen are more affluent, have higher educational levels (the highest percentage of estrogen users is found among postmenopausal gynecologists), exercise more often, have lower body weights, use more alcohol, visit physicians more often, and undergo more screening tests. Although many epidemiologists do not believe that these factors have the power to account for the observed survival benefit, only prospective, randomized, placebo-controlled trials, such as the Heart and Estrogen/Progestin Replacement Study secondary prevention trial and the Womens' Health Initiative primary prevention trial, will provide a definitive answer to this question *(2)*. The second question is this: If indeed there is a cardiovascular benefit,

From: *Contemporary Endocrinology: Hormones and the Heart in Health and Disease*
Edited by: L. Share © Humana Press Inc., Totowa, NJ

Table 1
Estrogen: Possible Mechanisms for Cardioprotection

Related to lipoprotein metabolism
  Increased hepatic clearance of LDL
  Increased synthesis of apolipoprotein A_1 and A_2, decreased clearance of HDL
  Increased synthesis of VLDL and triglycerides[a]
Related to endothelial function
  Increased release of NO
  Increased expression of genes that encode for NO synthase (controversial)
  Decreased release of endothelin I decreased response to endothelin I
  Increase release of PGI_2
  Decreased formation of thromboxane A_2
  Increased endothelial proliferation
  Increased endothelial cell migration
  Increased capillary tube formation
  Decreased endothelial cell apoptosis
Related to oxidation
  Antioxidant properties
  Decreased formation of oxygen-derived free radicals
Related to coagulation
  Decreased plasma fibrinogen
  Decreased plasminogen activator inhibitor
  Antiplatelet effect
  Increased fibrinolysis
  Decreased antithrombin III[a]
  Decreased protein C[a]
Related to carbohydrated metabolism
  Increased insulin sensitivity
  Decreased blood glucose
  Decreased blood insulin
Related to ion channels
  Calcium channel blockade
  Potassium channel opening
Related to arterial wall
  Vasodilation (decreased vasospasm)
  Decreased myointimal proliferation
  Decreased uptake of LDL

[a]Potentially adverse effect.

what are the mechanisms by which estrogen exerts this effect on the heart and blood vessels? This chapter will attempt to summarize the extensive investigation that has taken place in this field in recent years (Table 1).

THE ESTROGEN RECEPTOR AND RECEPTOR-MEDIATED EFFECTS

Much of the understanding of the physiologic effects of estrogen comes from studies of estrogen target organs, the breast and the female genital tract, in which specific estrogen receptors (ERs) have been identified. However, it is now clear that estrogens have an affect on many body tissues, and, in fact, specific ERs have been found in several tissues, including the vascular system, where ERs have been identified in endothelial cells (ECs) and in vascular smooth muscle cells (VSMCs) *(3–6)*.

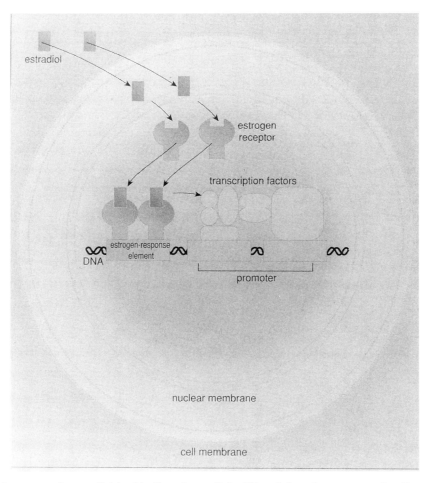

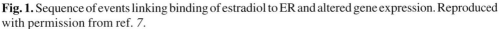

Fig. 1. Sequence of events linking binding of estradiol to ER and altered gene expression. Reproduced with permission from ref. 7.

Estrogen is a steroid hormone produced in the ovaries, testes, and adrenals (7). It is secreted into the blood stream, where it travels to target tissues. Because estrogen is lipid-soluble, it freely passes through cell membranes and nuclear membranes. Within the nucleus, estrogen binds to a specific ER (Fig. 1). The receptor has specific sites, one of which binds its ligand, estrogen; the other binds to DNA. Two ER complexes form a dimer, which then binds to a specific estrogen response element on chromosomal DNA. The dimer interacts with transcription factors on an adjacent promoter region, which then changes the behavior of the gene, activating, suppressing, or altering the transcription of mRNA, which, in turn, alters translation to proteins that influence cell physiology.

Recent studies have discovered that more than one type of ER exists. The previously identified receptors in heart, uterus, and elsewhere have been designated ER-α. The second receptor, which to date has been identified in prostate, brain, and blood vessels, is called ER-β (8,9). Much work remains to be done to uncover the distribution and function of the two types of receptors.

ER-α is believed to mediate inhibition of the migration and growth of VSMCs, regulation of gene expression in vascular tissues, protection from vascular injury, and inhibition of atherosclerotic plaque growth.

NONGENOMIC EFFECTS
OF ESTROGEN IN THE CARDIOVASCULAR SYSTEM

Studies in experimental animals and in humans have demonstrated vascular effects of estradiol (E_2) occurring in a few minutes, which is believed to be too short a time period to be mediated by the sequence of ER-mediated events outlined earlier. This has led to studies of the nongenomic effects of estrogen on the blood vessel wall *(10)*.

E_2, in micromolar concentrations, will relax segments of human umbilical arteries in vitro within 5 min *(11)*. In studies of the isolated rabbit heart with coronary spasm induced by vasopressin, E_2 caused prompt vasodilation *(12)*. Precontracted segments of human coronary arteries are promptly relaxed by 17β-estradiol *(13)*.

In a classic experiment, Harder and Coulson *(14)* isolated coronary arteries from dogs and measured electrical properties of the vascular membrane. Fifteen min after addition of diethylstilbestrol, they observed a hyperpolarizing response, which, they concluded, was caused by opening potassium channels. Compounds with this property are now being developed as antihypertensive agents.

Jiang et al. *(15)*, in studies of isolated guinea pig cardiac myocytes, examined the effect of 17β-estradiol on contraction, calcium (Ca) current, and intracellular free Ca concentration, and concluded that E_2, in micromolar concentrations, acted as voltage-dependent Ca channel blocking agent, which contributed to its vasodilating properties. Because experimental results were similar whether or not ECs were present, they concluded that E_2 has vasodilator effects that are endothelial-independent.

EFFECT OF ESTROGEN ON ENDOTHELIAL FUNCTION

It is now recognized that ECs comprise the largest organ in the body, and play an extremely important role in the function of the cardiovascular system. Endothelium contributes to the regulation of vascular tone by releasing two relaxing factors, nitric oxide (NO) and prostaglandin I_2, and two constricting factors, endothelin and thromboxane A_2 *(16)*. NO is derived from L-arginine by the action of NO synthase, and contributes to the maintenance of resting vascular tone in healthy subjects, as well as to the increases in blood flow during exercise via flow-mediated vasodilitation *(17)*.

Healthy ECs also prevent the adherence of platelets, which initiates thrombus formation, and monocytes, which initiates the growth of atherosclerotic plaques. In addition, ECs inhibit the migration and proliferation of VSMCs and the uptake of low-density lipoprotein (LDL), which contributes to the growth of atherosclerotic plaques *(16)*.

A number of disorders that are known to be associated with atherosclerosis have been found to have an adverse effect on endothelial function. These include cigarette smoking, hypertension, diabetes mellitus, hypercholesterolemia, and estrogen deficiency *(16)*.

An early event in the impairment of endothelial function is the expression of adhesion molecules on the EC surface *(18)*. These molecules attach to receptor sites on monocytes and lymphocytes, which cause them to adhere to the EC and migrate between the cells into the blood vessel wall, where they become macrophages capable of injesting oxidized LDL, becoming foam cells, necrosing because of the toxic effects of oxidized LDL, and forming a lipid pool. If this pool continues to expand, the thin fibrous cap which overlies the pool can rupture, expose thrombogenic material, and lead to intra-arterial thrombus formation, which occludes the coronary artery and causes a myocardial infarction (MI).

Expression of adhesion molecules by ECs is inhibited by 17β-estradiol. In studies using cultured human umbilical vein ECs, Caulin-Glaser et al. *(19)* examined the effect of 17β- and 17α-estradiol on expression of adhesion molecules after activation by cytokine, interleukin I (IL-1). They found that 17β-estradiol inhibited IL-1-mediated membrane E-selectin and vascular cell adhesion molecule-1 induction and intercellular adhesion molecular-1 hyperinduction by 60–80%. This effect was specific to 17β-estradiol; 17α-estradiol had no effect, and it was receptor mediated, because the specific ER antagonist, ICI 164,384, blocked the effect of 17β-estradiol. Thus, one mechanism by which estrogen might prevent cardiovascular events is by preventing one of the first steps in initiation of the atherosclerotic plaque.

The effects of estrogen on endothelial release of relaxing factor or NO has received extensive study. Acetylcholine (ACh) and several other vasoactive compounds stimulate the endothelium to release a relaxing factor, NO *(17,20)*, which in turn stimulates the enzyme guanyl cyclase to form more cyclic guanine monophosphate. Interactions with Ca result in vasodilatation. Ludmer et al. *(21)* used quantitative coronary arteriography to study endothelial function in patients with and without coronary artery disease. Graded concentrations of ACh and nitroglycerin were infused into the left anterior descending artery of eight patients with severe coronary artery disease, four patients with angiographically normal coronary vessels, and six patients with mild atherosclerosis occluding less than 20% of the vessel diameter. In normal arteries, ACh resulted in dose-dependent dilatation. In eight patients with severe coronary artery disease, ACh resulted in a dose-dependent constriction to about 30% of the initial diameter. However, in normal subjects, the maximum dose of ACh caused an 11% increase in vessel diameter. In the subjects with mild disease, 5 of the 6 vessels studied displayed constriction after ACh. The response to ACh was contrasted with the response to nitroglycerin, a nonendothelium-dependent vasodilator that dilated all vessels studied. The authors concluded that endothelial function was impaired in atherosclerotic vessels.

Williams et al. *(22)* conducted a similar study in nonhuman primates. Twelve cynomolgus macaque monkeys underwent bilateral ovariectomy. They were fed a high-fat diet for 30 mo. Six monkeys were treated for the final 26 mo with subcutaneous 17β-estradiol. Six monkeys served as a control group, and received vehicle. Coronary arteriography was performed under anesthesia and coronary artery diameter was measured at rest and after intracoronary infusions of ACh and nitroglycerin.

ACh ($1 \times 10^{-6} M$) caused constriction of coronary arteries to about 50% of their initial diameter in the estrogen-deficient monkeys, but resulted in 25% dilatation in the estrogen treated monkeys. ERT was also associated with reduced atherosclerotic plaque extent. However, size of plaque did not explain the altered vasomotion.

Herrington et al. *(23)* studied the effect of ERT on ACh response in women undergoing coronary arteriography. Endothelial function was assessed in 19 vessel segments from seven postmenopausal women with mild coronary artery disease. Intracoronary infusions of ACh were given in doses of 10^{-8}, 10^{-7}, and $10^{-6} M$. The percent change in coronary diameter was measured at baseline, and again after each infusion, by quantitative coronary arteriography. The responses of three women who were receiving ERT were compared with the diameter changes observed in seven segments from four women not receiving ERT. Dose-dependent relaxation was observed in the women receiving ERT, and dose-dependent vasoconstriction was seen in the four women not receiving estrogen therapy.

A more detailed study was reported by Reis et al. *(24)* in 15 postmenopausal women undergoing coronary arteriography. These investigators measured changes of coronary flow, resistance, and cross-sectional area in response to ACh before, and 15 min after, ethinyl estradiol, 35 µg, was given intravenously. The effect of estrogen on baseline parameters was compared to the response to placebo infusion in 33 women. This study found that estrogen altered basal coronary vasomotor tone in 22 women, increasing flow by about 23%. This was accompanied by a 15% decrease in coronary vascular resistance and a 20% increase in the cross-sectional area of the larger epicardial vessels. Administration of placebo to 11 women resulted in no change in these measurements. Estrogen attenuated the vasoconstrictor responses to ACh in women with coronary disease. Seven women were selected who manifested a decrease in coronary flow in response to ACh of about 34%. Coronary resistance rose by 39%. Seven additional women were selected who had an abnormal decrease in cross-sectional area of the epicardial vessels in response to ACh. These changes were not seen after the administration of estrogen. There was a statistically significant difference in the ACh-induced flow resistance and cross-sectional area responses at baseline and after estrogen administration. The authors concluded that estrogen decreases basal coronary vasomotor tone and attenuates abnormal coronary vasomotor responses to ACh in postmenopausal women.

Gilligan et al. *(25)* studied the short-term effects of estrogen on coronary artery and microvascular resistance in 20 postmenopausal women. They found no effect of intracoronary infusion of E_2 in physiologic doses on basal coronary tone. However, E_2 acutely potentiated endothelium-dependent vasodilation in both large coronary conductance arteries and coronary microvascular resistance arteries.

Collins et al. *(26)* compared the responses to intracoronary E_2 in postmenopausal women and men with atherosclerosis. After 20 min, intracoronary E_2 attenuated ACh-induced coronary artery constriction in nine postmenopausal women but not in seven men of similar age.

Blumenthal et al. *(27)* have found that long-term estrogen replacement reduces the response of coronary arteries to acute iv doses of estrogen (35 µg).

Thus, there is compelling evidence in both nonhuman primates and in human subjects to show that endothelial function is impaired during estrogen deficiency states, and that this impairment is diminished or corrected by the administration of estrogen, resulting in vasodilatation or less vasoconstriction in response to pressor stimuli. This potentially favorable effect on vascular tone is very likely to play a significant role in the cardioprotective effect of estrogen.

Estrogen has been found to have a number of other endothelial effects that are potentially important in the prevention of cardiovascular disease.

Morales et al. *(28)* studied the effect of 17β-estradiol on human umbilical vein EC behavior in vitro, and on angiogenesis in vivo. They found that 17β-estradiol caused ECs to increase their attachment to various surfaces, to increase cell proliferation by 3–5-fold, to increase migration into wounded areas by threefold, and to increase the organization of ECs into tubular networks. The effect on wound coverage and on tube formation were blocked by ICI 182,780.

Kim-Schulze et al. *(29)* also found that E_2 promoted proliferation of human umbilical vein ECs, and that the effect was receptor mediated, because it could be blocked by ICI 182,780.

In an interesting series of experiments, Spyridopoulos et al. *(30)* have demonstrated that E_2 protects ECs from apoptosis. They exposed human umbilical vein ECs to tumor necrosis factor-α, and reported that E_2 affected a dose-dependent, receptor-mediated inhibition of tissue necrosis factor-α-induced EC apoptosis, which may play a role in the preservation of endothelial integrity; this may, in turn, contribute to the atheroprotective effect.

A large body of evidence has accumulated to show that estrogen inhibits proliferation of vascular smooth muscle and reduces the myointimal proliferation that takes place after vascular injury. Many of these studies have used the rat carotid injury model. Chen et al. *(31)* have shown that estrogen replacement reduces myointimal proliferation after balloon injury to the carotid arteries of oophorectomized rats.

Iafrati et al. *(32)* have studied the effect of 17β-estradiol on the response to carotid injury in ER-α-deficient mice, and found that 17β-estradiol still inhibited the response to injury. They concluded that estrogen inhibits vascular injury by a novel mechanism that is independent of ER-α and probably involves other mechanisms.

EFFECT OF ESTROGEN ON VASCULAR VASOMOTOR TONE AND BLOOD FLOW

Estrogen increases uterine blood flow in animals *(33,34)* and in humans *(35)*. A fall in systemic vascular resistance has been reported in the ewe *(33)*. Estrogen increases aortic blood flow and cardiac output *(36)*. Intravenous estrogen increases resting coronary blood flow *(25)*, and improves or restores the vasodilatory effects of ACh in postmenopausal women *(24)*.

Intra-arterial 17β-estradiol, in a dose intended to increase venous E_2 to 300 pg/mL, did not vasodilatate the brachial artery, but enhanced the response to ACh *(37)*. These results are consistent with the findings of Sullivan et al. *(38)*, in which neither iv injection of conjugated equine estrogen in a dose of 25 mg nor 21 d of oral therapy at a daily dose of 0.625 mg caused vasodilitation of the forearm vessels.

Less is known about the effect of progestins on vascular resistance or reactivity, although most evidence suggests that progestins are vasoconstrictors and antagonize the effects of estrogens. Anderson et al. *(39)* noted that E_2 alone increased uterine blood flow in the ewe, and supplemental progesterone blunted the increase in blood flow seen with E_2. Batra et al. *(40)* studied the effects of estrogens and progestins on blood flow in the lower urinary tract of the rabbit, and observed that E_2 increased blood flow to the uterus, vagina, and urethra, and that progesterone treatment reduced the effect of estrogen. MaLauglin et al. *(41)* measured vascular reactivity in the hind limb of the pregnant ewe, and found that pregnancy and progesterone were associated with increased vascular reactivity to phenylephrine, but with decreased reactivity to angiotensin II. Laugel et al. *(42)* studied the effect of estrogen and progesterone on cochlear blood flow in the rat, and noted that progesterone pretreatment increased the pressor response to angiotensin II. In contrast, estrogen treatment decreased the pressor effects of phenylephrine and nicotine, but combined progesterone and estrogen increased blood pressure (BP) responses to phenylephrine *(43)*. Doppler studies in postmenopausal women showed that transdermal estrogen replacement increased uterine arterial flow, and that vaginal progesterone did not blunt this increase *(35)*. Another study, using similar techniques, found that the uterine artery pulsatility index fell with estrogen replacement, but was highest in estrogen users with progesterone added every month *(44)*. Another study found that pulsatility index fell by 47% with estrogen replacement, but only 34% when progestins were added *(45)*. Sullivan et al. *(38)* found that the addition of progestin increased forearm vascular resistance, decreased venous compliance, and increased pressor responsiveness to cold.

EFFECT OF ESTROGENS ON MYOCARDIUM

There are few studies of the effect of estrogen on cardiac performance. Schuer et al. *(46)* found that ovariectomy resulted in weight gain and decreased cardiac function in female rats. Estrogen or estrogen plus progesterone restored function.

Beyer, Yu, and Hoffmeister *(47)* studied the acute dose-dependent effects of iv 17β-estradiol on hemodynamics in the rat, and on isovolumic left ventricular generating capacity. They found that high doses of E_2 (200 ng/kg) decreased myocardial contractility, although cardiac output increased because of reduced total peripheral resistance. In studies of the effects of E_2 benzoate on anoxic resistance, Martin et al. *(48)* observed that the isolated right heart of gonadectomized, estrogenized female rats maintained the ability to generate evoked tension during 10 min of anoxia 2–3-fold better than gonadectomized rats that did not receive estrogen.

Delyani et al. *(49)* studied the effects of acute administration of 17β-estradiol on myocardial reperfusion in the cat. After 90 min of occlusion of the left anterior descending coronary artery, either 17β- or 17α-estradiol was given intravenously, and the heart reperfused 30 min later. In animals receiving 17β-estradiol, there was less cardiac necrosis, less myocardial polymorphonuclear neurophil infiltration, and less adherence of neutrophils to coronary endothelium than in the cats receiving 17α-estradiol. Hale and Kloner *(50)* also reported that 17β-estradiol reduced infarct size in rabbits, although there was no increase in myocardial blood flow, and no effect on systemic hemodynamics.

In studies of dogs subjected to 15 min of ischemia, animals pretreated with 17β-estradiol for 2 wk had fewer ventricular arrhythmias during reperfusion, maintained higher BP, and had more rapid systolic shortening and greater increase in coronary artery flow in response to ACh than those receiving vehicle *(51)*.

In studies of postmenopausal women, using Doppler echocardiography, Pines et al. *(36)* observed that there were significant increases in peak aortic flow velocity, mean acceleration, and ejection time after 2.5 mo of hormone replacement therapy (HRT), which they attributed to both increased inotrophism and vasodilatation. In later publications, they reported that each of these parameters continued to decline with time after menopause *(52)*. In a recent study, they reported that left ventricular cavity size and mass decreased with estrogen use, as did the increment in BP during dynamic or isometric exercise *(53)*. In contrast, Sbarouni et al. *(54)* found that iv conjugated estrogen, in doses of 0.625–1.25 mg, decreased heart rate and cardiac output, effects which they attributed to estrogen's Ca-blocking effect.

Myocardial contractility determines the extent and velocity of cardiac contraction from a given resting or end diastolic fiber length. The extent of contraction is dependent on the loading characteristics of the heart, i.e., preload and afterload *(55)*. Because of these circumstances, myocardial contractility is difficult to measure in humans or whole animals by noninvasive techniques. Isolated papillary muscles and isolated, perfused beating hearts are two models that allow precise control of preload and afterload. Using an isolated beating heart preparation, Sullivan et al. *(56)* found that 17β-estradiol had no significant effect on myocardial contractility in well-oxygenated hearts at baseline, during ischemia, reperfusion, or anoxia. However, they noted a trend toward longer preservation of contractility during ischemia in estrogenized hearts. It is possible that the higher doses of 17β-estradiol would have a greater effect. In contrast, Kolodgie et al. *(57)* reported that estrogen replacement in ovariectomized rats improved contractility after ischemia and reperfusion.

Large doses of sublingual E_2 have been found to increase exercise treadmill time to ischemia in women with ischemic heart disease *(58)*. However, another study found that chronic estrogen replacement did not significantly increase treadmill time *(59)*. In women without coronary disease, estrogen replacement did not improve exercise capacity *(60)*.

OTHER POTENTIAL MECHANISMS OF CARDIOPROTECTION BY ESTROGEN REPLACEMENT THERAPY

Analysis of data from observational studies initially suggested that the cardioprotective effect of estrogen was caused by estrogen-induced changes in serum lipoproteins *(61)*. After menopause, LDL levels rise while high-density lipoproteins (HDL) levels decline *(62)*, thus worsening the LDL:HDL ratio, which accelerates the development of atherosclerotic disease. Estrogen replacement results in lower levels of total cholesterol, decreased levels of LDL cholesterol, increased levels of HDL cholesterol, and increased levels of triglycerides *(62,63)*. However, recent epidemiologic estimates and experimental results suggest that no more than 25–35% of the cardioprotective effect of ERT can be explained by changes in serum lipids *(64)*.

Other mechanisms that have been considered have been the effect of ERT on lipoprotein (a) levels, which climb after menopause, and which are lowered toward normal by ERT or HRT *(65)*. ERT has also been found to impede the oxidation of LDL cholesterol *(66)*, which in turn could result in less cholesterol accumulating in arterial walls. In the nonhuman primate, ERT decreases the rate at which LDL is taken up by the blood vessel wall in postmenopausal animals fed a high-fat diet. Postmortem studies have demonstrated less extensive atherosclerosis in estrogen-treated postmenopausal monkeys, even when serum lipid levels do not change substantially *(67)*. ERT has also been shown to increase endothelial production of postaglandin I2, a vasodilating, platelet-repelling compound that should oppose the development of atherosclerosis, and to decrease formation of thromboxane A_2 *(68)*.

ERT has additional potentially favorable effects on carbohydrate metabolism, i.e., increased insulin sensitivity, and decreased plasma insulin and glucose levels *(69)*. Insulin resistance has been associated with high triglycerides, low HDL cholesterol, hypertension, and premature atherosclerosis.

Estrogen lowers BP, although perhaps not sufficiently to have clinically important effects on the development of atherosclerosis *(70)*.

The results of studies of the effects of ERT on components of the coagulation system are inconsistent *(71)*. After menopause, levels of fibrinogen and plasminogen activator inhibitor increase, and both have been found by epidemiologic studies to be associated with an increased risk of coronary heart disease. ERT lowers fibrinogen and lowers platelet activator inhibitor levels; however, it also lowers levels of antithrombin III and protein C, factors which oppose clot formation. Thus, there may be no net favorable or unfavorable effect of estrogen replacement. Estrogen replacement also enhances fibrinolytic activity.

CLINICAL EFFECTS OF ESTROGEN DEFICIENCY AND REPLACEMENT

In 1953, Wuerst et al. reported the results of a postmortem study showing that women who had both ovaries removed had significant coronary stenosis as often as men of the same age, but women with intact ovaries had fewer lesions until 10–15 yr after menopause *(72)*. The Framingham Study observed that the incidence of cardiovascular disease increased about fourfold in women who underwent menopause under the age of 40, and about twofold if menopause occurred after age 50 *(73)*.

Controversy continues about the effect of natural menopause on cardiovascular risk. It is clear that the risk of cardiovascular disease increases with age, but the magnitude of the contribution of the loss of ovarian function to this result remains a matter of debate. Although the Framingham Study found that the risk of cardiovascular disease increased in women who underwent natural menopause, other epidemiologic studies have not shown an increased risk *(74)*.

More than 35 observational studies have examined the effect of ERT on cardiovascular events and on all-cause mortality *(1,75)*. There have been 13 case-control studies using either hospital- or population-based controls. Ten of 13 studies found that women receiving estrogen had fewer cardiovascular events than those who did not. However, only one study was statistically significant. There have been 17 prospective cohort studies, using either internal or external controls. Sixteen of these studies found a protective effect of estrogens. The exception was the Framingham Study, which found an increased risk of cardiovascular disease in estrogen users, which might be explained by different ages and end points *(76)*.

Four laboratories have performed cross-sectional studies to examine the effect of ERT on the extent of coronary stenosis *(77–80)*. In all four studies, significantly less coronary disease was found in women who used estrogen replacement.

In one study, the effect of ERT on all-cause mortality in women who underwent coronary angiography was examined over a period of up to 10 yr *(81)*. Women who did not have coronary artery disease at baseline had a high survival rate, regardless of whether ERT was used. Five-yr survival was 98% in women who had never used ERT and in those who had used estrogen at some time since angiography. By 10 yr, survival was 91% in the never users and 98% in the ever users, a difference that did not reach statistical significance. Women who had coronary disease and used estrogens had a significantly better survival rate. The survival rate of women who had mild-to-moderate coronary disease was 85%; the group that used estrogen had a survival of 96%. The difference was greatest in the women with severe coronary artery disease, with 5-yr survival of 81% in the never users and 97% in the users, a difference that increased to 60% survival in the never users and 97% in the users at 10 yr ($p = 0.007$). In this study, Cox's multiproportional hazards model was used to estimate survival as a function of multiple covariables, and estrogen use was found to have a significant effect on survival that was independent of other risk factors.

Data from two other large prospective cohort studies support the concept that ERT is most effective for the secondary prevention of cardiovascular disease. The Lipid Research Clinics Study *(82)*, which included a cohort of 2270 women followed for an average of 8.5 yr, observed a mortality rate of 12.8/10,000 in estrogen users, who did not have clinical evidence of cardiovascular disease at baseline; the mortality rate was 30.2/10,000 in estrogen nonusers, which is a reduction of 58%. In women with prevalent cardiovascular disease, a 79% reduction was observed, with a death rate of 13.8/10,000 in the users and 66.3/10,000 in the women who did not use estrogen.

The Leisure World Study *(83)*, which included 8881 postmenopausal women followed over an average of 7.5 yr, found an all-cause mortality rate of 21.8/1000 for women without

RELATIVE RISK

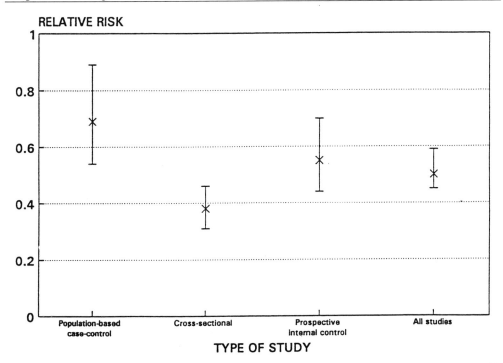

TYPE OF STUDY

Fig. 2. Relative risk of heart disease in women who are currently using estrogen. Reproduced with permission from ref. *1*.

a history of angina or myocardial infarction (MI) who used estrogen, and 26.7/1000 if they had not used estrogen, which is a reduction of about 18%. In those women who had a history of MI or angina pectoris, all-cause mortality was 41.7/1000 in the estrogen nonusers and 27.5/1000 in the estrogen users, or a reduction of 34%.

A meta-analysis by Grodstein and Stampfer *(1)* of all of the studies cited above found an overall reduction of risk to 0.64 (95% CI, 0.59–0.68) when estrogen users were compared to those who had never used estrogen replacement. A relative risk of 0.50 (95% CI, 0.45–0.59) was found in current users of estrogen (Fig. 2). Thus, the data are consistent that ERT is associated with a lower cardiovascular and total mortality rate, especially in current estrogen users.

Most of these studies have used estrogen alone. To avoid the risk of abnormal endometrial proliferation and endometrial cancer, estrogen is frequently given with a progestin. Because the addition of a progestin attenuates the increase in HDL cholesterol that follows estrogen administration, and the effect on HDL is believed to play an important role in the improved cardiovascular outcome, concern has arisen that the benefits observed in earlier studies are not relevant to current practice. Few studies have addressed this issue. Five studies have either used HRT (i.e., estrogen plus a progestin) or have compared groups who used HRT with those that have used estrogen alone. In the only published randomized trial of HRT, that of Nachtigall et al. *(84)*, medroxyprogesterone acetate was added to conjugated equine estrogen, and used to treat 84 pairs of hospitalized women. In this study, the risk of MI was lowered to 0.33. However, the result was not statistically significant. Hunt et al. *(85)*, conducted a prospective cohort study in the United Kingdom that involved 4544 women. In this study, the relative risk of death caused by cardiovascular disease in women using hormone replacement was reduced to 0.37 (95% CI, 0.15–0.58). In a population-based, case-control study, Thompson found no significant differences in the rate of MI or stroke in women receiving hormone replacement *(86)*. In contrast, a Swedish study observed approximately equal reductions in the risk of first MI or stroke when women who received ERT were compared to those receiving estrogens plus progestin *(87)*. In the Puget Sound area, Psaty et al. *(88)* found that ERT lowered the relative risk of MI to 0.69 (95% CI, 0.02–0.47). Women who were receiving estrogen plus progestin had a similar reduction of risk to 0.68 (95% CI, 0.38–1.22).

Recently, 16-year follow-up data from the 59,337 participants of the Nurses' Health Study showed that the relative risk for major coronary heart disease was 0.39 (95% CI, 0.19–0.78) when women who used estrogen and progestin were compared with women who did not receive HRT. The relative risk in those who used estrogens alone was 0.60 (95% CI, 0.43–0.83) *(89)*. Therefore, although the evidence is limited, that available so far does not suggest that the addition of progestins eliminates the effect of ERT on cardiovascular risk.

REFERENCES

1. Grodstein F, Stampfer M. Epidemiology of coronary heart disease and estrogen replacement in post-menopausal women. Prog Carciovasc Dis 1995;38:199–210.
2. Rich-Edwards JW, Hennekens CH. Postmenopausal hormones and coronary heart disease. Curr Opin Cardiol 1996;11:440–446.
3. Colburn P, Buonassis V. Estrogen-binding sites in endothelial cell cultures. Science 1978;201:817–819.
4. Orimo A, Inoue S, Ikegami A, Hosoi T, Akeshela M, Ouchi Y. Vascular smooth muscle cells as target for estrogen. Biochem Biophys Res Commun 1993;195:730–736.
5. Karas RH, Patterson BL, Mendelsohn ME. Human vascular smooth muscle cells contain functional estrogen receptor. Circulation 1994;89:1943–1950.
6. Venkov CD, Rankin AB, Vaughan DE. Identification of authentic estrogen receptor in cultured endothelial cells: a potential mechanism for steroid hormone regulation of endothelial function. Circulation 1996;94:727–733.
7. McLachlan JA, Arnold SF. Environmental estrogens. Am Sci 1996;84:452–461.
8. Kuiper GGJM, Enmark E, Pelto-Huikko M, Nilsson S, Gustafsson JA. Cloning of a novel estrogen receptor expressed in rat prostate and ovary. Proc Natl Acad Sci USA 1996;93:5925–5930.
9. Mosselman S, Polman J, Dijkema R. ERβ: identification and characterization of a novel human estrogen receptor. FEBS Lett 1996;392:49–53.
10. Farhat MY, Abi-Younes S, Ramwell PW. Non-genomic effects of estrogen and the vessel wall. Biochem Pharmacol 1996;51:571–576.
11. De Sa M, Meirelles R. Vasodilating effect of estrogen on the human umbilical artery. Gynecol Invest 1977;8:307–313.
12. Raddino R, Manca C, Poli E, Bolognesi R, Visioli O. Effects of 17β-estradiol on the isolated rabbit heart. Arch Int Pharmaco-dyn 1986;281:57–65.
13. Mügge A, Riedel M, Barton M, Kuhn M, Lichtlen PR. Endothelium independent relaxation of human coronary arteries by 17β-oestradiol in vitro. Cardiovasc Res 1993;27:1939–1942.
14. Harder D, Coulson P. Estrogen receptors and effects of estrogen on membrane electrical properties of coronary vascular smooth muscle. J Cell Physiol 1979;100:375–382.
15. Jiang C, Poole-Wilson PA, Sarrel PM, Mochizuki S, Collins P, MacLeod KT. Effect of 17β-oestradiol on contraction, Ca^{2+} current and intracellular free CA^{2+} in guinea-pig isolated cardiac myocytes. Br J Pharmacol 1992;106:739–745.
16. Vane JR, Anggard EE, Botting RM. Regulatory functions of the vascular endothelium. N Engl J Med 1990;323:27–36.
17. Ignarro LJ, Byrns RE, Buga GM, Wood KS, Byrns RE, Chaudhuri G. Endothelium-derived relaxing factor produced and released from artery and vein is nitric oxide. Proc Natl Acad Sci USA 1987;84:9265–9269.
18. Ross R. Medical progress: the pathogenesis of atherosclerosis—an update. N Engl J Med 1986;314:488–500.

19. Caulin-Glaser T, Watson CA, Pardi R, Bender JR. Effects of 17β-estradiol on cytokine-induced endothelial cell adhesion molecule expression. J Clin Invest 1996;98:36–42.

20. Furchgott RF, Cherry PD, Zawadzki J, Jothianandan D. Endothelial cells as mediators of vasodilation of arteries. J Cardiovasc Pharmacol 1984;6(Suppl 2):S336–S343.

21. Ludmer PL, Selwyn AP, Shook TL, Wayne RR, Mudge GH, Alexander RW, Ganz P. Paradoxical vasoconstriction induced by acetylcholine in atherosclerotic coronary arteries. N Engl J Med 1986;315: 1046–1051.

22. Williams JK, Adams MR, Klopfenstein HS. Estrogen modulates responses of atherosclerotic coronary arteries. Circulation 1990;81:1680–1687.

23. Herrington DM, Braden GA, Williams JK, Morgan TM. Endothelial-dependent coronary vasomotor responsiveness in postmenopausal women with and without estrogen replacement therapy. Am J Cardiol 1994;73:951–952.

24. Reis SE, Gloth ST, Blumenthal RS, Resar JR, Zacur HA, Gerstenblith G, Brinker JA. Ethinyl estradiol acutely attenuates abnormal coronary vasomotor responses to acetylcholine in postmenopausal women. Circulation 1994;89:52–60.

25. Gilligan DM, Quyyum AA, Cannon RO. Effects of physiological levels of estrogen on coronary vasomotor function in postmenopausal women. Circulation 1994;89:2545–2551.

26. Collins P, Rosano GMC, Sarrel PM, Ulrich L, Adamopoulos S, Beale CM, et al. 17β-estradiol attenuates acetylcholine-induced coronary arterial constriction in women but not men with coronary heart disease. Circulation 1995;92:24–30.

27. Blumenthal RS, Brinker JA, Resar JR, Gloth ST, Zacur HA, Coombs V, et al. Long-term estrogen therapy abolishes acute estrogen-induced coronary flow augmentation in postmenopausal women. Am Heart J 1997;133:323–328.

28. Morales DE, McGowan KA, Grant DS, Maheshwari S, Bhartiya D, Cid MC, et al. Estrogen promotes angiogenic activity in human umbilical vein endothelial cells in vitro and in a murine model. Circulation 1995;91:755–763.

29. Kim-Schulze S, McGowan KA, Hubchak SC, Cid MC, Martin MB, Kleinman HK, et al. Expression of an estrogen receptor by human coronary artery and umbilical vein endothelial cells. Circulation 1996; 94:1402–1407.

30. Spyridopoulos I, Sullivan AB, Kearney M, Isner JM, Losordo DW. Estrogen-receptor-mediated inhibition of human endothelial cell apoptosis. Estradiol as a survival factor. Circulation 1997;95: 1505–1514.

31. Chen SJ, Li H, Durand J, Oparil S, Chen YF. Estrogen reduces myointimal proliferation after balloon injury of rat carotid artery. Circulation 1996;93:577–584.

32. Iafrati MD, Karas RH, Aronovitz M, Kim S, Sullivan TR Jr, Lubahn DB, et al. Estrogen inhibits the vascular injury reponse in estrogen receptor α-deficient mice. Nature Med 1997;3:545–548.

33. Magness RR, Rosenfeld CR. Local and systemic estradiol-17β: effects on uterine and systemic vasodilation. Am J Physiol 1989;256:E536–E542.

34. Clewell WH, Stys S, Meschia G. Stimulus summation and tachyphylaxis in estrogen response in sheep. Am J Obstet Gynecol 1980;138:485–493.

35. deZiegler D, Bessis R, Frydman R. Vascular resistance of uterine arteries: physiological effects of estradiol and progesterone. Fertil Steril 1991;55:775–779.

36. Pines A, Fisman EZ, Levo Y, Averbuch M, Lidor A, Drory Y, et al. Effects of hormone replacement therapy in normal postmenopausal women: measurements of Doppler-derived parameters of aortic flow. Am J Obstet Gynecol 1991;164:806–812.

37. Gilligan DM, Badar DM, Parrza JA, Quyyumi AA, Cannon OR 3rd. Acute vascular effects of estrogen in postmenopausal women. Circulation 1994;90:786–791.

38. Shala B.A, Sullivan JM. Patient with congestive heart failure. In: Messerli F, ed. The ABC's of Antihypertensive Therapy, 2nd ed. Author's Publishing House, New York, 1999.

39. Anderson SG, Hackshaw BT, Still JG, Greiss FC Jr. Uterine blood flow and its distribution after chronic estrogen and progesterone administration. Am J Obstet Gynecol 1977;127:138–142.

40. Batra S, Bjellin L, Iosif S, Martensson I, Sjogren C. Effect of oestrogen and progesterone on the blood flow in the lower urinary tract of the rabbit. Acta Physiol Scand 1985;123:191–194.

41. McLaughlin MK, Quinn P, Farnham JG. Vascular reactivity in the hind limb of the pregnant ewe. Am J Obstet Gynecol 1985;152:593–598.

42. Laugel GR, Wright JW, Dengerink HA. Angiotensin II and progesterone effects on laser Doppler measures of cochlear blood flow. Acta Otolaryngol 1988;106:34–39.

43. Laugel GR, Dengerink HA, Wright JW. Ovarian steroid and vasoconstrictor effects on cochlear blood flow. Hear Res 1987;31:245–251.

44. Pirhonen JP, Vuento MH, Makinen JI, Salmi TA. Long-term effects of hormone replacement therapy on the uterus and on uterine circulation. Am J Obstet Gynecol 1993;168:620–630.

45. Hillard TC, Bourne TH, Whitehead MI, Crayford TB, Collins WP, Campbell S. Differential effects of transdermal estradiol and sequential progestogens on impedance to flow within the uterine arteries of postmenopausal women. Fertil Steril 1992;58:959–963.

46. Scheuer J, Malhotra A, Schaible TF, Capasso J. Effects of gonadectomy and hormonal replacement on rat hearts. Circ Res 1987;61:12–19.

47. Beyer ME, Yu G, Hoffmeister HM. Hemodynamic and inotropic effects of estrogen in vivo. Circulation 1996;94:I–278.

48. Martin LG, Brenner GM, Jarolim KL, Banschbach MW, Coons DL, Wolfe AK. Effects of sex steroids on myocardial anoxic resistance (43537). Proc Soc Exp Biol Med 1993;202:288–294.

49. Delyani JA, Murohara T, Nossuli TO, Lefer AM. Protection from myocardial reperfusion injury by acute administration of 17β-estradiol. J Mol Cell Cardiol 1996;28:1001–1008.

50. Hale SL, Kloner RA. Estradiol, administered acutely, protects ischemic myocardium in both female and male rabbits. J Am Coll Cardiol 1995;25:189A.

51. Kim YD, Chen B, Beauregard J, Kouretas P, Thomas G, Farhat MY, et al. 17β-estradiol prevents dysfunction of canine coronary endothelium and myocardium and reperfusion arrhythmias after brief ischemia/reperfusion. Circulation 1996;94:2901–2908.

52. Pines A, Fisman EZ, Drory Y, Levo Y, Shemesh J, Ben-Ari E, Ayalon D. Menopause-induced changes in Doppler-derived parameters of aortic flow in healthy women. Am J Cardiol 1992;69:1104–1106.

53. Pines A, Fisman EZ, Shapira I, Drory Y, Weiss A, Eckstein N, et al. Exercise echocardiography in postmenopausal hormone users with mild systemic hypertension. Am J Cardiol 1996;78:1385–1389.

54. Sbarouni E, Kyriakides ZS, Antoniadis A, Kremastinois DT. Acute hemodynamic effects of estrogen administration in postmenopausal women. Am J Cardiol 1997;80:532–535.

55. Opie LH. Regulation of myocardial contractility. J Cardiovasc Pharmacol 1995;26(Suppl 1):S1–S9.

56. Sullivan JM, Miller LA, Upmalis DH. Effect of 17β-estradiol on contractility of the isolated, beating rat heart. Menopause. (submitted)

57. Kolodgie FD, Farb A, Litovsky SH, Narula J, Jeffers LA, Lee SJ, Virmani R. Myocardial protection of contractile function after global ischemia by hysiologic estrogen replacement in the ovariectomized rat. J Mol Cell Cardiol 1997;29:2403–2414.

58. Rosano GMC, Sarrel PM, Poole-Wilson PA, Collins P. Beneficial effect of oestrogen on exercise-induced myocardial ischaemia in women with coronary artery disease. Lancet 1993;342:1330–1336.

59. Sbarouni E, Kyriakides ZS, Nikolaou N, Kremastinos DT. Estrogen replacement therapy and exercise performance in postmenopausal women with coronary artery disease. Am J Cardiol 1997;79:87–89.

60. Lee M, Giardina EG, Homma S, DiTullio MR, Sciacca RR. Lack of effect of estrogen on rest and treadmill exercise in postmenopausal women without known cardiac disease. Am J Cardiol 1997;80: 793–797.

61. Walsh BW, Schiff I, Rosner B, Greenberg I, Ravnikar V, Sacks FM. Effects of postmenopausal estrogen replacement on the concentrations and metabolism of plasma lipoproteins. N Engl J Med 1991;325: 1196–1204.

62. Sacks FM, Walsh BW. Effect of reproductive hormones on serum lipoproteins: unresolved issues in biology and clinical practice. Ann NY Acad Sci 1990;592:272–285.

63. Colvin PL, Auerbach BJ, Case LD, Hazzard WR, Applebaum-Bowden D. Dose-response relationship between sex hormone-induced change in hepatic triglyceride lipase and high-density lipoprotein cholesterol in postmenopausal women. Metabolism 1991;40:1052–1056.

64. Bush TL. Epidemiology of cardiovascular disease in postmenopausal women. Ann NY Acad Sci 1990; 592:263–271.

65. Sacks FM, McPherson R, Walsh BW. Effect of postmenopausal estrogen replacement on plasma Lp(a) lipoprotein concentrations. Arch Intern Med 1994;154:1106–1110.

66. Sack MN, Rader DJ, Cannon RO 3rd. Oestrogen and inhibition of oxidation of low-density lipoproteins in postmenopausal women. Lancet 1994;343:269–270.

67. Adams MR, Williams JK, Clarkson TN, Jayo MJ. Effects of oestrogens and progestogens on coronary atherosclerosis and osteoporosis of monkeys. Baillieres Clin Obstet Gynaecol 1991;5:915–934.

68. Fogelberg M, Vesterqvist O, Diczfalusy U, Henriksson P. Experimental atherosclerosis: effects of oestrogen and atherosclerosis on thromboxane and prostacyclin formation. Eur J Clin Invest 1990;20:105–110.

69. Barrett-Connor E, Laakso M. Ischemic heart disease risk in postmenopausal women. Effects of estrogen use on glucose and insulin levels. Artheriosclerosis 1990;10:531–534.

70. Fowlkes L, Sullivan JM. Estrogens, blood pressure and cardiovascular disease. Cardiol Rev 1995;3: 106–114.

71. Nabulsi AA, Folsom AR, White A, Patsch W, Heiss G, Wu KK, Szklo M. Association of hormone-replacement therapy with various cardiovascular risk factors in postmenopausal women. N Engl J Med 1993;328:1069–1075.

72. Wuest JH Jr, Dry TJ, Edwards JE. The degree of coronary atherosclerosis in bilaterally oophorectomized women. Circulation 1953;7:801–809.

73. Lerner DJ, Kannel WB. Patterns of coronary heart disease morbidity and mortality in the sexes: a 26-year follow-up of the Framingham population. Am Heart J 1986;113:383–390.

74. Rich-Edwards JW, Manson JE, Hennekens CH, Buring JE. Primary prevention of coronary heart disease in women. N Engl J Med 1995;332:1758–1766.

75. Stampfer MJ, Colditz GA. Estrogen replacement therapy and coronary heart disease: a quantitative assessment of the epidemiologic evidence. Prev Med 1991;20:47–63.

76. Wilson PW, Garrison RJ, Castelli WP. Postmenopausal estrogen use, cigarette smoking, and cardiovascular morbidity in women over 50: the Framingham Study. N Engl J Med 1985;313:1038–1043.

77. Sullivan JM, Vander-Zwaag R, Lemp GF, Hughes JP, Maddock V, Kroetz FW. Postmenopausal estrogen use and coronary atherosclerosis. Ann Intern Med 1988;108:358–363.

78. Gruchow HW, Anderson AJ, Barboriak JJ, Sobocinski KA. Postmenopausal use of estrogen and occlusion of coronary arteries. Am Heart J 1988;115:954–963.

79. McFarland KF, Boniface ME, Hornung CA, Earnhardt W, Humphries JO. Risk factors and noncontraceptive estrogen use in women with and without coronary disease. Am Heart J 1989;117:1209–1214.

80. Hong MK, Romm PA, Reagan K, Green CE, Rackley CE. Effects of estrogen replacement therapy on serum lipid values and angiographically defined coronary artery disease in postmenopausal women. Am J Cardiol 1992;69:176–178.

81. Sullivan JM, Vander-Zwaag R, Hughes JP, Maddock V, Kroetz FW, Ramanathan KB, Mirris DM. Estrogen replacement and coronary artery disease— effect on survival in postmenopausal women. Arch Intern Med 1990;150:2557–2562.

82. Bush TL, Barrett-Connor E, Cown LD, Criqui MH, Wallace RB, Suchindran CM, et al. Cardiovascular mortality and noncontraceptive use of estrogen in women: results from the Lipid Research Clinics Program Follow-up Study. Circulation 1987;75:1102–1109.

83. Henderson BE, Paganini-Hill A, Ross RK. Decreased mortality in users of estrogen replacement therapy. Arch Intern Med 1991;151:75–78.

84. Nachtigall LE, Nachtigall RH, Nachtigall RD, Beckman EM. Estrogen replacement therapy II: a prospective study in the relationship to carcinoma and cardiovascular and metabolic problems. Obstet Gynecol 1979;54:74–79.

85. Hunt K, Vessey M, McPherson K. Mortality in a cohort of long-term users of hormone replacement therapy: an updated analysis. Br J Obstet Gynaecol 1990;97:1080–1086.

86. Thompson SG, Meade TW, Greenberg G. Use of hormonal replacement therapy and the risk of stroke and myocardial infarction in women. J Epidemiol Commun Health 1989;43:173–178.

87. Falkeborn M, Persson I, Adami HO, Bergstrom R, Eaker E, Lithell H, et al. Risk of acute myocardial infarction after oestrogen and oestrogen-progestogen replacement. Br J Obstet Gynecol 1992;99:821–828.

88. Psaty BM, Heckbert ST, Atkins D, Lemaitre R, Koepsell TD, Wahl PW, et al. Risk of myocardial infarction associated with the combined use of estrogens and progestins in postmenopausal women. Arch Intern Med 1994;154:1333–1339.

89. Grodstein F, Stampfer MJ, Manson JE, Colditz GA, Willett WC, Rosner B, et al. Postmenopausal estrogen and progestin use and the risk of cardiovascular disease. N Engl J Med 1996;335:453–461.

14 Androgen and Estrogen Effects on Plasma Lipids in Men

Carrie J. Bagatell and William J. Bremner

CONTENTS

ANDROGEN PHYSIOLOGY
EPIDEMIOLOGICAL STUDIES
EXPERIMENTALLY DECREASED AND INCREASED ANDROGEN LEVELS
    AND LIPIDS IN MEN
SUMMARY AND CONCLUSIONS
REFERENCES

It is widely appreciated that premenopausal women have a lower risk for coronary artery disease (CAD) than do men, and that this risk increases in postmenopausal women *(1,2)*. The effects of estrogens on plasma lipids and other factors affecting coronary risk in women have been studied extensively, and are reviewed elsewhere *(3–5)*. The contributions of gonadal steroids to coronary risk in men have received less attention. This chapter reviews the effects of androgens and estrogen on plasma lipids and relates these data to the increased coronary risk associated with male gender.

ANDROGEN PHYSIOLOGY

Androgens are 19-carbon steroid rings that have the capacity to initiate and maintain the development of male reproductive organs, secondary sexual characteristics, and reproductive function. Testosterone (T) is the most abundant circulating androgen in the human male. Smaller amounts of dihydrotestosterone (DHT) and adrenal androgens are also present in plasma. Adrenal androgens bind weakly to the androgen receptor, and have weaker biological effects than other androgens. At the cellular level, T may be reduced to DHT, a more potent androgen that may account for many androgenic effects, particularly in the prostate and in skin. T may also be aromatized to estradiol (E_2) by the aromatase enzyme complex. Aromatization may account for some of the differences in the physiological effects (including lipid-related effects) of T itself vs those of its alkylated derivatives.

T is degraded quickly by the liver; the half-life of native T is approximately 10 min *(6)*. In order to produce clinically useful preparations, T must be altered chemically.

From: *Contemporary Endocrinology: Hormones and the Heart in Health and Disease*
Edited by: L. Share © Humana Press Inc., Totowa, NJ

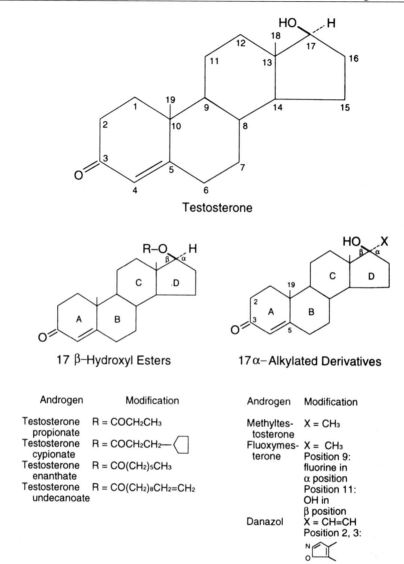

Fig. 1. Structures of testosterone and its derivatives. Reprinted with permission from ref. *5a*.

Esterfication at the 17-hydroxy position is a common modification. The resultant compound is more hydrophobic than native T, and it is released gradually from oily vehicles. After injection, T is hydrolyzed from the ester, and is metabolically identical to the endogenous hormone. Hydrolysis of the esterified preparation produces fluctuating serum T levels. Supraphysiological T levels are achieved in the first few days after an injection, and fall toward or below baseline before the next shot. T enanthate and T cypionate are commonly used in clinical settings (Fig. 1). One ester preparation, T undecanoate (Fig. 1), has a very long aliphatic side chain, and is somewhat absorbable into the lymphatics, thereby initially avoiding the liver. T undecanoate can therefore be administered both parenterally and orally. However, it has lower bioavailability than injected esters *(6)*, and it must be taken several times each day. Although this compound is used in Europe, it is not available in the United States.

In the past few years, T patches have also been released for prescription usage. Both scrotally applied and nonscrotally applied vehicles are available. These forms of delivery offer more constant T levels and avoid the inconvenience of im injection. However, they are more expensive than other formulations.

T may also be alkylated at the 1 or 17 positions, giving rise to androgens that are more resistant to hepatic metabolism (Fig. 1). Many of these androgens are sufficiently resistant to degradation that they can be administered orally, and they form the basis of many anabolic steroids. Their metabolites are unlike those of endogenous androgens, and some of their physiologic effects differ from those of T esters. The alkylated androgens can cause hepatic dysfunction, and their clinical utility is therefore limited.

EPIDEMIOLOGICAL STUDIES

Plasma Lipids During Puberty, Adulthood, and Aging

Gender-related differences in plasma lipids and lipoproteins emerge around the time of puberty, when T levels increase in boys and E_2 levels increase in girls. Cross-sectional studies in boys have demonstrated that plasma high-density lipoprotein (HDL) levels decrease during puberty, and that low-density lipoprotein (LDL) cholesterol and triglycerides increase (7–9). In girls, plasma HDL and LDL levels change very little, and plasma triglycerides increase only slightly (26,27). Longitudinal studies show similar results (10–12). In general, adult males have lower levels of HDL cholesterol and higher levels of LDL cholesterol and triglycerides than do premenopausal women (13).

Cross-sectional data demonstrate that, after the age of 50, mean levels of HDL cholesterol increase slightly in men, and there is a decrease in the rate of rise in LDL cholesterol levels (14,15). T levels decrease with age in men (16,17), and this may contribute to the observed trends in lipid levels. An alternative explanation is that men with very low HDL and/or very high LDL cholesterol levels die of early cardiovascular disease.

Epidemiological Correlations Between Androgens and Lipids in Men

Over 20 cross-sectional reports of the relationships between androgens and plasma lipids have been published (18–39). Most of these studies report a positive association between serum T levels and plasma HDL levels. In only two studies (22,27) were higher T levels associated with lower levels of HDL; in three additional studies (19,24,37), there was no relationship. An inverse relationship between serum T and plasma triglycerides was observed in most of these reports.

EXPERIMENTALLY DECREASED AND INCREASED ANDROGEN LEVELS AND LIPIDS IN MEN

Suppression of Endogenous Androgens

Endogenous androgen production is markedly reduced by surgical castration or by hormonal suppression of T production. Furman et al. (40) reported that castrated men had higher levels of α-lipoproteins and lower levels of β-lipoproteins than intact men of similar ages. The development of gonadotropin releasing hormone (GnRH) analogs has offered investigators a means to suppress androgens experimentally. GnRH agonists initially stimulate the pituitary secretion of follicle-stimulating hormone and luteinizing hormone (LH), but, after a period of days to weeks, downregulation of the receptors occurs, and gonadotropin secretion decreases dramatically *(41)*. Because testicular production of T is dependent on LH stimulation, T levels decrease to near-castrate levels after a few weeks of agonist administration. GnRH antagonists also suppress gonadotropin and T secretion. However, their effect is immediate, with complete T suppression occurring within a few days after the initiation of the antagonist *(41)*.

GnRH agonists are used clinically in the management of advanced prostate cancer and other hormone-dependent conditions. In men with advanced prostate cancer, administration of GnRH agonist, together with an antiandrogen, significantly increased HDL cholesterol, with no change in very low density lipoprotein or LDL cholesterol *(42)*. The same investigators also reported *(43)* that men who underwent orchiectomy for their disease showed no change in HDL cholesterol, but apoprotein B (APO[B]) levels increased. They speculated that the more complete suppression of E_2 levels in the orchidectomized men accounted for the disparity in the lipid levels in the two groups.

These studies were conducted in older men with a co-existing illness, and the results may not be generalizable to the male population at large. However, studies of healthy men also suggest that suppression of endogenous androgens increases HDL cholesterol. Goldberg et al. *(44)* reported that, in volunteers receiving GnRH agonist for 7–10 wk with no androgen replacement, T levels fell profoundly; HDL cholesterol, apo A1, and Apo (B) levels increased. A second group of men in this study received agonist plus partial T replacement; their T levels were maintained at approximately one-half the baseline level. Modest increases in HDL cholesterol were noted toward the end of the treatment period. Byerley et al. *(45)* used a GnRH agonist to suppress androgens in normal men and then administered T at two different doses, resulting in serum T levels at the low and high ends of the normal male range. Plasma lipids were similar in the two groups of subjects, despite their differing T levels. These data suggest that the relationship between serum T levels and plasma HDL is not a linear one. That is, there may be a threshold below which serum T levels must fall in order to effect an increase in plasma HDL cholesterol.

The authors have used the GnRH antagonist, Nal-Glu, to study androgen effects on lipoproteins in healthy young men *(46)*. Initially 15 healthy men were studied. During the 6-wk treatment period, each man received either Nal-Glu sc daily, plus sesame oil placebo im weekly (Nal-Glu alone); Nal-Glu sc daily plus T enanthate, 100 mg im weekly; or placebo sc and im injections. Serum T and E_2 levels in men receiving Nal-Glu alone fell significantly within 3 d after the experimental regimen began; they reached the castrate range after 1–2 wk, and remained suppressed during the rest of the treatment period. Mean HDL cholesterol concentrations increased by 26% during the treatment period in these men ($p < 0.05$). Mean levels of HDL_2 and HDL_3 cholesterol increased by 63 and 17%, respectively, during the treatment period ($p < 0.05$), and mean apo A1 concentration increased by 17% ($p < 0.05$). Plasma lipids did not change significantly in the other treatment groups.

The authors later studied additional men in each of the treatment groups (total of 9 or 10 men per group). These data were similar with the larger number of men (Fig. 2). It was also found that administration of Nal-Glu, together with T, 50 mg/wk, resulted in no change in plasma lipoproteins (Fig. 2; Table 1). Pavlou et al. *(47)* reported that administration of Nal-Glu, together with subphysiological T replacement (25 mg im weekly) for 20 wk, resulted in a 25% increase in HDL cholesterol.

Few studies to date have reported on the effects of androgen suppression on lipoprotein (a) (Lp[a]). Henriksson et al. *(48)* reported a 20% increase in Lp(a) in a group of

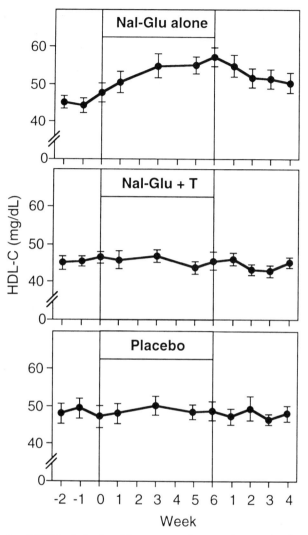

Fig. 2. Plasma levels of HDL cholesterol in groups of men who received one of the following regimens for 6 wk: Nal-Glu GnRH antagonist plus no androgen replacement (**top panel**; $n = 9$); Nal-Glu plus T enanthate 50 mg im weekly (**middle panel**; $n = 10$); or placebo injections of Nal-Glu and testosterone (**bottom panel**; $n = 9$). Reprinted with permission from ref. *46a*.

Table 1
Levels of T and E_2 and Resulting Changes in HDL and HDL_2
Cholesterol in Studies Using Nal-Glu GnRH Antagonist in Healthy Men

Regimen	T level	E_2 level	HDL	HDL_2
Nal-Glu alone	↓↓↓	↓↓↓	↑↑	↑↑
Nal Glu + TE 50 mg weekly	↓	↓	No change	No change
Nal Glu + TE 100 mg weekly	No change	No change	No change	No change
Nal Glu + TE 100 mg weekly + Teslac	No change	↓↓↓	↓	↓↓

prostate cancer patients 6 mo after orchietomy, with no change in either HDL or LDL levels. In contrast, Arrer et al. *(49)* demonstrated a 48% reduction in Lp(a) in men with prostate cancer who received the GnRH agonist, buserelin, for 8 wk. Several of the 12 patients in the study had significantly elevated baseline Lp(a) levels, and the decreases in Lp(a) induced by buserelin were greatest in those patients. Neither HDL nor LDL cholesterol levels were affected, but apo B levels decreased with treatment. Denti et al. *(50)* reported a small but statistically significant increase in Lp(a) in a subgroup of patients receiving another GnRH agonist, goserelin, for 3 mo. The group as a whole showed no significant change in Lp(a) during therapy, but a subgroup of patients, who had slightly lower Lp(a) levels before treatment than did the other patients, showed a small but significant increase in Lp(a) after agonist administration.

Because all of these studies were small and the results were not stratified by patient Lp(a) isoforms, it is unknown whether patients in these studies had different Lp(a) isoforms that may have responded differently to androgen deprivation.

Androgen Administration in Delayed Puberty

Kirkland et al. *(9)* administered T enanthate for 3 mo to 14 boys, ages 13–16 yr, with delayed puberty. Each boy received a 100-mg injection once during the first month, and 200-mg injections monthly during the second and third months. Serum T levels reached the normal adult male range, and plasma HDL levels decreased by a mean of 7.4 mg/dL (0.2 mmol/L) after a 100-mg T injection, and by 13.7 mg/dL (0.35 mmol/L) after a 200-mg injection. The investigators then followed 12 of the boys during spontaneous puberty that followed the T injections. As serum T levels increased to the adult range, plasma HDL levels decreased by a mean of 12.0 mg/dL (0.30 mmol/L). Thus, increasing T levels during puberty appear to be directly linked to the decrease in HDL cholesterol observed during the same time period. The association is probably complex, because increased androgen production is also associated with increases in body mass, changes in body composition, and a variety of metabolic variables *(51)*.

Androgen Administration in Hypogonadal Men

Androgens are used therapeutically in postpubertal men with hypogonadism, and several groups have examined their effects on plasma lipids in hypogonadal men of varying ages. Sorva et al. *(52)* studied 13 young men with hypopituitarism and severe androgen deficiency who were treated with T enanthate. Plasma lipids and postheparin plasma hepatic lipase and lipoprotein lipase activities were measured before and after 1 and 4 wk of weekly T injections. Serum T levels after 1 wk were within the normal male range, and plasma HDL and apo A1 levels had decreased nonsignificantly. After 4 wk, plasma HDL and LDL cholesterol and apo A1 levels had decreased, although only the decrease in apo A1 was statistically significant. Postheparin plasma hepatic lipase and lipoprotein lipase activities increased significantly after 1 wk, although only hepatic lipase activity remained increased after 4 wk. These findings support the data of Kirkland et al. *(9)* and suggest that androgens stimulate postheparin plasma hepatic lipase activity, which in turn increases the catabolism of HDL cholesterol. In contrast, Jones et al. *(53)* studied 10 men with Klinefelter's syndrome who were receiving T ester implants. Blood samples were drawn 4–6 mo after implantation of a capsule (baseline), and then 1 and 4 wk after insertion of a new capsule. Serum T levels increased from 18.4 ± 4.0 to 34.1 ± 3.2 nmol/L after 4 wk, and a small increase in LDL cholesterol was observed, but

HDL and apo A1 and apo A2 did not change. However, plasma lipids in the hypogonadal state were not reported, and it is possible the pre- and postinjection values in these men were somewhat lower than the true baseline levels.

More recently, Ozata et al. *(54)* administered T injections or gonadoptropins to hypogonadal men with testicular or hypothalamic dysfunction. In both groups, T levels reached the normal male range after 3 mo of treatment. The authors reported no change in HDL cholesterol, apo A1, Lp(a), or triglycerides, but levels of LDL cholesterol and the HDL_2 subfraction increased significantly.

Although T levels do not decline uniformly with age in men, some elderly men do exhibit symptoms of hypogonadism. Recently, the possibility of androgen replacement in such men has been evaluated. In a double blind, crossover study, Tenover *(55)* administered T enanthate, 100 mg/wk, or placebo, for 3 mo, to 13 elderly men with mild but symptomatic hypogonadism. Mean serum T levels increased from 11.6 ± 0.4 to 19.7 ± 0.7 nmol/L during T administration. Mean plasma HDL levels and apo A1 levels decreased from 49 ± 3 to 44 ± 2 mg/dL and 135 ± 6 to 118 ± 6 mg/dL, respectively, and mean LDL levels decreased from 128 ± 7 to 113 ± 5 mg/dL ($p < 0.05$). In contrast, Morley et al. *(56)* reported no change in plasma HDL levels in older, hypogonadal males who were treated with T enanthate, 200 mg every 2 wk for 3 mo. LDL levels were not reported, but total cholesterol levels fell significantly. These studies were small and of limited duration, and longer and larger studies will be needed to better evaluate the lipid-related effects of androgen replacement in the elderly. Cardiovascular disease is a major cause of morbidity and mortality in older men, and these data will be important in evaluating the practicality of androgen replacement on a widespread basis.

Androgen Supplementation

EXOGENOUS TESTOSTERONE

In addition to their use as hormone replacement therapy, androgens are being explored as potential hormonal male contraceptive agents, alone *(57–59)*, or in combination with other hormonal agents *(47,57,60,61)*. In order to be acceptable to a large number of men, a potential regimen must be highly effective and reversible, and side effects, including adverse effects on other physiological systems, must be minimized. Anabolic steroids are being used by large numbers of athletes, from high-school age to the professional level. The metabolic effects of supplemental androgens are therefore of considerable importance.

The effects of exogenous androgens on plasma lipids vary considerably with type of androgen administered (aromatizable or nonaromatizable), and with the route of administration (oral vs parenteral). The lipid responses to both T esters and alkylated androgens have been examined under a variety of experimental paradigms.

Friedl et al., Thompson et al., and Zmuda et al. *(62–64)* administered T enanthate (200–280 mg im weekly) to normal men for 3–6 wk periods. Friedl et al. *(62)* reported that plasma HDL levels decreased by approx 5%, and LDL levels did not change. Thompson et al. *(63)* and Zmuda et al. *(64)* reported decreases in plasma HDL of 9 and 16% ($p < 0.05$ in each case), respectively. In the former study, LDL cholesterol levels decreased by 16% ($p < 0.05$), with no change in plasma triglycerides.

The authors have administered T enanthate (200 mg im weekly) to healthy men for up to 20 wk *(65)*, and found that HDL cholesterol levels decreased significantly within the first 4 wk of treatment. This suppression persisted until the period of T administration was completed; at the end of the treatment period, mean plasma HDL levels were 13% below baseline. Apo A1 and the HDL_2 and HDL_3 subfractions were also significantly suppressed during T treatment; LDL cholesterol and triglycerides did not change. Similar changes were observed by Meriggiola et al. *(66)* during 6 mo of T administration.

Bhasin et al. *(67)* have administered T enanthate, 600 mg weekly, or placebo for 10 wk to 43 healthy men. Some of the men also underwent a strength training program, and others remained sedentary. There was a trend for HDL cholesterol to decrease in all of the groups, but the decrease was significant only in a group receiving placebo. Neither LDL cholesterol nor triglycerides changed significantly in any of the men.

The reasons for the variability of HDL suppression under differing paradigms are unclear. The duration of treatment does not appear to be a major factor. The subjects' baseline HDL levels may affect the degree of HDL suppression seen during T administration, however. In the authors' study, and in the study of Zmuda et al. *(64)*, baseline levels were somewhat higher than in the studies of Bhasin et al. *(67)*, Friedl et al. *(62)*, and Thompson et al. *(63)*, and the degree of HDL suppression was somewhat greater in subjects with higher baseline HDL levels. The mechanisms underlying this effect are not known.

Despite the lack of change in LDL cholesterol generally observed with androgen administration, recent data demonstrate that androgens have a suppressive effect on Lp(a) *(68–71)*. In the authors' study *(68)*, and in the study of Zmuda et al. *(69)*, Lp(a) decreased significantly in response to T (mean decrease of 37% in the authors' study) in subjects whose baseline Lp(a) levels were elevated; in subjects with low baseline Lp(a) levels, little change was observed (Fig. 3). Anderson et al. *(70)* reported a reduction in Lp(a) of 25% in response to exogenous T; the magnitude of the decrease was similar, whether or not baseline Lp(a) levels were elevated. At present, it is unknown whether the reduction in Lp(a) induced by T administration has any effect on an individual's risk for CAD, particularly in the face of concurrent decreases in HDL cholesterol.

NONAROMATIZABLE ANDROGENS

Nonaromatizable androgens induce profound decreases in HDL cholesterol, particularly the HDL_2 density fraction, and in apo A1 and apo A2 *(62,63,72–75)*. Concurrently, LDL levels increase by 30–40% *(86,91,92)*. In two recent studies *(62,63)*, the effects of parenteral T enanthate and oral, nonaromatizable agents were compared directly. The marked suppression of total HDL, HDL_2, and apo A1, and the increase in plasma LDL observed with nonaromatizable androgens contrasted sharply with the more moderate suppression of these parameters by testosterone enanthate (Fig. 4).

Nonaromatizable androgens usage is associated with decreased plasma triglycerides in normal men *(75)*, and in hyperlipidemic subjects *(76,77)*. Lp(a) levels decrease by 65–80% in women treated with danazol *(78)* or stanozolol *(79)*, even though LDL levels increase concurrently. The clinical significance of decreased Lp(a), in the face of increased LDL and/or decreased HDL levels, is unknown, however, especially in subjects whose baseline Lp(a) levels are low.

Estrogen and Plasma Lipoproteins in Men

Total serum estradiol levels in normal men are nearly 1000-fold lower than are total serum T levels; the normal range for E_2 is approx 10 to 40 pg/mL; the normal range for serum T is approx 2.80 to 10 ng/mL. However, although endogenous E_2 levels in men are very low, it has been demonstrated that circulating E_2 in men is important in maintaining

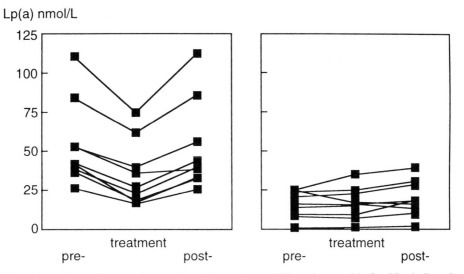

Fig. 3. Lp(a) levels in 19 men who received T enanthate, 200 mg im weekly for 20 wk. Reprinted with permission from ref. *68.*

HDL levels, particularly the HDL_2 subfraction, in normal men *(80)*. Using the same approach as in the studies cited above, the authors administered Nal-Glu together with T enanthate, 100 mg im weekly, to healthy men for 6 wk. Another group of men received Nal-Glu together with the same dosage of T; in addition, they were given testolactone (Teslac, Bristol-Meyers) orally. Testolactone is an aromatase inhibitor and inhibits the conversion of T to E_2 in peripheral tissues. Thus, the men who received Teslac (Squibb, Princeton, NJ) had normal T levels, but markedly suppressed E_2 levels. After 6 wk of treatment, plasma HDL, especially the HDL_2 subfraction, was suppressed significantly in men who received Teslac; these parameters were not suppressed significantly in the other men (Table 1).

As discussed shortly, when T is given exogenously, aromatization to E_2 appears to be important in mitigating the androgen's suppressive effect on HDL cholesterol. This process may not be as important in mediating the suppression of Lp(a) observed with T administration, however. Zmuda et al. *(69)* have shown that exogenous, supraphysiological doses of T alone suppress Lp(a) to approximately the same extent, whether or not aromatization is inhibited by testolactone.

Administration of E_2 to men suppresses endogenous T production, and therefore, studies of E_2 administration to men have been largely limited to studies of men receiving E_2 as therapy for prostate cancer. Several studies *(43,71,81–83)* have demonstrated that E_2 administration is associated with significantly increased levels of HDL cholesterol, apo A1, and triglycerides, along with significantly decreased LDL cholesterol. Because of the concurrent androgen suppression in these studies, it is unknown what percentage of the observed changes in lipoproteins results from an effect of E_2 itself, and what percentage results from T suppression.

Two reports of E_2 effects on Lp(a) have been published to date. Both studies were conducted by the same researchers, using elderly men with prostate cancer as subjects. The studies differ, in that in the first study *(48)* combined oral and parenteral E_2 therapy was administered, but in the second study *(71)*, parental E_2 alone was administered. Lp(a)

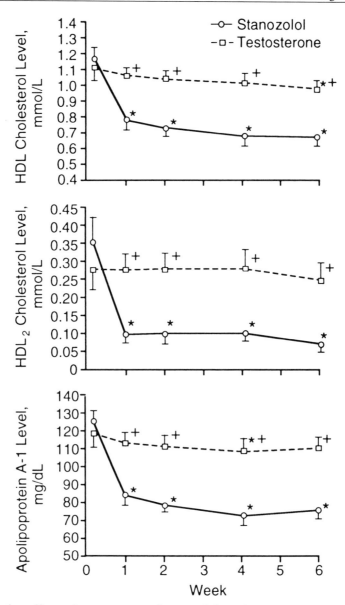

Fig. 4. Contrasting effects of testosterone and stanozolol on plasma lipoprotein levels. Reprinted with permission from ref. *63*.

levels decreased by nearly 50% in patients receiving both oral and parenteral E_2, but there was no change in Lp(a) in men receiving only parenteral hormone. Basal Lp(a) levels were higher in the latter group. Serum T levels were suppressed to similar, very low levels in both groups. The authors speculated that the more potent effect of oral estrogen on the liver contributed to its greater effect on Lp(a).

Ironically, these theoretically beneficial changes in plasma lipids have not resulted in improved survival nor in decreased cardiovascular morbidity and mortality. In patients with prostate cancer, administration of high-dose diethylstilbestrol and other estrogens has been associated with an increased incidence of cardiac complications *(84,85)*. In the Coronary Drug Project, conjugated estrogen was administered to patients with previous myocardial infarctions at doses of 5.0 and 2.5 mg/d. Both treatment arms of this study were discontinued because of the increased incidence of nonfatal cardiovascular incidents in patients receiving the higher dosage, and because of increased overall mortality in men receiving the lower dosage *(86,87)*. It is likely that in both clinical paradigms the thromboembolic properties of estrogen outweighed the beneficial effects of its lipid-lowering properties.

Mechanisms of Action

The decreases in HDL cholesterol, HDL_2, and apo A1 induced by androgens appear to be mediated at least in part by hepatic lipase. This enzyme contributes to the catabolism of HDL, and converts lipoprotein particles from the HDL_2 density fraction to the HDL_3 fraction *(88)*. Postheparin plasma hepatic lipase activity increases during administration of both T enanthate and anabolic steroids *(62,63,73–76)*, resulting in enhanced catabolism of HDL particles *(74)*. This increase is greater with nonaromatizable androgens *(62,63)*. An increase in postheparin plasma hepatic lipase activity precedes the decrease in HDL_2 cholesterol seen with use of stanozolol *(89)*, suggesting a causal relationship. Use of norgestrel, an androgenic progestin, is also associated with a dose-response relationship between hepatic lipase activity and plasma HDL_2 *(90)*. The triglyceride-lowering effect of anabolic steroids may also be mediated by increased hepatic lipase activity. Although lipoprotein lipase may also contribute to HDL metabolism, only one study has demonstrated increased lipoprotein lipase activity during androgen administration *(63)*.

The factors underlying the differing effects of the two types of androgens on HDL and postheparin plasma hepatic lipase activity have not been defined completely, but it is likely that differences in their routes of administration and their metabolic pathways contribute to the observed differences. Orally administered agents are absorbed into the portal circulation and are resistant to hepatic metabolism, and high hepatic concentrations of androgen can be demonstrated shortly after dosing. Hepatic lipase is found in highest concentration in the liver, and it is likely that high local concentrations of androgens stimulate its activity. At present, no androgen is available in both oral and injectable form, and so a direct test of the effects of route of administration is not possible.

Several studies strongly suggest that aromatization of T to E_2 accounts in part for the lesser suppression of HDL cholesterol by T esters. Estrogens, particularly oral estrogens, increase HDL cholesterol levels, particularly the HDL_2 density fraction *(91)*. This effect is caused in part by estrogen suppression of hepatic lipase activity, resulting in decreased catabolism of HDL particles *(92)*. When aromatizable androgens such as T enanthate are administered, plasma levels of both androgens and estrogens increase, and the net effect on postheparin plasma hepatic lipase activity is a mild stimulation. The role of aromatization in the regulation of plasma HDL has been demonstrated in studies by Friedl et al. *(62)* and Zmuda et al. *(64)*, in which T enanthate was administered to healthy volunteers for 3–12 wk. A separate group of volunteers received T enanthate at the same dosage, plus testolactone orally 4 times daily. Because testolactone inhibits conversion of T to E_2, E_2 levels in these men did not increase in response to T injection. In both studies, plasma HDL and apo A1 levels were suppressed, and postheparin plasma hepatic lipase activity increased more in the men who received T plus testolactone than in the men who received only T. The authors' study of physiological levels of E_2 in the regulation of HDL cholesterol in men *(80)* also demonstrates the importance of aromatization in moderating the suppression of HDL resulting from administration of T enanthate.

The mechanisms underlying the suppression of Lp(a) by both aromatizable and nonaromatizable androgens and by estrogen is unknown. Data in transgenic mice suggest that steroid hormones reduce Lp(a) gene expression (93), and the mechanism of suppression may be related to a general chemical property of gonadal steroids.

Significance

Could the physiological regulation of HDL cholesterol by androgens contribute to the difference in the incidence of CAD between men and premenopausal women? The magnitude of increase in HDL cholesterol induced by androgen deficiency is similar to the gender difference in HDL cholesterol levels between men and premenopausal women. In the Lipid Research Clinics prevalence study (15), HDL cholesterol levels at the fiftieth percentile were 22% (0.26 mmol/L) higher in women aged 30–34 than in men of the same age. As noted, there is a strong inverse relationship between plasma levels of HDL cholesterol and risk of CAD in epidemiological studies. It is therefore possible that suppression of HDL cholesterol induced by physiologic levels of androgens contributes to the known increased risk of coronary disease in men. Whether this risk is altered by androgen suppression of Lp(a) in some individuals is unknown.

Androgens and Nonlipid Risk Factors for Coronary Artery Disease

In addition to lipoproteins, a wide variety of factors contribute to overall risk for atherosclerotic disease. Full discussion of these factors and their androgen modulation is beyond the scope of this chapter. However, the net effect of androgen administration to hypogonadal men, particularly elderly men, may be influenced by T regulation of some of these other parameters.

Several studies suggest that T administration reduces both sc and visceral fat depots in the abdomen (94–96). Excess abdominal fat, especially in the visceral compartment, has been clearly linked to increased risk for CAD (97,98). Nonaromatizable androgens increase platelet aggregation (99) and have been implicated in case reports of myocardial infarction and cerebrovascular disease in young men (100,101). In contrast, recent work suggests that T enanthate decreases platelet aggregation (102). Through these mechanisms, in certain individuals, androgen administration may reduce risk for atherosclerotic disease.

Estrogen effects directly on the vasculature are well described and are believed to account for a significant portion of the overall reduction in cardiac risk attributed to estrogen usage (103,104). Much less is known about the direct effects of androgens on vascular structures, and data from human studies are lacking. Reports using animal models suggest that, like estrogens, androgens are vasodilators (105,106). However, androgens may stimulate intimal smooth muscle proliferation (107). Although one study in rabbits failed to demonstrate any proatherosclertotic effects of T administration (108), a study in cynomolgus monkeys reported that female monkeys treated with T implants developed significantly greater atherosclerosis than did control animals (105). It is unknown whether these data are generalizable to humans, and whether cardiac risk in an individual man is affected by androgen status.

SUMMARY AND CONCLUSIONS

Both androgens and estrogens are modulators of plasma lipoproteins in men. The effects of these two steroids on HDL cholesterol are opposite: Androgens generally have a suppressive effect on HDL; estrogens increase HDL cholesterol levels. In general, androgens have little effect on levels of triglycerides and LDL cholesterol, but estrogens decrease LDL levels and increase triglycerides. Both androgens and estrogens suppress Lp(a).

Males have a greater risk for CAD than do premenopausal women, and it is likely that androgens, primarily via their effect on HDL cholesterol, contribute to this increased risk. Estrogens are believed to be protective against the development of atherosclerosis in women. In men, high estrogen levels may increase risk of coronary events, probably because of estrogen's thrombogenic properties. However, physiologic levels of E_2 appear to have a beneficial effect on HDL cholesterol, particularly HDL_2 cholesterol. Similarly, the mildly supraphysiologic levels of E_2 that result from administration of exogenous aromatizable androgens mitigate the suppressive effect of androgen on HDL cholesterol.

The risk of an individual developing atherosclerosis is dependent on several factors in addition to lipoprotein levels. The effects of androgen administration on these factors have not yet been clearly elucidated. Nevertheless, the authors recommend that androgen replacement regimens and potential male contraceptive formulations be evaluated carefully for their effects on plasma lipoproteins, and agents that have the fewest adverse effects on plasma lipoproteins should be used preferentially.

REFERENCES

1. Castelli WP. Epidemiology of coronary heart disease: the Framingham study. Am J Med 1984;76A: 4–12.
2. Knopp RH. Effects of postmenopausal estrogen therapy on the incidence of arteriosclerotic vascular disease in women. Obstet Gynecol 1988;72:295–305.
3. Knopp RH, Zhu X, Bonet B, Bagatell CJ. Effect of sex steroid hormones and lipoproteins, clotting, and the arterial wall. Semin Reprod Endocrinol 1996;14:15–27.
4. Sacks FM, Gerhard M, Walsh BW. Sex hormones, lipoproteins, and vascular reactivity. Curr Opin Lipidol 1995;6:161–165.
5. Knopp RH, Zhu X, Bonet B. Effects of estrogens on lipoprotein metabolism and cardiovascular disease in women. Atherosclerosis 1994;110:S83-S91.
5a. Bagatell CJ, Bremner WJ. Androgens in men: uses and abuses. N Engl J Med 1996;334:707–714.
6. Wu FWC. Testicular steroidogenesis. Ballieres Clin Endocrinol Metab 1992;6:373–403.
7. Beaglehole R, Trost DC, Tamir I, Kwiterovich P, Glueck CJ, Insull W, Christensen B. Plasma high-density lipoprotein cholesterol in children and young adults. The Lipid Research Clinics Program Prevalence study. Circulation 1980;62(Suppl 4):83–92.
8. Berenson GS, Srinivasan SR, Cresanta JL, Foster TA, Webber LS. Dynamic changes in serum lipoproteins in children during adolescence and sexual maturation. Am J Epidemiol 1981;113:157–170.
9. Kirkland RT, Keenan BS, Probstfield JL, Patsch W, Lin TL, Clayton GW, et al. Decrease in plasma high-density lipoprotein cholesterol levels at puberty in boys with delayed adolescence. JAMA 1987; 257:502–507.
10. Freedman DS, Cresanta JL, Srinivian SR, Webber LS, Berenson GS. Longitudinal serum lipoprotein changes in white males during adolescence: the Bogalusa Heart Study. Metabolism 1985;34:396–403.
11. Morrison JA, Laskarzewski PM, Rauh JL, Brookman R, Mellies M, Frazer M, et al. Lipids, lipoproteins, and sexual maturation during adolescence: the Princeton maturation study. Metabolism 1979; 28:641–648.
12. Stozicky F, Slaby P, Volenikova L. Longitudinal study of serum cholesterol apolipoproteins and sex hormones during puberty. Acta Pediatr Scand 1991;80:1139–1144.
13. Crook D, Seed M. Endocrine control of plasma lipoprotein metabolism: effects of gonadal steroids. Ballieres Clin Endocrinol Metab 1990;4:851–875.
14. Heiss G, Tamir I, Davis CE, Tyroler HS, Rifkind BM, Schonfeld G, et al. Lipoprotein-cholesterol distributions in selected North American population: the Lipid Research Clinics Program Prevalence Study. Circulation 1980;61:302–315.
15. Lipid Research Clinics. Population Studies Data Book, vol. 1: the Prevalence Study. Dept. of Health and Human Services, 1980.

16. Gray A, Feldman HA, McKinlay JB, Longcope C. Age, disease, and changing sex hormone levels in middle-aged men: the Massachusetts male aging study. J Clin Endocrinol Metab 1991;73:1016–1025.

17. Vermeulen A. Androgens in the aging male. J Clin Endocrinol Metab 1991;73:221–224.

18. Barrett-Connor E, Khaw KT. Endogenous sex hormones and cardiovascular disease in men: a prospective population based study. Circulation 1988;78:539–545.

19. Duell PB, Bierman EL. Relationship between sex hormones and high-density lipoprotein cholesterol levels in healthy adult men. Arch Int Med 1990;150:2317–2320.

20. Norday A. Sex hormones and high density lipoproteins in healthy males. Atherosclerosis 1979;34:431–436.

21. Dai WS, Gutai JP, Kuller LH, Laporte RE, Falvo-Gerard L, Caggiula A. Relation between high-density lipoprotein cholesterol and sex hormone concentrations in men. Am J Cardiol 1984;53:1259–1263.

22. Semmens J, Rouse I, Beilin LJ, Masarec JRL. Relationship of plasma HDL-cholesterol to testosterone, estradiol, and sex-hormone binding globulin levels in men and women Metabolism 1983;32:28–32.

23. Heller RF, Wheeler MJ, Micalleff J, Miller NE, Lewis B. Relationship of high density lipoprotein cholesterol with total and free testosterone and sex hormone binding globulin. Acta Endocrinol (Copenhagen) 1983;104:253–256.

24. Kiel DP, Plymate SR. Sex hormones and lipoproteins in men. Am J Med 1989;87:35–39.

25. Khaw KT, Barrett-Connor E. Endogenous sex hormones, high density lipoprotein cholesterol and other lipoprotein fractions in men. Arteriosclerosis Thromb 1991;11:489–494.

26. Lichtenstein M, Yarnell JWG, Elwood PC, Beswick AD, Sweetnam PM, Marks V. Sex hormones, insulin, lipids and prevalent ischemic heart disease. Am J Epidemiol 1987;12:647–657.

27. Stefanick ML, Williams PT, Krauss RM, Terry RB, Vranizan KM, Wood PD. Relationships of plasma estradiol, testosterone, and sex hormone-binding globulin with lipoproteins, apolipoproteins, and high density lipoprotein subfractions in men. J Clin Endocrinol Metab 1987;64:723–729.

28. Freeman DS, O'Brien TR, Flanders WD, DeStafano F, Barboriak JJ. Relation of serum testosterone levels to high density lipoprotein cholesterol and other characteristics in men. Arteriosclerosis Thromb 1991;11:307–315.

29. Mendoza SG, Osuna A, Zerpa A, Gartside PS, Gleuck CJ. Hypertriglyceridemia and hypoalphalipoproteinemia in azoospermic and oligospermic young men: relationships of endogenous testosterone to triglyceride and high density lipoprotein cholesterol metabolism. Metabolism 1981;30:481–489.

30. Barrett-Connor E. Lower endogenous androgen levels and dyslipidemia in men with non-insulin dependent diabetes mellitus. Ann Int Med 1992;117:807–811.

31. Hamalainen E, Tikkanen H, Harkonen M, Naveri H, Aldercreutz, H. Serum lipoproteins, sex hormones and sex hormone binding globulin in middle-aged men of different physical fitness and risk of coronary heart disease. Atherosclerosis 1987;67:155–162.

32. Lindholm J, Winkel P, Brodthagen U, Gyntelberg F. Coronary risk factors and plasma sex hormones. Am J Med 1982;73:648–651.

33. Gutai J, LaPorte R, Kuller L, Dai W, Falvo-Gerard L, Caggiula A. Plasma testosterone, high density lipoprotein cholesterol and other lipoprotein fractions. Am J Cardiol 1981;48:896–901.

34. Miller GJ, Wheeler MJ, Price SGL, Beckles GLA, Kirkwood BR, Carson DC. Serum high density lipoprotein subclasses, testosterone and sex-hormone binding globulin in Trinidadian men of African and Indian descent. Athersclerosis 1985;55:251–258.

35. Deutscher S, Bates MW, Caines MJ, LaPorte RE, Puntereri A, Taylor FH. Determinants of lipid and lipoprotein level in elderly men. Atherosclerosis 1986;60:221–229.

36. Dioyssiou-Asteriou A, Katimertzi M. Endogenous testosterone and serum apolipoprotein (a) levels. Atherosclerosis 1993;100:123–126.

37. Oppenheim DS, Greenspan SL, Zervas N, Schoenfeld DA, Klibanski A. Elevated serum lipids in hypogonadal men with and without hyperprolactinemia. Ann Int Med 1989;111:288–292.

38. Hamalainen E, Aldercreutz, H, Ehnholm C, Puska P. Relationship of serum lipoproteins and apoproteins to sex hormones and to the binding capacity of sex hormone binding globulin in healthy Finnish men. Metabolism 1986;35:535–541.

39. Yarnell JWG, Beswick AD, Sweetnam PM, Riad-Fahmy D. Endogenous Sex hormones and ischemic heart disease in men: the Caerphilly prospective study. Arteriosclerosis Thromb 1993;13:517–520.

40. Furman RH, Howard RP, Imagawa R. Serum lipid and lipoprotein concentrations in castrate and noncastrate male subjects. Circulation 1956;14:490.

41. Karten MJ, Rivier JE. Gonadotropin releasing hormone analog design. Structure function studies toward the development of agonists and antagonists: rationale and perspective. Endocr Rev 1986;7:44–66.

42. Moorjani S, Dupont A, Labrie F, Lupien PJ, Brun D, Gagne C, et al. Increase in plasma high-density lipoprotein concentration following complete androgen blockage in men with prostatic carcinoma. Metabolism 1987;36:244–250.

43. Moorjani S, Dupont A, Labrie F, Lupien PJ, Gagne C, Brun D, et al. Changes in plasma lipoproteins during various androgen suppression therapies in men with prostatic carcinoma: effects of orchiectomy, estrogen and combination treatment with luteinizing hormone-releasing hormone agonist and flutamide. J Clin Endocrinol Metab 1988;66:614–621.

44. Goldberg RB, Rabin D, Alexander A, Doelle N, Getz GS. Suppression of plasma testosterone leads to an increase in serum total and high density lipoprotein cholesterol and apoproteins A1 and AII. J Clin Endocrinol Metab 1985;60:203–207.

45. Byerley L, Lee WN, Swerdloff RS, Buena F, Nair SK, Buchanan TA, et al. Effect of modulating serum testosterone levels in the normal male range on protein, carbohydrate, and lipid metabolism in men: implications for testosterone replacement therapy. Endocr J 1993;1:253–262.

46. Bagatell CJ, Knopp RH, Vale WW, Rivier JE, Bremner WJ. Physiologic levels of testosterone suppress HDL cholesterol levels in normal men. Ann Int Med 1992;116:967–973.

46a. Bagatell CJ, Bremner WJ. Androgen and progestagen effects on plasma lipids. Prog Cardiovasc Disc 1995;38:255–271.

47. Pavlou SN, Brewer K, Lindner J, Farley MG, Bastias C, Rogers BJ, et al. Combined administration of a gonadotropin releasing hormone antagonist and testosterone in men induces reversible azoospermia without loss of libido. J Clin Endocrinol Metab 1991;73:1360–1369.

48. Henriksson P, Angelin B, Berglund L. Hormonal regulation of serum Lp(a) levels. Opposite effects of estrogen treatment and orchidectomy in males with prostatic carcinoma. J Clin Invest 1992;89:1166–1171.

49. Arrer E, Jungwirth A, Mack D, Frick J, Patsch W. Treatment of prostate cancer with gonadotropin releasing hormone analogue: effect on lipoprotein (a). J Clin Endocrinol Metab 1996;81:2508–2511.

50. Denti L, Pasolinii G, Cortellini P, Ferretti S, Sanfelici L, Ablondi F, Valenti G. Effects of androgen suppression by gonaotropin releasing hormone agonist and flutamide on lipid metabolism in men with prostate cancer: focus on lipoprotein (a). Clin Chem 1996;42:1176–1181.

51. Mooradian AD, Morley JE, Korenman SG. Biological effects of androgens. Endocr Rev 1987;7:1–28.

52. Sorva R, Kuusi T, Taskinen M-R, Perheentupa J, Nikkila EA. Testosterone substitution increases the activity of lipoprotein lipase and hepatic lipase in hypogonadal males. Atherosclerosis 1988;69:191–197.

53. Jones DB, Higgins B, Billet JS, Price WH, Edwards CRW, Beastall GH, et al. The effect of testosterone replacement on plasma lipids and lipoproteins. European J Clin Invest 1989;19:438–441.

54. Ozata M, Yildirimkaya M, Bulur M, Yilmaz K, Bolu E, Corakci A, Gundogan A. Effects of gonaotropin and testosterone treatments on lipoprotein (a), high density lipoprotein particles, and other lipoprotein levels in male hypogonadism. J Clin Endocrinol Metab 1996;81:3372–3378.

55. Tenover JS. Effects of testosterone supplementation in the aging male. J Clin Endocrinol Metab 1992;75:1092–1098.

56. Morley JE, Perry M, Kaiser FE, Kraenzle D, Jensen J, Houston K, et al. Effects of testosterone replacement therapy in older hypogonadal males: a preliminary study. J Am Geriat Soc 1993;41:149–152.

57. Paulsen CA, Bremner WJ, Leonard J. Male contraception: clinical trials, In: Mishell DR, ed. Advances in Fertility Research. Raven, New York. 1982, pp. 157–170.

58. Matsumoto A. Effects of chronic testosterone administration in normal men: safety and efficacy of high-dosage testosterone and parallel dose-dependent suppression of luteinizing hormone, follicle-stimulating hormone, and sperm production. J Clin Endocrinol Metab 1990;70:282–287.

59. World Health Organization Task Force on Male Fertility. Contraceptive efficacy of testosterone-induced azoospermia in normal men. Lancet 1990;336:955–959.

60. Bagatell CJ, Matsumoto AM, Christensen RB, Rivier JE, Bremner WJ. Comparison of a gonadotropin releasing hormone antagonist plus testosterone (T) versus T alone as potential male contraceptive regimens. J Clin Endocrinol Metab 1993;77:427–432.

61. Bebb RA, Anawalt BD, Christensen RB, Paulsen CA, Matsumoto AM. Combined adminstration of levonorgestrel and testosterone induces more rapid and effective suppression of spermatogenesis than testosterone alone: a promising male contraceptive approach. J Clin Endocrinol Metab 1996;81:757–762.

62. Friedl KE, Hannan CJ, Jones RE, Kettler TM, Plymate SR. High-density lipoprotein is not decreased if an aromatizable androgen is administered. Metabolism 1990;39:69–77.

63. Thompson PD, Cullinane EM, Sady SP, Chevenevert C, Saritelli AL, Sady MA, et al. Contrasting effects of testosterone and stanozolol on serum lipoprotein levels. JAMA 1989;261:1165–1168.

64. Zmuda JN, Fahrenbach MC, Younkin BT, Bausserman LL, Terry RB, Catlin DH, et al. Effect of testosterone aromatization on high-density lipoprotein cholesterol level and post-heparin lipolytic activity. Metabolism 1993;42:446–450.

65. Bagatell CJ, Heiman JR, Matsumoto A, Rivier JE, Bremner WJ. Metabolic and behavioral effects of high dose, exogenous testosterone (T) in normal men. J Clin Endocrinol Metab 1994;79:561–567.

66. Meriggiola MC, Marcovina S, Paulsen CA, Bremner WJ. Testosterone enanthate at the dose of 200 mg/week decreases HDL-cholesterol levels in healthy men. Int J Androl 1995;18:237–242.

67. Bhasin S, Storer TW, Berman N, Callegari C, Clevenger B, Phillips J, et al. Effects of supraphysiologic doses of testosterone on muscle size and strength in normal men. N Engl J Med 1996;335:1–7.

68. Marcovina SM, Lippi G, Bagatell CJ, Bremner WJ. Testosterone induced suppression of lipoprotein (a) in normal men; relation to basal lipoprotein (a) level. Atherosclerosis 1996;122:89–95.

69. Zmuda JM, Thompson PD, Dickenson R, Bausserman LL. Testosterone decreases lipoprotein (a) in men. Am J Cardiol 1996;77:1244–1247.

70. Anderson RA, Wallace EM, Wu FC. Effect of testosterone enanthate on serum lipoproteins in men. Contraception 1995;52:115–119.

71. Berglund L, Carlstrom K, Reinhard S, Gottlieb C, Eriksson M, Angelin B, Henrikkson P. Hormonal regulation of serum liporotein (a) levels: effects of parenteral administration of estrogen or testosterone in males. J Clin Endocrinol Metab 1996;81:2633–2637.

72. Alen M, Rahlika P, Marniemi J. Serum lipids in power athletes self-administering testosterone and anabolic steroids. Int J Sports Med 1985;6:139–144.

73. Kantor MA, Bianchini A, Bernler D, Sady SP, Thompson PD. Androgens reduce HDL_2-cholesterol and increase hepatic triglyceride lipase activity. Med Sci Sports Exerc 1985;144:62–65.

74. Haffner SM, Kushwaha RS, Foster DM, Applebaum-Bowden D, Hazzard W. Studies on the metabolic mechanism of reduced high density lipoproteins during anabolic steroid therapy. Metabolism 1983;32: 413–420.

75. Taggart HM, Applebaum-Bowden D, Haffner S, Warnick GR, Cheung MC, Albers JJ, et al. Reduction in high density lipoproteins by anabolic steroid (stanozolol) therapy for postmenopausal osteoporosis. Metabolism 1982;31:1147–1152.

76. Hazzard WR, Haffner SM, Kushwaha RS, Applebaum-Bowden D, Foster DM. Preliminary report: kinetic studies on the modulation of high-density lipoprotein, apolipoprotein, and subfraction metabolism by sex steroids in a post-menopausal woman. Metabolism 1984;33:779–784.

77. Gleuck CJ, Swanson F, Fishbak J. Effects of oxandrolone on plasma triglycerides and post-heparin lipolytic activity in patients with types II, IV, and V hyperlipoproteinemia. Metabolism 1971;20:691–702.

78. Crook D, Sidhu M, Seed M, O'Donnell MO, Stevenson JC. Lipoprotein (a) levels are reduced by danazol, an anabolic steroid. Atherosclerosis 1992;92:41–47.

79. Albers JJ, Taggart HM, Applebaum-Bowden D, Haffner S, Chestnut CH, Hazzard WR. Reduction of lecithin-cholesterol acyltransferase, apoprotein D and the Lp(a) lipoprotein with the anabolic steroid, stanozolol. Biochim Biophys Acta 1984;795:293–296.

80. Bagatell CJ, Knopp RH, Bremner WJ. Physiological levels of estradiol stimulate plasma high density lipoprotein2 cholesterol levels in normal men. J Clin Endocrinol Metab 1994;78:855–861.

81. Erikson M, Berglund L, Rudling M, Henriksson P, Angelin B. Effect of estrogen on low density lipoprotein metabolism in males. J Clin Invest 1989;84:802–810.

82. Bulusu NV, Leis S, Das S, Clayton WE. Serum lipid changes after estrogen therapy in prostatic carcinoma. Urology 1982;20:147–150.

83. Rossner S, Hedlund P-O. Jogestrand T, Sawe U. Treatment of prostatic cancer: effets of serum lipoproteins and the cardiovascular system. J Urol 1985;133:53–57.

84. Blackard CE, Doe RP, Mellinger GT, Byar DP. Incidence of cardiovascular disease and death in patients receiving diethylstilbestrol for carcinoma of the prostate. Cancer 1970;25:249–256.

85. Veterans Administration Co-operataive Urological Research Group. Treatment and survival of patients with cancer of the prostate. Surg Gynecol Obstet 1967;124:1011–1017.

86. Coronary Drug Project Research Group. Coronary Drug Project; Initial findings leading to modifications of its research protocol. JAMA 1970;214:1303–1313.

87. Coronary Drug Project Research Group. Coronary Drug Project; Findings leading to discontinuation of the 2.5 mg/day estrogen group. JAMA 1973;226:652–657.

88. Eisenberg S. High density lipoprotein metabolism. J Lipid Res 1984;25:1017–1058.

89. Applebaum-Bowden D, Haffner SM, Hazzard W. The dyslipoproteinemia of anabolic steroid therapy: increase in hepatic triglyceride lipase precedes the decrease in high density lipoprotein2 cholesterol. Metabolism 1987;36:949–952.

90. Colvin PL, Auerback BJ, Case LD, Hazzard WR, Applebaum-Bowden D. Dose-response relationship between sex-hormone induced change in hepatic triglyceride lipase and high-density cholesterol in postmenopausal women. Metabolism 1991;40:1052–1056.

91. Sacks FM,Walsh BW. Effects of reproductive hormones on serum lipoproteins: unresolved issues in biology and clinical practice. Ann NY Acad Sci 1990;592:273–285.

92. Applebaum-Bowden D, Goldberg AP, Pyalisto OJ, Brunzell JD, Hazzard WR. Effect of estrogen on post-heparin hepatic lipase. J Clin Invest 1977;59:601–608.

93. Frazer KA, Narla G, Zhang JL, Rubin EM. Apoliprotein (a) gene is regulated by sex hormones and acute phase inducers in YAC transgenic mice. Nature Genet 1995;9:424–431.

94. Katznelson L, Finkelstein JS, Schoenfeld DA, Rosenthal DI, Anderson EJ, Klibanski A. Increase in bone density and lean body mass during testosterone administration in men with acquired hypogonadism. J Clin Endocrinol Metab 1996; 81:4358–4365.

95. Marin P, Holmang S, Jonsson L, Sjostrom L, Kvist H, Holm G, Lindstedt G, Bjorntorp P. The effects of testosterone treatment on body composition and metabolism in middle-aged obese men. Int J Obes Relat Metab Disord 1992;16:991–997.

96. Marin P, Holmang S, Gustafsson C, Jonsson L, Kvist H, Elander A, et al. Androgen treatment of abdominally obese men. Obes Res 1993;1:245–251.

97. Despres J-P, Moorjani S, Lupien PJ, Tremblay A, Nadeau A, Bouchard C. Regional distribution of body fat, plasma lipoproteins, and cardiovascular disease. Arteriosclerosis 1990;10:497–511.

98. Peiris AN, Sothmann MS, Hoffmann RG, Hennes M, Wilson CR, Gustafson AB, Kissebah AH. Adiposity, fat distribution, and cardiovascular risk. Ann Int Med 1989;110:867–872.

99. Ferenchik G, Schwartz D, Ball M, Schwartz K. Androgenic-anabolic steroid abuse and platelet aggregation: a pilot study in weight lifters. Am J Med Sci 1992;302:78–82.

100. McNutt RA, Ferenchik GS Kirlin PC, Hamlin NJ. Acute myocardial infarction in a 22 year old world class weight lifter using anabolic steroids. Am J Cardiol 1992;62:164.

101. Frankle MA, Eichberg R, Zachariah SB. Anabolic androgenic steroids and a stroke in an athlete: case report. Arch Phys Med Rehabil 1988;69:632–633.

102. Nguyen T, Goldschmidt-Clermont PJ, Bray PF, Dobs A. Effect of exogenous testosterone administration on platelet aggregation as a marker of clotting function. Program of the 79th Annual Meeting of the Endocrine Society, Minneapolis, MN, June 11–14, 1997, p. 214.

103. Collins P, Shay J, Jiang C, Moss J. Nitric oxide accounts for dose-dependent estrogen-mediated relaxation following acute estrogen withdrawal. Circulation 1994;90:1964–1968.

104. Wagner JD, Clarkson TB, St. Clair RW, Schwenke DC, Shively CA, Adams MR. Estrogen and progesterone replacement therapy reduces LDL accululation in the coronary arteries of surgically postmenopausal cymolgus monkeys. J Clin Invest 1991;88:1995–2002.

105. Adams RN, Williams K, Kaplan JR. Effect of androgens on coronary artery atherosclerosis and atherosclerosis-related impairment of vascular responsiveness. Arterioscler Thromb Vasc Biol 1995; 15:562–570.

106. Yue P, Chatterjee K, Beale C, Poole-Wilson PA, Collins P. Testosterone relaxes rabbit coronary arteries and aorta. Circulation 1995;91:1154–1160.

107. Fujimoto R, Morimoto I, Morita E, Sugimoto H, Ito Y, Sumiya E. Androgen receptors, 5 alpha reductase activity and androgen dependent proliferation of vascular smooth muscle cells. J Steroid Biochem Molec Biol 1994;50:169–174.

108. Larsen BA, Nordestgaard BG, Stender S, Kjeldsen K. Effect of testosterone on atherogenesis in cholesterol-fed rabbits with similar plasma cholesterol levels. Atherosclerosis 1993;99:79–86.

INDEX